LUNG CANCER
Natural History, Prognosis, and Therapy

CONTRIBUTORS

A. Philippe Chahinian
Jacques Chrétien
Elias G. Elias
Paul Lo Gerfo
Lucien Israel
Bowen Keller

Mary J. Matthews
Olivier Monod
Clifton F. Mountain
Carlos A. Perez
Philip Rubin
Oleg S. Selawry

LUNG CANCER

Natural History, Prognosis, and Therapy

EDITED BY

Lucien Israel, M.D.

Centre Hospitalier
Universitaíre Lariboisiere
Paris, France

A. Philippe Chahinian, M.D.

Department of Neoplastic Diseases
Mt. Sinai School of Medicine
of The City University of New York
New York, New York

ACADEMIC PRESS   New York San Francisco London   1976

A Subsidiary of Harcourt Brace Jovanovich, Publishers

ACADEMIC PRESS, INC.
111 Fifth Avenue, New York, New York 10003

United Kingdom Edition published by
ACADEMIC PRESS, INC. (LONDON) LTD.
24/28 Oval Road, London NW1

Library of Congress Cataloging in Publication Data

Main entry under title:

Lung cancer : natural history, prognosis, and therapy.

    Includes bibliographical references.
    1.   Lungs–Cancer.   I.   Israel, Lucien.
II.   Chahinian, A. Philippe.   [DNLM: 1.   Lung neoplasms.
WF658 L963]
RC280.L8L78   616.9$'$94$'$24   75-30468
ISBN 0–12–375050–4

Contents

Chapter 8 Nonspecific Causes of Death in Lung Cancer
A. Philippe Chahinian

Chapter 9 The Logical Basis of Radiation Treatment
Policies in the Multidisciplinary
Approach to Lung Cancer
Philip Rubin, Carlos A. Perez, and Bowen Keller

Chapter 10 Problems of Best Supportive
Therapy in Lung Cancer
Lucien Israel

Chapter 11 On Chemotherapy of Lung Cancer
Oleg S. Selawry

Chapter 12   Palliative Surgery in Lung Cancer
Olivier Monod

Chapter 13   The Role of Anticoagulation Chemotherapy
in Lung Carcinoma
Elias G. Elias

Chapter 14   Nonspecific Immune Stimulation
with Corynebacteria in Lung Cancer
Lucien Israel

Chapter 15   Presentation of the Current EORTC Lung
Group Protocols for Immunostimulation with
BCG in Lung Cancer
Lucien Israel

List of Contributors

Numbers in parentheses indicate the pages on which the author's contributions begin.

A. Philippe Chahinian, M.D. (1, 63, 95, 151), Department of Neoplastic Diseases, Mt. Sinai School of Medicine of the City University of New York, New York, New York

Jacques Chrétien, M.D. (1), Respiratory Diseases, Hospital Intercommunal, Creteil, France

Elias G. Elias, M.D. (259),* Department of General Surgery, Roswell Park Memorial Institute, Buffalo, New York

Paul Lo Gerfo, M.D. (81), Department of Surgery, Columbia University College of Physicians and Surgeons, New York, New York

Lucien Israel, M.D. (63, 95, 141, 199, 273, 281, 285, 295, 301), Centre Hospitalier Universitaire Lariboisiere, Paris, France

Bowen Keller, M.D. (159), Division of Radiation Oncology, Strong Memorial Hospital, Rochester, New York

Mary J. Matthews, M.D. (23), National Cancer Institute, Veterans Administration Medical Oncology Service, Washington, D.C., and George Washington University School of Medicine, Washington, D.C.

Olivier Monod, M.D. (241), Department of Thoracic Surgery, Centre Chirurgical du Val d'Or, Saint Cloud, France

Clifton F. Mountain, M.D. (107), Section of Thoracic Surgery, The University of Texas System Cancer Center, M. D. Anderson Hospital and Tumor Institute, Houston, Texas

Carlos A. Perez, M.D. (159), Division of Radiation Oncology, Washington University School of Medicine, St. Louis, Missouri

* Present address: Department of Surgery, University of Maryland School of Medicine, Baltimore, Maryland.

xi

Philip Rubin, M.D. (159), Division of Radiation Oncology, Strong Memorial Hospital, Rochester, New York

Oleg S. Selawry, M.D. (205), Division of Thoracic Oncology, Department of Oncology, Comprehensive Cancer Center for Florida, University of Miami School of Medicine, Miami, Florida

Preface

Lung cancer is one of the leading causes of death from malignant disease, and its incidence is increasing dangerously throughout the world. Cytotoxic agents and combined strategies, which have already enabled appreciable progress against some solid tumors such as breast cancer and ovarian cancer, have not, unfortunately, produced the same results against lung cancer. Far from being discouraging, this situation presents a challenge which should encourage greater effort in the analysis and refinement of existing concepts.

I have had occasion to meet fellow workers who are diligently engaged in achieving this goal. I asked them to contribute to this monograph which aims to provide an account of the knowledge acquired by several specialists through extensive personal experience; draw attention to methodologic progress, conceptual debates, and controversial points resulting from this experience; and encourage criticism, cooperation, and further investigation by other teams working in this field.

I have chosen to present papers from reknowned specialists in their fields in order to provide readers with recent, well-established data. My contributions are concerned with problems, speculations, and criticisms of current therapeutic strategies.

Due to the present frequency and widespread extension of this disease in all the advanced countries, this book should be of interest not only to specialists of respiratory diseases, but also to oncologists, surgeons, radiotherapists, immunologists, and internists. Only their combined efforts and interest can improve the prognosis of lung cancer.

I would like to extend my sincere thanks to all the authors who have contributed to this work with preciseness and independence of thought. I would like also to thank Dr. P. Chahinian whose help in editing this work was invaluable. We are indebted to Dr. R. Edelstein and Dr. M. L.

Slankard for reviewing our manuscripts. Finally, I would like to gratefully acknowledge the cordial and efficient assistance of the staff of Academic Press.

LUCIEN ISRAEL

Chapter 1

Present Incidence of Lung Cancer: Epidemiologic Data and Etiologic Factors

A. Philippe Chahinian and Jacques Chrétien

The history of lung cancer merges with that of its etiology. In 1420, shortly after the opening of the Schneeberg mines in Saxony (renowned today not only for their richness in various metals but also for radon) Theophrastus Paracelsus described the *Bergkrankheit* (or mountain sickness) in miners. It was only in 1879 that Harting and Hesse recognized the malignant nature of this disease, which they erroneously termed pulmonary sarcoma [89]. The accurate diagnosis of lung cancer was established in 1913 [15]. It is true that at that time the disease was extremely rare, since Adler was able to collect no more than 374 cases in the world medical literature [89]! Nevertheless, the role of cigarette smoking was already suspected.*

* For more details, the reader can refer to "Lung Cancer" by Selawry and Hansen [81a].

Since then, the incidence of lung cancer has increased incessantly, until today it has reached an alarming level. This dramatic and exceptional progression is one of the most striking facts in cancerology. Lung cancer causes more deaths among the male populations of all industrialized countries, than any other form of cancer, with almost 70,000 deaths in the United States alone in 1972 [87].

I. PRESENT INCIDENCE

Tables I and II show the annual mortality rate for lung cancer for each sex in most industrialized countries. For Doll, the morbidity rate may be assessed by multiplying the mortality rate by 1.20; this coefficient clearly shows the disastrous prognosis associated with the disease. Even more striking than the present-day absolute levels is the increase in incidence: lung cancer is on the rise in all countries, Great Britain being the record holder [21]. However, it is difficult to make statistical comparisons between countries in view of the disparity in age groups, information contained in death certificates, and accuracy of epidemiologic surveys [21]. In fact, all these factors contribute to an underestimation of the true incidence of the disease. The absolute incidence has nearly doubled every 10 years over the past few decades. This rise is a real one and cannot be attributed to improved diagnostic procedures, population increase, longer life span, or more accurate death registers [21, 48].

However, the most recent statistics reveal that this increase is slowing down in some male populations, namely, in the United States (in Caucasians), Great Britain, Finland, Denmark, and Japan [81]. In view of this finding, it may be hoped that the incidence of lung cancer is becoming

TABLE I
Primary Bronchogenic Carcinoma[a, b]

Year	France Male	Female	Great Britain Male	Female	Germany Male	Female	Italy Male	Female
1955	20.6	5.5	69.3	10.6	34.4	6.0	15.6	4.1
1960	27.7	5.6	85.6	13.2	48.4	7.3	23.9	5.2
1965	35.0	6.4	95.7	17.0	56.9	9.0	34.0	6.2

[a] From Council of Europe [21].
[b] Mortality rate per 100,000 in four European countries.

TABLE II

Lung Cancer Death Rates per 100,000 Population in the United States[a]

Year	Male	Female
1958	31.9	5.5
1960	35.3	5.7
1965	43.0	7.7
1970	53.4	11.9

[a] SOURCE: "Vital Statistics of the United States," U.S. Department of Health, Education and Welfare. Data kindly provided by Edwin Silverberg, American Cancer Society, New York.

stable or even decreasing [81], and this change should be appreciable after 1980 [53].

II. EPIDEMIOLOGIC DATA

A. Age and Lung Cancer

Generally speaking, the incidence of lung cancer in the male population is highest around the age of 65 and around the age of 75 in the female population. Beyond these ages, the incidence decreases. In fact, these data, derived from conventional mortality tables, are inaccurate since they are based on deaths of persons of different age groups studied at the same time [21]. Correct analysis can be made only through the study of cohort mortality tables, that is by following groups of people born in the same period. This method reveals that the decrease in incidence is illusory and that, in fact, the mortality rate continues to increase with age [21]. Furthermore, the most marked increase in mortality rate occurs in the oldest section of the population. This factor alone can account for the more advanced age at which maximum death rate is observed in the female population, since increase in mortality rate due to lung cancer is a more recent phenomenon among females than among males [21]. These findings suggest the involvement of some carcinogenic processes with a cumulative effect and a long latent period.

In contrast, lung cancer is rare before the age of 40, accounting for approximately 2% of all cases [1]. The absolute number of cases for this age group has remained stable in all countries, and the epidemiologic profile of the disease seems unremarkable [1]. For example, male predominance is still observed, but to a lesser degree. It even appears that the incidence is decreasing in this age group in the United States and in Great Britain [81], possibly as a result of environmental changes.

B. Sex and Lung Cancer

Male predominance is a constant feature of lung cancer, but the sex ratio (ratio of the number of male cases to the number of female cases) is presently changing. In the United States, the sex ratio reached its peak in 1960 (6.8 : 1) and has fallen consistently since to less than 5 : 1 in the Caucasian population [81]. This phenomenon is not due to a decrease in the male mortality rate but to a more rapid rise in the female mortality rate. This rise in female mortality became appreciable only after 1960 [13, 94]. Since then, the mortality rates for women have risen and are increasing at more than an exponential pace, as determined in the United States (in Caucasians), in Great Britain (peak sex ratio = 6.2 in 1960 as against 4.9 in 1969), and in Denmark [81]. A continued decrease in the sex ratio is likely over the next few decades because of an increasing incidence in the female population [13].

C. Geographical Distribution

Lung cancer is encountered predominantly in highly industrialized regions. The first striking increase in the incidence of the disease was reported immediately following World War I in the large industrial cities of Germany [89]. All other factors being equal, the death rate is usually 2 to 5 times greater in cities than in rural areas. Moreover, there is a correlation with the density of population and with the degree of urban concentration. Thus, the mortality rate due to lung cancer in conurbations is 20% higher than in small towns [21].

D. Occupation and Social Class

The poorest classes are the most severely affected. Mainly unskilled laborers are affected, with skilled workers affected to a lesser extent [21]. Analysis of this data is complex and is connected with the study of etiologic factors, such as smoking, occupational hazards, and environment.

E. Ethnic Factors

In the United States, the mortality rate due to lung cancer in both men and women is increasing approximately twice as fast for nonwhites as for whites [62]. This phenomenon emphasizes the important role of environmental factors in the causation of the disease [49]. The importance of the environment is even more obvious in studies of migratory populations. In the United States, the mortality rate due to lung cancer has decreased for British and German immigrants, whereas it has increased for Italian and Scandinavian immigrants [48]. In Italian and Scandinavian immigrants the incidence of lung cancer has tended to approach that recorded in the United States. It would thus appear that variations between different ethnic groups might, in fact, be related to environmental factors and personal habits.

III. ETIOLOGIC FACTORS

The 60 to 90 m² of respiratory epithelium are an ideal target for atmospheric carcinogens carried by the 12 m³ of air daily inhaled by man. The large number of etiologic factors involved makes their study a complex one. Their analysis must take into account the interactions between numerous carcinogens, some of which have yet to be identified. These interactions may produce simple additive effects or synergistic effects. Furthermore, some factors are *initiators,* modifying the genetic apparatus and giving rise to a potential tumor cell. Others are *promoters*, inactive by themselves but able to stimulate the initiated cell, and thus contribute to tumor induction and proliferation [17, 18].

A. Tobacco

On this point, all epidemiologic investigations are in agreement [21]. In all countries, the increased incidence of lung cancer follows the increase in cigarette smoking. This strong relationship is based on the following evidence.

1. STATISTICAL EVIDENCE

The marked rise in the incidence of lung cancer coincided with a notable increase in cigarette consumption. In Finland, for example, annual cigarette production reached one million units a year as early as 1880, while in Norway production began only in 1886. In 1930 the incidence of lung cancer in Finland far exceeded that in Norway [51].

The following three statistical surveys were decisive.

   a. The survey by Doll and Hill [25] involving 40,000 British doctors followed for 4 years. Of 36 cases of lung cancer, 25 involved smokers. The

TABLE III

**Distribution of Lung Cancer (in %) according to the Mean Number
of Cigarettes Smoked Daily[a, b]**

Sex	Nonsmoker	No. of cigarettes smoked daily			
		< 5	5	15	25 or more
Male	0.3	4.6	35.9	35	24.3
Female	40.6	13.7	22.0	9.5	14.2

[a] From Doll and Hill [25a].
[b] Subjects from 45 to 74 years of age.

risk for heavy smokers (more than 25 cigarettes a day) is 20 times greater than for nonsmokers. Table III shows this relationship, which is striking in males and less so in females.

b. In their survey in the United States, Hammond and Horn [40] reported an identical correlation after investigating the mortality rate (Table IV).

c. Denoix, Schwartz, and Anguera [23] reached the same conclusions in France.

Generally speaking, the risk is proportional to the quantity of tobacco consumed. Cigarettes are the chief hazard. The risk is not nil for pipe smokers or cigar smokers, although the risk is 3 times and 10 times less, respectively, than cigarette smokers. Some cigarette filters are reputed to reduce the risk by about one-third [105].

With equal consumption, other factors influencing the risk are inhalation of the smoke, which is more pronounced in cigarette smokers than cigar or pipe smokers [22], earlier initiation of smoking, speed of combustion and number of puffs per cigarette, the habit of keeping a cigarette in the mouth or relighting a stubbed-out cigarette, the length of the butt, and associated alcoholism [17, 23].

TABLE IV

**Lung Cancer Death Rate per 100,000 according to the
Number of Cigarettes Smoked Daily[a, b]**

Nonsmoker	No. of cigarettes smoked daily		
	10–20	20–40	Over 40
3.4	54.3	143.9	217.3

[a] From Hammond and Horn [40].
[b] Data based on 187,783 men.

2. HISTOLOGICAL EVIDENCE

Through a systematic study of the bronchial epithelium of smokers, Auerbach *et al.* [5, 5a, 5b] quantified the histological abnormalities encountered. Three characteristics were noted: loss of bronchial cilia, basal epithelial hyperplasia, and nuclear abnormalities [5, 5a]. The occurrence of all these three types of change together was never seen among specimens from nonsmokers and was seen in 9.3% of histological sections from men who smoked one to two packs of cigarettes a day, in 11.4% of sections from those who smoked two or more packs a day, and in 15.0% of sections from those who died of lung cancer [5].

In young cigarette smokers below the age of 40, early pathologic changes affect the small bronchioles and include a respiratory bronchiolitis with clusters of brown-pigmented macrophages, edema, fibrosis, and epithelial hyperplasia in the adjacent bronchiolar and alveolar walls [68].

3. EXPERIMENTAL EVIDENCE

Smoke condensate is a complete carcinogen and appears to be carcinogenic in a wide variety of animal species and tissues [104]. Over 1200 substances have been counted in cigarette smoke, which contains both initiators (polynuclear aromatic hydrocarbons such as benzo[*a*]pyrene, formed by pyrosynthesis) and promoters (phenol and derivatives) [104]. Numerous radioactive elements may also be found (polonium-210, carbon-14, potassium-40, radium) as well as many contaminants (arsenic, nickel, molds, additives) [17]. The presence of nitrosamines is still controversial [17, 104].

In view of the large number of these substances, one can readily estimate the complexity of the carcinogenic mechanism. It appears that the determining influence is exerted by the particulate phase of cigarette smoke, since it is this phase that deposits on the carinæ between dividing bronchi and bronchioles, the most common sites for cancer [17, 48]. The gaseous phase may penetrate as far as the alveolar sacs, but the incidence of alveolar cancer is not higher in smokers than nonsmokers [17]. The direct toxic effect consists of changes in bronchial elimination processes: the mucociliary apparatus is damaged and the macrophages are affected, thus making the bronchial tree more vulnerable to other forms of aggression [17, 43].

Polycyclic aromatic hydrocarbons combine with cellular DNA during the S phase of the cycle [78]. Other aromatic hydrocarbons may be metabolized in lung tissue by microsomal enzymes [73].

The manner in which the tobacco is manufactured is also important. Air-cured, low sugar tobaccos, such as cigar tobacco, burley tobacco, Maryland tobacco, and certain pipe tobaccos, appears to be less hazardous and less likely to produce lung cancer than flue-cured, high sugar tobaccos [32, 104].

Moreover, all these factors, combined with the ciliotoxic effect of tobacco, promote local infection with recurrent cell desquamation–regeneration cycles. Thus chronic bronchitis is often related to tobacco and often complicated by lung cancer [89]. As for attendant alcoholism, it is assumed that it impairs liver metabolism of polycyclic hydrocarbons, especially benzo[a]pyrene [48].

Immunologic disturbances have also been incriminated. *In vivo* antibody titers against the influenza virus A2 after natural infection or vaccination are lower in adult smokers than in nonsmokers [35]. Carcinoembryonic antigen titers are increased in smokers of more than 15 cigarettes daily [93]. *In vitro,* cigarette smoke or its gaseous phase extracts exert an effect on both lymphoid cells (decreased blastic transformation by phytohemagglutinin [24], decreased immunoglobulin synthesis in cell cultures [77]) and macrophages (depression of phagocytic activity [38], decreased adenosine triphosphate activity [65], increase in acid hydrolase activity, and presence of an intracytoplasmic autofluorescent substance [58]).

4. Special Features

a. *In nonsmokers* lung cancer does exist, but two features make it distinct: the considerably lower incidence of the disease and the different histological distribution. Thus, Kreyberg [51] has demonstrated the role of tobacco chiefly in squamous cell carcinoma and to a lesser degree in oat cell carcinoma (type I) (Table V). Tobacco has little if any influence on adenocarcinomas and bronchioloalveolar cancers (type II). In nonsmokers, the predominant cell type is adenocarcinoma [42, 106]. Thus, cigarette smoking is reputed to be responsible for 95% of squamous cell carcinomas and 90% of oat cell carcinomas [42]. Squamous cell carcinoma is rarely encountered in nonsmokers [103]. According to Harris [42], the histological distribution is the same for both sexes, while Kreyberg [51] reported a male predominance for squamous cell carcinoma (ratio 5 : 1) mainly related to occupational factors. The amount of smoking somewhat modifies the histologic pattern. The percentage of small cell carcinomas of the lung increases with cigarette smoking while the other histologic groups show little increase with the amount of smoking [5c].

b. *Cessation of smoking* induces a return to a normal bronchial epithelium and the risk of lung cancer becomes identical to that of nonsmokers after an average of 13 years* [105]. In a prospective survey of British doctors, Doll and Pike found a 25% decrease in the mortality rate

---

* It is difficult to conclude from that study whether the risk in each individual decreases actually or stays constant from the point he stops smoking. For Doll [R.

TABLE V

Mean Tobacco Consumption and Risk of Lung Cancer Compared to Nonsmokers according to Histological Type[a]

Histologic type	Men		Women	
	Mean tobacco consumption[b] (gm/24 hr)	Risk	Mean tobacco consumption[b] (gm/24 hr)	Risk
Kreyberg type I				
Squamous cell	21	× 25	14	× 16
Anaplastic oat cell	22	× 20	21	× 6.6
Kreyberg type II				
Primary adenocarcinoma	16	× 3	10	× 1
Bronchiolo-alveolar	19	× 1	8	× 1

[a] From Kreyberg [51].
[b] One cigarette equals 1 gm of tobacco.

due to lung cancer in 12 years, during which the number of cigarette smokers decreased by almost 50% within this group [27]. Although some of the data mentioned in the report of the Royal College of Physicians [88] have been criticized from a statistical standpoint [86], it may be reasonably concluded that "it helps to stop smoking" [31].

c. *Induction time* for cancer related to cigarette smoking has been calculated to be approximately 30 years [13]. By following various cohorts according to the age of onset and importance of cigarette smoking, the highest incidence of lung cancer occurred at the age of 61–62 years for subjects who began smoking before the age of 25, and at 67–68 years for those who began smoking after the age of 25 [101]. Using theoretical calculations, Burch [14] estimated the mean age of appearance of lung cancer to be 61.9 years for "early smokers," as against 65.4 years for "late smokers."

d. *In women* the incidence of cigarette smoking is rising constantly, and a gradual increase in the ratio between Kreyberg's type I and type II is taking place. This factor appears to be decisive in explaining the present increase of lung cancer incidence in women [102], the gradual drop in the

Doll, The age distribution of cancer: Implications for models of carcinogenesis. *J. Roy. Statistic. Soc. (A)* **134,** 133 (1971)], the risk may fall slightly at first and then rise again slowly, in keeping with the increase in risk in nonsmokers.

male to female ratio, and the proportionally greater increase in women than in men [13]. It has been predicted, however, that the incidence of lung cancer in women will not reach the maximum level observed in men because of the consumption of filter cigarettes with lower tar yields [102]. Also, high risk occupational factors associated with smoking are less prevalent in women [51]. Furthermore, in the United States, women smoke fewer cigarettes per day (mean of 17) than men (mean of 22) [37]. However, women do not find it easier to quit smoking than men do. From 1966 to 1970 the smoking rate among men fell sharply from 51.9 to 42.3%, while among women the rate fell from 33.7 to 30.5% [37].

e. However, *numerous etiological problems* have yet to be solved. Thus, for example, in animals, the upper respiratory tract is just as sensitive as the lower respiratory tract to the carcinogenic effect of tobacco [89]. In man, however, although the relationship between cancer of the larynx and cigarette smoking appears to be established, the incidence of cancer of the larynx has remained practically stable since 1910 [91]. Experimentally there is a threshold above which carcinogenesis occurs even when tobacco consumption is discontinued [89]. In man, on the other hand, cellular abnormalities, seen in 93% of bronchial sections from heavy smokers by Auerbach *et al.* [5b], regressed after cessation of smoking and dropped to 6% of sections after 5 years of nonsmoking as compared to 1.2% of sections from nonsmokers.

B. Air Pollution

The incidence of lung cancer in urban areas suggests that air pollution might be involved, but this notion in fact encompasses several complex facts. There are many sources of pollution including domestic heating systems, industrial combustion, and motor vehicle fumes. The last apparently plays a minor role because an unduly high incidence of lung cancer has not been reported in highly exposed individuals [6, 21, 28].

Pollutants released divide into two phases: a *gaseous phase* (CO, CO_2, SO_2, hydrocarbons, etc.) and a *solid phase* made up of particles of cinders, soot, smoky charcoal, and various types of ash, which adsorbs gases, transports them, and enhances their effects. The impingement of these particles in the bronchial tree, namely, at bronchial and bronchiolar divisions, depends on their size, with maximum retention occurring for particles 1 μm in diameter [48].

The detected carcinogens are almost identical to those found in tobacco (perhaps because they are the only ones known): aliphatic hydrocarbons and aromatic hydrocarbons including benzo[*a*]pyrene which serves as a reference. However, there are many other factors, such as traces of radioactive substances, metals (nickel, lead, chromium, etc.), and arsenic compounds [89].

There are two distinct major forms of urban air pollution [20]: (a) *The oxidizing form* (e.g., found in Los Angeles) which consists mainly of primary pollutants (hydrocarbons and nitrogen oxides) and photochemical reaction pollutants (ozone, nitrogen dioxides, aldehydes, and organic nitrates). This type of pollution has not been incriminated in the genesis of lung cancer [12] or chronic bronchitis [20]. (b) *The reducing type* (e.g., found in London) which consists mainly of carbonaceous, particulate matter, and sulfur dioxide. This type of pollution is associated with a high incidence of chronic bronchitis [52], which promotes bronchial cell changes and sensitizes the epithelium to other forms of aggression [4, 89]. Chronic bronchitis favors the onset of lung cancer [74]. In nonsmokers, its effect is weak [52]. The risk of lung cancer when chronic bronchitis and cigarette smoking are combined is reputedly higher than the sum of the two individual risks [52]. However, for an equal consumption of tobacco the incidence of chronic bronchitis in urban areas is higher in men than in women, and this suggests the involvement of constitutional or occupational factors [52]. Among the "urban factors," a major role has been attributed to smoky coal-burning domestic heaters [28, 81, 92]. The substantial aggravating role of associated cigarette smoking should, however, be emphasized [7, 28].

C. Occupational Factors

Metallurgy and mining are the main occupations involved. Experimentally, apart from radioactive minerals, an impressive number of metals have proved to be carcinogenic in animals (e.g., nickel and silver mainly, but also chromium, cadmium, beryllium, cobalt, selenium, steel) [96]. The mechanism of carcinogenesis is a complex one and involves a dual effect: a chemical effect by dissolution in the serum and bonding with various low molecular weight proteins that allow diffusion into tissues, formation of radicals, and alteration of redox and enzyme systems [100] and a physical effect that depends on the size and shape of the particles (Oppenheimer effect) [69]. Moreover, these factors combine with smoking, pneumoconiotic pulmonary changes and highly polluted air. Here again the interaction of factors prevails.

1. RADIOACTIVE MINERALS

The historical example of the Schneeberg and Joachimstahl radium mines is a significant one. All types of radiation may be carcinogenic [45]. The lung cancer risk is increased from 3- to 30-fold depending on the degree of exposure. The latent period (interval between beginning of exposure and onset of lung cancer) is not shorter than 10 years, the mean value being 16 to 17 years [89]. In this regard it is relevant to mention the increased incidence of lung cancer among survivors of the Hiroshima and Nagasaki bombings and certain cases of therapeutic irradiation [2, 19].

Experimentally, *radon* induces lung tumors in 100% of rats. These tumors are either adenocarcinomas (two-thirds) or squamous cell carcinomas (one-third) [71]. In man, however, over half the cases are undifferentiated carcinomas, similar but not identical to anaplastic oat cell carcinomas [79]. The tobacco cofactor also plays a part, mainly for the squamous cell type [79].

The role of *uranium*, which is weakly radioactive, is the object of various investigations that take into account the appearance of lung cancer, the exposure level [WLM (working level-months)],* exposure conditions, and the involvement of cofactors, with tobacco being one of the most important in the opinion of most investigators [79]. However, Lundin et al. [54] have shown that both smoking and nonsmoking uranium miners had respiratory cancer rates that were higher than those of their counterparts in the general population (4-fold increase). Although there is a great excess of lung cancer among cigarette smoking miners (about a 10-fold increase), suggesting a multiplicative model [81], smoking alone cannot account for this increase [54]. Moreover, at each level of estimated radiation exposure in uranium mines, a significant excess of respiratory cancer has been observed 10 or more years after the start of uranium mining, even at low WLM [54].

2. NICKEL

As early as 1933, it was shown that nickel refining techniques could induce respiratory cancers. Experimentally, the inhalation of nickel powder, and especially nickel–carbonyl, induces lung adenomas in rats. Nickel itself inhibits RNA synthesis by combining with DNA. Nickel–carbonyl, used in some refining techniques in England, inhibits the induction of pulmonary benzopyrene hydrolases that convert 3,4-benzopyrene into noncarcinogenic hydroxylated derivatives, thus prolonging the retention of this hydrocarbon [95]. In this respect, it is noteworthy that a decrease in the incidence of lung cancer has been recorded, undoubtedly because of the technical changes made in this refining process after 1925 (use of arsenic-free sulfuric acid, less dusty calciners, and personal protection)

---

* 1 WLM is any combination of radon daughters in 1 liter of air which results in the ultimate release of 1.3×10^5 MeV of α energy [44].

[30]. Before 1925, the mortality rate due to lung cancer varied from 5 to 10 times that encountered in the general population, while deaths resulting from nasal cancer varied from about 100 to 900 times the expected numbers [26, 30]. Among the men first employed after 1925, there were 8 deaths from lung cancer (compared to 6.2 expected) and no deaths from nasal cancer. However, the conclusion that the hazard was not due specifically to the carbonyl process was supported by the occurrence of cases of lung cancer (23-fold increase) and nasal sinus cancer (250-fold increase) in men employed in refineries using the electrolytic process [70]. The average interval between the start of employment and manifestation of the disease was 31.6 years, and there was no apparent correlation between risk and duration of exposure [70]. Traces of nickel are also present in tobacco smoke.

3. CHROMIUM

The incidence of lung cancer in industries handling chromates and chromium is approximately 4 to 15 times greater than in the general population. The mean latent period is 15 years. The role of chromium is unknown. Exposed subjects have a substantially higher blood chromium level than controls, but lung tumors and the livers of affected subjects contain less chromium than normal lung or liver tissue [66].

4. ASBESTOS

Asbestos has now become a universally recognized carcinogen since the first reports dating back to 1935 [56]. Among asbestos workers, one death out of five is due to lung cancer, one out of ten to pleural or peritoneal mesotheliomas, and one out of ten to gastrointestinal carcinomas [85]. Lung cancer is found at autopsy in 13% of cases of asbestosis, and there is no correlation with the severity of the latter [63]. The mean risk is six to ten times greater, with a latent period of between 20 and 30 years [82].

Differences in the physical properties and chemical composition of the various types of asbestos indicate that there should be differences in their carcinogenic potential [33]. Men exposed to chrysotile asbestos have a respiratory cancer mortality rate 2.4 times higher than controls, whereas those exposed to a combination of chrysotile and crocidolite asbestos have a mortality rate 5.3 times higher than controls [33]. For amosite asbestos, the death rate due to respiratory cancers is more than 10 times higher than in controls [84].

Experimentally, various types of asbestos are carcinogenic in animals. The mechanism appears to be a complex one: asbestos fibers contain natural mineral oils and various metals (e.g., iron and magnesium). During industrial handling, the fibers adsorb various impurities, including nickel, chromium, and cobalt, which are themselves carcinogenic, as well as aromatic hydrocarbons and 3,4-benzopyrene that comes mainly from jute bags [41].

Tobacco is an important cofactor. The risk of lung cancer for heavy smokers exposed to asbestos is 92 times greater than for nonsmokers not exposed to asbestos [83]. This effect has suggested a multiplicative hypothesis with smoking [9, 83]. The number of asbestos bodies in the lungs appears to be correlated with the consumption of tobacco [64].

Asbestos is far more than a simple occupational hazard [11]. Pollution due to asbestos fibers is increasing steadily and proportionally to its growing use. Thus, ferruginous bodies are found in the lungs of 100% of city dwellers in France [10]. The atmosphere in New York contains 10×10^{-9} to 50×10^{-9} gm of asbestos per cubic meter of air, which corresponds to millions of submicroscopic fibrils [85]. One can only hope that effective prophylactic measures will be quickly introduced, as has been the case recently in New York, with the interdiction of high-power projection of insulating substances in the building of skyscrapers [57].

5. IRON

The role of iron and siderosis is not as clear and was first suggested as recently as 1947 [6]. Thus, in France the incidence of lung cancer among iron miners in the Lorraine region is 3.3% as against 1.5% in the reference population [6]. Hematite (ferric oxide + silica) is the incriminated agent. The carcinogens are presumably iron–carbohydrate complexes of the iron–dextran type rather than iron and its oxides [96].

Moreover, the atmospheric level of radon in hematite mines appears to play a role: when this concentration is low or nil, the increase in risk is extremely slight (1.7 in Cumberland). The risk is multiplied by ten in the Colorado mines where radon levels are higher [29].

Recently, it has been demonstrated that when monkeys inhale hematite particles less than 5 μm diameter, these particles can penetrate directly into the bronchial cells, inducing vacuolation in their apical cytoplasm and partial loss of cilia [59].

6. COAL

Lung cancer does not appear to be unduly common in coal miners and has even been reported to be less common than usual in the case of anthracosilicosis [3]. Various hypotheses have been put forward: protective effect of thiol radicals, enhancement of immune mechanisms by silica, obstruction of lymphatic ducts due to accumulation of dust [3]. However, this viewpoint is not universally acknowledged. Scarano et al. [80] demonstrated a 7-fold increase in the incidence of lung cancer in Pennsylvania miners with anthracosilicosis, the squamous cell type being by far the most prevalent. It should be mentioned, however, that uranium deposits exist in these places.

Coal-transforming industries (combustion, distillation, gas factories) are major producers of 3,4-benzopyrene [46, 92]. The risk to workers in these industries is more than doubled, with a mean latent period of 20 to 24 years. The effect of road tarring is still questioned despite experimental data [6].

7. OTHER OCCUPATIONAL FACTORS

a. *Arsenic* and its inorganic compounds induce cutaneous hyperkeratosis and skin cancer. Their role in certain lung cancers is probable, since it has been demonstrated by the cases of lung cancer in wine-growers who use these compounds as insecticides or in patients treated for many years with arsenic-containing drugs [89]. The arsenic concentration in the bronchial mucosa of affected subjects is higher than that of controls [6].

b. *Beryllium,* which is carcinogenic in animals [99], probably has a similar effect in man.

c. *Many other occupational factors* have been incriminated, namely, in newspaper workers [39, 67], African gold miners [75], haloethers and chloromethyl methyl ether workers [34]. This list is undoubtedly far from complete.*

D. Individual Factors

1. GENETIC FACTORS

Some reports have indicated that susceptibility to lung cancer is inherited. Tokuhata demonstrated familial clustering that could be dissociated from environmental factors [97]. Recently, Kellerman et al. [47] suggested that this susceptibility was associated with genetically higher cellular levels of *aryl hydrocarbon hydroxylase* activity. This inducible membrane-bound enzyme is involved in the metabolism of chemical carcinogens, particularly polycyclic hydrocarbons which are converted into chemically more reactive compounds.

---

* A recent example is the carcinogenic potential of vinyl chloride. A 60% excess of lung cancer has been reported in vinyl chloride workers. [65a].

2. ENDOCRINE FACTORS

Results of investigations in this field are sparse and involve mainly the steroid hormones.

a. *In male patients* with lung cancer, serum cortisol levels are abnormally high in 40% of cases, with less diurnal variation and with adrenal hyperplasia. Moreover, in 90% of cases, it has been shown that the androsterone : etiocholanolone ratio is low, while the 17-OH steroid : androsterone ratio is high. These changes are reported to persist after surgical removal of the lung tumor [72].

b. *In female patients*, the lower incidence of lung cancer may be partly accounted for by occupational differences and different habits. However, cytologic studies on bronchial aspiration material have shown structural cell variations related to the various phases of the menstrual cycle: gradual ascension of the nucleus and increase in the cell mucopolysaccharide content. These cyclic fluctuations, which are absent in males and aged females, might afford women some degree of protection against inhaled irritants and carcinogens [16].

3. BRONCHOPULMONARY DISORDERS

a. The so-called *"scar-cancer"* is a classical notion. Histologically these tumors are usually mucin-secreting adenocarcinomas, although squamous cell and undifferentiated large cell carcinomas have also been known to occur [60]. Among the "scars" incriminated are old infarcts, gunshot wounds, stab wounds, metallic foreign bodies, and granulomatous infections such as tuberculosis [60].

b. The association between *tuberculosis and lung cancer* is reported to be between 7 and 30% depending on the particular geographic area and the population being surveyed [90]. In many cases, tuberculosis occurs concomitantly with lung cancer [50, 61], and this might be accounted for by a lowering of immune defense mechanisms. In cases where tuberculosis precedes cancer by several years, one might well ask if the two did not really occur together, since the "birth" of cancer precedes its clinical expression by several years. Moreover, the mean age of tuberculous patients has increased from 49 to 61 years, and this might explain the association with lung cancer [8]. However, apart from the problems raised by scar-cancers, antituberculous drugs may be directly responsible. In animals, isoniazid is a potential carcinogen [76] and induces pulmonary adenomas in mice [98]. The major metabolite of isoniazid in man (1-acetyl-2-isonicotinoylhydrazine) greatly increases the incidence of lung tumors in mice [98]. It is still too early to assess the impact of this drug in man with accuracy, since it was introduced only in 1952. It is noteworthy, moreover, that rifampicin is endowed with immunodepressant properties [36].

c. Cases of lung cancer occurring on *bronchiectasis or pulmonary dystophies* are rare, and a statistically significant relationship has not been established [6].

d. *Virus-like inclusions* have recently been found in the tumor cell cytoplasm of two anaplastic carcinomas and three adenocarcinomas [55]. These data are not sufficient to conclude that a virus was, in fact, responsible.*

An analysis of immune deficiencies in lung cancer patients is given elsewhere in this book.

IV. CONCLUSION

The various risk factors and hazards that account for the high incidence of lung cancer have been discussed. They are chiefly the result of our industrialized society. The number of factors continues to increase each day, and the list is still far from complete. The mechanisms of action of most of these factors have, as yet, been barely explored. Closer contact between medical centers and industrial medicine and a more thorough knowledge of statistical epidemiology will undoubtedly allow advances in the next few years.

However, at the present time, simple but effective preventive measures are readily available: the fight against smoking, protection of susceptible professions, and antipollution measures should be given fullest attention if the alarming rise in the incidence of lung cancer is to be curbed.

REFERENCES

1. Akoun, G., Depierre, A., and Brocard, H., Le cancer bronchique primitif avant quarante ans. *Sem. Hop.* **45,** 2148 (1969).
2. Archer, V. E., Lung cancer among populations having lung irradiation. *Lancet* **2,** 1261 (1971).
3. Ashley, D. J., Lung cancer in miners. *Thorax* **23,** 87 (1968).
4. Ashley, D. J., Environmental factors in the aetiology of lung cancer and bronchitis. *Brit. J. Prev. Soc. Med.* **23,** 258 (1969).
5. Auerbach, O., Stout, A. P., Hammond, E. C., and Garfinkel, L., Changes in

* Recently, Gabelman *et al.* [35a] have isolated an RNA tumor virus, related to the Woolly monkey virus, using cocultivation of a cell line derived from a patient with an adenocarcinoma of the lung and concomitant chronic lymphocytic leukemia, and passed with a nonproducer rat cell line.

bronchial epithelium in relation to cigarette smoking and in relation to lung cancer. *N. Engl. J. Med.* **265,** 253 (1961).

5a. Auerbach, O., Stout, A. P., Hammond, E. C., and Garfinkel, L., Changes in bronchial epithelium in relation to sex, age, residence, smoking and pneumonia. *N. Engl. J. Med.* **267,** 111 (1962).

5b. Auerbach, O., Stout, A. P., Hammond, E. C., and Garfinkel, L., Bronchial epithelium in former smokers. *N. Engl. J. Med.* **267,** 119 (1962).

5c. Auerbach, O., Garfinkel, L., and Parks, V. R., Histologic type of lung cancer in relation to smoking habits, year of diagnosis and site of metastases. *Chest* **67,** 382 (1975).

6. Bariéty, M., Delarue, J., Paillas, J., and Rullière, R., "Les Carcinomes Bronchiques Primitifs." Masson, Paris, 1967.

7. Bates, D. V., Air pollutants and the human lung. *Amer. Rev. Resp. Dis.* **105,** 1 (1972).

8. Berroya, R. B., and Polk, J. W., Concurrent pulmonary tuberculosis and primary carcinoma. *Thorax* **26,** 384 (1971).

9. Berry, G., Newhouse, M., and Turok, M., Combined effect of asbestos exposure and smoking on mortality from lung cancer in factory workers. *Lancet* **2,** 476 (1972).

10. Bignon, J., Goni, J., Bonnaud, G., Jaurand, M. C., Dufour, G., and Pinchon, M. C., Incidence of pulmonary ferruginous bodies in France. *Environ. Res.* **3,** 430 (1970).

11. Brouet, G., Bignon, J., Bonnaud, G., and Goni, J., Incidence sur la santé de la pollution atmosphérique par l'asbeste ou autres particules fibreuses. *Rev. Tuberc. Pneumol.* **35,** 461 (1971).

12. Buell, P., Dunn, J. E., and Breslow, L., Cancer of the lung and Los Angeles-type air pollution. *Cancer* **20,** 2139 (1967).

13. Burbank, F., U.S. lung cancer death rates begin to rise proportionately more rapidly for females than for males: A dose-response effect? *J. Chronic Dis.* **25,** 473 (1972).

14. Burch, P. R. J., Smoking and cancer. *Lancet* **1,** 939 (1973).

15. Chahinian, P., and Chrétien, J., Fréquence actuelle du cancer bronchique. Données épidémiologiques et facteurs étiologiques. *Rev. Prat.* **23,** 1113 (1973).

16. Chalon, J., Loew, D. A., and Orkin, L. R., Tracheobronchial cytologic changes during the menstrual cycle. *J. Amer. Med. Ass.* **218,** 1928 (1971).

17. Chrétien, J., Hirsch, A., Harf, A., and Thiéblemont, M., Le rôle du tabac en pathologie respiratoire. *Rev. Tuberc. Pneumol.* **36,** 243 (1972).

18. Chrétien, J., Hirsch, A., and Thiéblemont, M., "Pathologie Respiratoire du Tabac." Masson, Paris, 1973.

19. Cihak, R. W., Radiation and lung cancer. *Hum. Pathol.* **2,** 525 (1971).

20. Cohen, C. A., Hudson, A. R., Clausen, J. L., and Knelson, J. H., Respiratory symptoms, spirometry and oxidant air pollution in non-smoking adults. *Amer. Rev. Resp. Dis.* **105,** 251 (1972).

21. Council of Europe, "Lung Cancer in Western Europe," 2nd ed. Council of Europe, Strasbourg, 1972.

22. Cowie, J., Stillet, R. W., and Ball, K. P., Carbon monoxide absorption by cigarette smokers who change to smoking cigars. *Lancet* **1,** 1033 (1973).

23. Denoix, P. F., Schwartz, D., and Anguera, G., L'enquête française sur l'étiologie du cancer broncho-pulmonaire. Analyse détaillée. *Bull. Ass. Fr. Cancer* **26,** 1085 (1958).

24. Desplaces, A., Charreire, J., and Izard, C., Action de la phase gazeuse de fumée de cigarette sur la transformation lymphoblastique du petit lymphocyte humain. *Rev. Eur. Etud. Clin. Biol.* **16**, 822 (1971).
25. Doll, R., and Hill, A. B., Mortality in relation to smoking: Ten years' observations of British doctors. *Brit. Med. J.* **1**, 1399 (1964).
25a. Doll, R., and Hill, A. B., A study of the aetiology of carcinoma of the lung. *Brit. Med. J.* **2**, 1271 (1952).
26. Doll, R., Morgan, L. G., and Speizer, F. E., Cancers of the lung and nasal sinuses in nickel workers. *Brit. J. Cancer* **24**, 623 (1970).
27. Doll, R., and Pike, M. C., Trends in mortality among British doctors in relation to their smoking habits. *J. Roy. Coll. Physicians, London* **6**, 216, (1972).
28. Editorial, Polluted air. *Lancet* **1**, 875 (1970).
29. Editorial, Lung cancer in haematite miners. *Lancet* **2**, 758 (1970).
30. Editorial, A cancer prevented. *Lancet* **1**, 787 (1971).
31. Editorial, Does it help to stop smoking? *Lancet* **1**, 238 (1972).
32. Editorial, Sugar in tobacco: Theory and fact. *Lancet* **1**, 187 (1973).
33. Enterline, P. E., and Henderson, V., Type of asbestos and respiratory cancer in the asbestos industry. *Arch. Environ. Health* **27**, 312 (1973).
34. Figueroa, W. G., Raszkowski, R., and Weiss, W., Lung cancer in chloromethyl methyl ether workers. *N. Engl. J. Med.* **288**, 1096 (1973).
35. Finklea, J. F., Hasselblad, V., Riggan, W. B., Nelson, W. C., Hammer, D. I., and Newill, V. A., Cigarette smoking and hemagglutination inhibition response to influenza after natural disease and immunization. *Amer. Rev. Resp. Dis.* **104**, 368 (1971).
35a. Gabelman, N., Waxman, S., Smith, W., and Douglas, S. D., Appearance of C-type virus-like particles after cocultivation of a human tumor-cell line with rat (XC) cells. *Int. J. Cancer* **16**, 355 (1975).
36. Graber, C. D., Jebaily, J., Galphin, R. L., and Doering, E., Light chain proteinuria and humoral immunoincompetence in tuberculous patients treated with Rifampicin. *Amer. Rev. Resp. Dis.* **107**, 713 (1973).
37. Green, D. E., and Nemzer, D. E., Changes in cigarette smoking by women. An analysis, 1966 and 1970. *U.S., Pub. Health Serv., Pub. Health Monogr.* **88**, 631 (1973).
38. Green, G. M., and Carolin, D., The depressant effect of cigarette smoke on the "in vitro" antibacterial activity of alveolar macrophages. *N. Engl. J. Med.* **276**, 421 (1967).
39. Greenberg, M., A proportional mortality study of a group of newspaper workers. *Brit. J. Ind. Med.* **29**, 15 (1972).
40. Hammond, E. L., and Horn, D., Smoking death-rates report on forty-four months of follow-up of 187,783 men. *J. Amer. Med. Ass.* **166**, 1159 and 1294 (1958).
41. Harington, J. S., and Roe, F. J. C., Studies of carcinogenesis of asbestos fibers and their natural oils. *Ann. N.Y. Acad. Sci.* **132**, 439 (1965).
42. Harris, C. C., The epidemiology of different histologic types of bronchogenic carcinoma. *Cancer Chemother. Rep., Part 3* **4**, 59 (1973).
43. Heidendal, G. K., Fontana, R. S., and Tauxe, W. N., Radioactive xenon pulmonary studies in the smoker. *Cancer* **30**, 1358 (1972).
44. Holaday, D. A., Rushing, D. E., Coleman, R. D., Woolrich, P. F., Kusnetz, H. L., and Bale, W. F., Control of radon and daughters in uranium mines and calculations on biologic effects. *U.S., Pub. Health Serv., Publ.* **494** (1957).

45. Hutchinson, G. B., Late neoplastic changes following medical irradiation. *Radiology* **105,** 645 (1972).
46. Kawai, M., Amamoto, H., and Harada, K., Epidemiologic study of occupational lung cancer. *Arch. Environ. Health* **14,** 859 (1967).
47. Kellerman, G., Shaw, C. R., and Luyten-Kellerman, M., Aryl hydrocarbon hydroxylase inducibility and bronchogenic carcinoma. *N. Engl. J. Med.* **289,** 934 (1973).
48. Kotin, P., Carcinogenesis of the lung: Environmental and host factors. *In* "The Lung" (A. A. Liebow and D. E. Smith, eds.), pp. 203–225. Williams & Wilkins, Baltimore, Maryland, 1968.
49. Kovi, J., and Heshmat, M. Y., Incidence of cancer in Negroes in Washington D.C. and selected African cities. *Amer. J. Epidemiol.* **96,** 401 (1973).
50. Kreus, K. E., Hakama, M., and Saxen, E., Association of pulmonary tuberculosis and carcinoma of the lung. *Scand. J. Resp. Dis.* **51,** 276 (1970).
51. Kreyberg, L., Nonsmokers and the geographic pathology of lung cancer. *In* "The Lung" (A. A. Liebow and D. E. Smith, eds.), pp. 273–283. Williams & Wilkins, Baltimore, Maryland, 1968.
52. Lambert, P. M., and Reid, D. D., Smoking, air pollution and bronchitis in Britain. *Lancet* **1,** 853 (1970).
53. Langston, H. T., Lung cancer. Future projection. *J. Thorac. Cardiov. Surg.* **63,** 412 (1972).
54. Lundin, F. E., Jr., Lloyd, J. W., Smith, E. M., Archer, V. E., and Holaday, D. A., Mortality of uranium miners in relation to radiation exposure, hardrock mining and cigarette smoking. 1950 through September 1967. *Health Phys.* **16,** 571 (1969).
55. Lupulescu, A. P., and Brinkman, G. L., Cytoplasmic inclusion bodies in pulmonary tumors: An electron microscopic study. *Amer. J. Clin. Pathol.* **56,** 553 (1971).
56. Lynch, K. M., and Smith, W. A., Pulmonary asbestosis. Carcinoma of the lung in asbestos silicosis. *Amer. J. Cancer* **24,** 56 (1935).
57. Mackler, A. D., Nicholson, W. J., Rohl, A. N., and Selikoff, I. J., L'asbeste chrysotile dans l'air ambiant des centres urbains des Etats-Unis. *Rev. Tuberc. Pneumol.* **36,** 1193 (1972).
58. Martin, R. R., Altered morphology and increased acid hydrolase content of pulmonary macrophages from cigarette smokers. *Amer. Rev. Resp. Dis* **107,** 596 (1973).
59. Masse, R., Fritsch, P., Ducousso, R., Lafuma, J., and Chrétien, J., Rétention de particules dans les cellules bronchiques, relations possibles avec les carcinogènes inhalés. *C.R. Acad. Sci. Paris, Ser. D* **276,** 2923 (1973).
60. McFadden, R. R., and Dawson, P. J., Adenocarcinoma arising in a Ghon complex and presenting with massive pericardial effusion. *Chest* **62,** 520 (1972).
61. McQuarrie, D. G., Nicoloff, D. M., Nostrand, D. V., Rao, K., and Humphrey, E. W., Tuberculosis and carcinoma of the lung. *Dis. Chest* **54,** 427 (1968).
62. Medical News, "Alarming increase" in cancer mortality seen among blacks. *J. Amer. Med. Ass.* **221,** 345 (1972).
63. Merewether, E. R. A., Asbestosis and carcinoma of the lung. Annual report of Chief Inspector of factories, 79 Her Majesty's Stationery Office, London, 1947, quoted by Wright (G. W.). *Amer. Rev. Resp. Dis.* **100,** 467 (1969).
64. Meurman, L. O., Hormia, M., Isomaki, M., and Sutinen, S., Asbestos bodies in the lung of a series of Finnish lung cancer patients. *In* "Pneumoconiosis" (H. A.

Shapiro, ed.), p. 404. Oxford Univ. Press (Cape Town), London and New York, 1970.

65. Meyer, D. H., Cross, C. E., Ibrahim, A. B., and Mustafa, M. G., Nicotine effects on alveolar macrophage respiration and adenosine triphosphate activity. *Arch. Environ. Health* **22,** 362 (1971).

65a. Monson, R. R., Peters, J. M., and Johnson, M. N., Proportional mortality among vinyl-chloride workers. *Lancet* **2,** 397 (1974).

66. Morgan, J. M., Hepatic copper, manganese and chromium content in broncho-genic carcinoma. *Cancer* **29,** 710 (1972).

67. Moss, E., Scott, T. S., and Atherley S. R. C., Mortality of newspaper workers from lung cancer and bronchitis, 1952–66. *Brit. J. Ind. Med.* **29,** 1 (1972).

68. Niewoehner, D. E., Kleinerman, J., and Rice, D. B., Pathologic changes in the peripheral airways of young cigarette smokers. *N. Engl. J. Med.* **291,** 755 (1974).

69. Oppenheimer, B. S., Oppenheimer, E. T., Danishefsky, I., and Stout, A., Carcinogenic effect of metals in rodents. *Cancer Res.* **16,** 439 (1956).

70. Pedersen, E., Hogetveit, A. C., and Andersen, A., Cancer of respiratory organs among workers at a nickel refinery in Norway. *Int. J. Cancer* **12,** 32 (1973).

71. Perraud, R., Chameaud, J., Lafuma, J., Masse, R., and Chrétien, J., Cancer broncho-pulmonaire expérimental du rat par inhalation de Radon. Comparaison avec les aspects histologiques des cancers humains. *J. Fr. Med. Chir. Thorac.* **26,** 25 (1972).

72. Rao, L. G., Discriminant function based on steroid abnormalities in patients with lung cancer. *Lancet* **2,** 441 (1970).

73. Reid, W. D., Ilett, K. F., Glick, J. M., and Krishna, G., Metabolism and binding of aromatic hydrocarbons in the lung. Relationship to experimental bronchiolar necrosis. *Amer. Rev. Resp. Dis.* **107,** 539 (1973).

74. Rimington, J., Smoking, chronic bronchitis, and lung cancer. *Brit. Med. J.* **2,** 373 (1971).

75. Robertson, M. A., and Harington, J. S., The cancer pattern in African gold miners. *Brit. J. Cancer* **25,** 395 (1971).

76. Rosenkrantz, H. S., and Carr, H. S., Hydrazine antidepressants and isoniazid: Potential carcinogens. *Lancet* **1,** 1354 (1971).

77. Roszman, T. L., and Rogers, A. S., The immunosuppressive potential of products derived from cigarette smoke. *Amer. Rev. Resp. Dis.* **108,** 1158 (1973).

78. Ryser, H. J. P., Chemical carcinogenesis. *N. Engl. J. Med.* **285,** 721 (1971).

79. Saccomano, G., Archer, V. E., Auerbach, O., Kuschner, M., Saunders, R. P., and Klein, M. G., Histologic types of lung cancers among uranium miners. *Cancer* **27,** 515 (1971).

80. Scarano, D., Fadali, A. M. A., and Lemole, G. M., Carcinoma of the lung and anthracosilicosis. *Chest* **62,** 251 (1972).

81. Schneiderman, M. A., and Levin, D. L., Trends in lung cancer. Mortality, incidence, diagnosis, treatment, smoking and urbanization. *Cancer* **30,** 1320 (1972).

81a. Selawry, O. S., and Hansen, H. H., Lung cancer. *In* "Cancer Medicine" (J. F. Holland and E. Frei, III, eds.), p. 1473. Lea & Febiger, Philadelphia, Pennsylvania, 1973

82. Selikoff, I. J., Bader, R. A., Bader, M. E., Churg, J., and Hammond, E., Asbestosis and neoplasia. *Amer. J. Med.* **42,** 487 (1967).

83. Selikoff, I. J., Hammond, E. C., and Churg, J., Asbestos exposure, smoking and neoplasia. *J. Amer. Med. Ass.* **204,** 106 (1968).

84. Selikoff, I. J., Hammond, E. C., and Churg, J., Carcinogenicity of Amosite asbestos. *Arch. Environ. Health* **25**, 183 (1972).
85. Selikoff, I. J., Nicholson, W. J., and Langer, A. M., Asbestos air pollution. *Arch. Environ. Health* **25**, 1 (1972).
86. Seltzer, C. C., Critical appraisal of the Royal College of Physicians' report on smoking and health. *Lancet* **1**, 243 (1972).
87. Silverberg, E., and Holleb, A. I., Cancer statistics 1972. *Ca* **22**, 2 (1972).
88. "Smoking and Health Now," A report of the Royal College of Physicians, Pitman, London, 1971.
89. Spencer, H., "Pathology of the Lung," p. 778. Pergamon, Oxford, 1969.
90. Steinitz, R., Pulmonary tuberculosis and carcinoma of the lung, a survey from two population-based disease registers. *Amer. Rev. Resp. Dis.* **92**, 758 (1965).
91. Stell, P. M., Smoking and laryngeal cancer. *Lancet* **1**, 617 (1972).
92. Sterling, T. D., and Pollack, S. V., The incidence of lung cancer in the U.S. since 1955 in relation to the etiology of the disease. *Amer. J. Pub. Health* **62**, 152 (1972).
93. Stevens, D. P., and Mackay, I. R., Increased carcinoembryonic antigen in heavy cigarette smokers. *Lancet* **2**, 1238 (1973).
94. Sullivan, P. D., Christine, B., Connelly, R., and Barrett, H., Analysis of trends in age-adjusted incidence rates for 10 major sites of cancer. *Amer. J. Pub. Health* **62**, 1065 (1972).
95. Sunderman, F. W., Nickel carcinogenesis. *Dis. Chest* **54**, 41 (1968).
96. Sunderman, F. W., Metal carcinogenesis in experimental animals. *Food Cosmet. Toxicol.* **9**, 105 (1971).
97. Tokuhata, G. K., Familial factors in human lung cancer and smoking. *Amer. J. Pub. Health* **54**, 24 (1964).
98. Toth, B., and Shimizu, H., Lung carcinogenesis with 1-acetyl-2-isonicotinoyl-hydrazine, the major metabolite of isoniazid. *Eur. J. Cancer* **9**, 285 (1973).
99. Wagner, W. D., Groth, D. H., Holtz, J. L., Madden, G. E., and Stokinger, H. E., Comparative chronic inhalation toxicity of beryllium ores, bertrandite and beryl with production of pulmonary tumors by beryl. *Toxicol. Appl. Pharmacol.* **15**, 10 (1969).
100. Weinzierl, S. M., and Webb, M., Interaction of carcinogenic metals with tissue and body fluids. *Brit. J. Cancer* **26**, 279 (1972).
101. Weiss, W., Cigarette smoke as a carcinogen. *Amer. Rev. Resp. Dis.* **108**, 364 (1973).
102. Wynder, E. L., Etiology of lung cancer: Reflections on two decades of research. *Cancer* **30**, 1332 (1972).
103. Wynder, E. L., and Berg, J. W., Cancer of the lung among nonsmokers. Special reference to histologic patterns. *Cancer* **20**, 1161. (1967).
104. Wynder, E. L., and Hoffmann, D., "Tobacco and Tobacco Smoke: Studies in Experimental Carcinogenesis." Academic Press, New York, 1967.
105. Wynder, E. L., Mabuchi, K., and Beattie, E. J., The epidemiology of lung cancer. Recent trends. *J. Amer. Med. Ass.* **213**, 2221 (1970).
106. Yesner, R., Gelfman, N. A., and Feinstein, A. R., A reappraisal of histopathology in lung cancer and correlation of cell types with antecedent cigarette smoking. *Amer. Rev. Resp. Dis.* **107**, 790 (1973).

Chapter 2

Problems in Morphology and Behavior of Bronchopulmonary Malignant Disease

Mary J. Matthews

I. INTRODUCTION

Bronchopulmonary neoplasms include a wide spectrum of tumors of epithelial and mesenchymal derivation with benign or malignant potentials. This chapter will be limited to the four major types of epithelial tumors that comprise over 90% of primary pulmonary malignancies [19]. These include epidermoid, small cell, adeno-, and large cell carcinomas and their various subtypes.

A massive amount of information has accumulated in the literature concerning bronchogenic carcinoma [59]. Many aspects of its epidemiology and pathogenesis have been documented. There is an acute awareness in both medical and nonmedical communities of the majority of presenting signs and symptoms. Sophisticated techniques have been developed to diagnose these tumors and to evaluate localized or extensive disease. Multiple surgical, radiotherapeutic, and chemotherapeutic protocols have been activated to retard or abate the malignant process. Recently, adjuvant immunotherapeutic procedures have been recommended in an attempt to modify the course of the disease. Many of these protocols are cell-type oriented in the belief that there is a distinct correlation between the cell type of a tumor, its biologic behavior, and possible response to therapy. The prognostic implications are apparent.

Pathology, unfortunately, has had little input into these protocols, beyond providing diagnoses of malignancy via cytology or tissue biopsy. An increasing number of pathologists adhere to one of the classifications of lung cancer recommended by the World Health Organization since 1958. Other pathologists believe a tumor should be named by its most mature element. Another segment of the pathology community feels that a tumor should be named by its dominant component. A number of pathologists fail to subdivide anaplastic carcinomas or to distinguish between the small cell carcinoma with its intermediate forms and the large cell tumor.

No attempt is made to demean these concepts or question the validity of the resulting diagnoses. However, the plethora of concepts makes comparison of data and response to therapy difficult to evaluate. Confusion results when attempts are made to evaluate data presented in the literature on the basis of cell type. Multiple concepts also tend to dilute or alter recognition of the biologic behavior of tumors by cell type.

In 1958, a distinguished panel of pathologists (Yesner, Auerback, and Gerstl) was formed to evaluate surgical materials for the Veterans Administration Lung Cancer Chemotherapy Study Group (VALG) [69]. A slightly modified version of a tentative lung classification proposed by the World Health Organization (WHO) was used for their study. In spite of the undoubted expertise of this panel and their basic agreement on classification, unanimity of agreement on the diagnoses of poorly differentiated epidermoid and adenocarcinomas and the polygonal form of small cell carcinoma occurred in less than 50% of the cases. Unanimous agreement was reached in only 10% of the cases of large cell carcinoma [68].

The Working Party for Therapy of Lung Cancer (WP-L), sponsored by the National Cancer Institute, established a pathology committee in 1971 to resolve some of these difficulties in morphologic criteria. A lung cancer classification, as compatible as possible with the WHO Histological Classification of Lung Tumors, published by Kreyberg [34] and the VALG lung tumor classification [69], was agreed upon. This version was recommended for use by the Pathology Committee of the First International Workshop for Therapy of Lung Cancer, held in October, 1972, at Airlie, Virginia [42]. In Table I, the three classifications are compared.

This chapter will present a synopsis of current information concerning the embryogenesis and histogenesis of lung tumors. Such concepts seem basic to the understanding of pulmonary neoplasia. The morphology of lung tumors, including characteristic gross, light, and electron microscopic (EM) features, will be reviewed. This chapter will also include a largely retrospective study of bronchopulmonary malignancies undertaken to assess the validity of the WP-L classification and to determine if such a classification can provide preliminary information concerning the behavior of lung cancers according to cell type. The role of cytology in the diagnosis and treatment of lung cancer will be discussed. A prospective study, undertaken to determine the accuracy of typing of cytologic specimens as compared to tissue diagnoses, using the WP-L classification will be summarized.

II. EMBRYOLOGY

The lower respiratory tract originates as a ventral diverticulum of the foregut. The primordial laryngotracheal segment becomes separated from its dorsal component, the esophagus, by a mutually derived tracheoesophageal septum. The diverticulum elongates caudally to form lung buds and bronchopulmonary buds from which subsequent dichotomous branchings take place.

By the sixteenth to seventeenth week of intrauterine life, the basic units of the pulmonary conducting system have been formed, and the lung resembles a tubular or glandular structure [46]. Approximately 24 bronchial branchings have occurred. Each bronchus, down to and including terminal bronchioles, is invested in a poorly vascularized mesenchyme and is lined by cuboidal to columnar epithelium. Identified within these cells are vacuoles, glycogen, ciliary processes, and neurosecretory granules (*infra vide*) [13].

By the twenty-fourth to twenty-eighth week, the respiratory portion of the lung is identifiable. Bronchial mucous glands are formed and have the potential to secrete both acid and neutral glycoproteins [15]. Terminal bronchioles have subdivided to form respiratory bronchioles with sacculations representing future alveolar ducts and primitive air sacs and alveoli. The mesenchyme becomes vascularized, and capillaries intimately approach respiratory epithelial cells. Bronchioles are lined by glycogen-containing cuboidal epithelial cells. These cells proliferate over the distal airways,

TABLE I

Comparison of the World Health Organization (WHO), Veterans Administration Lung Cancer Chemotherapy Study Group (VALG), and Working Party for Therapy of Lung Cancer (WP-L) Classifications of Lung Cancer[a]

WHO	VALG	WP-L

I. Epidermoid carcinoma	1. Squamous cell carcinoma (10)
	  (a) With abundant keratin (1a)
	  (b) With intercellular bridges: epidermoid (1b)
	  (c) without keratin or bridges: squamoid (1c)
		10. Epidermoid carcinoma
		  11. Well differentiated
		  12. Moderately differentiated
		  13. Poorly differentiated

II. Small cell anaplastic carcinoma
  1. Fusiform
  2. Polygonal
  3. Lymphocyte-like
  4. Others
	2. Small cell undifferentiated carcinoma (20)
	  (a) with oat cell structure (2a)
	  (b) with polygonal cell structure (2b)
		20. Small cell anaplastic carcinoma
		  21. Lymphocyte-like (oat cell)
		  22. Intermediate cell (fusiform, polygonal, others)

III. Adenocarcinoma
  1. Bronchogenic
    a. Acinar
    b. Papillary
  2. Bronchioloalveolar
	3. Adenocarcinoma (30)
	  a. Acinar (3a)
	  b. Papillary (3b)
	  c. Poorly differentiated (3c)
		30. Adenocarcinoma
		  31. Well differentiated
		  32. Moderately differentiated
		  33. Poorly differentiated
		  34. Bronchio-papillary

IV. Large cell carcinoma
  1. Solid tumors with mucin
  2. Solid tumors without mucin
  3. Giant cell
  4. Clear cell
	4. Large cell undifferentiated carcinoma (40)	40. Large cell carcinoma
		  41. With stratification
		  43. With mucin production
		  42. Giant cell
		  44. Clear cell

[a] WHO data [34]; VALG data [67]; WP-L data [42].

giving rise to two distinct types of alveolar lining cells. The Type I pneumocyte is a thinned attenuated epithelial cell. The Type II pneumocyte produces lamellar osmiophilic bodies, the apparent source of surfactant. An adequate vascular bed is available for gas exchange, and surfactant production is sufficient at this point to permit survival of a premature infant [46].

In the last trimester and until approximately the eighth year of life, there is progressive dilatation of terminal air sacs and alveolar spaces and proliferation of epithelial and vascular components [46].

III. HISTOGENESIS

The tracheobronchial tree, down to the terminal bronchioles, is lined by pseudostratified columnar epithelial cells resting on a basal membrane. Some of the columnar cells are ciliated; others contain mucin globules or are covered by brush borders. Intervening between these cells are multipotential small basal (reserve) cells and granular basal (so-called Kulchitsky or K-type) cells. These basally located cells give the mucosa its pseudostratified appearance [60]. Tonofilamentous elements, potential precursors of keratin, have been identified in the short basal cells by EM. Although these cells predominantly serve as a reservoir for columnar epithelial cells, they retain the potential to form a simpler less complex cell, the squamous cell, in response to chronic injury.

Bensch et al. [7] and Terzakis et al. [64] have identified membrane bound granules in the granular basal cells of the bronchial mucous glands, bronchioles, and bronchi [6, 22]. These cells have pseudopodal cytoplasmic processes that extend along the basal membrane and interdigitate in the intercellular spaces of adjoining columnar cells. The pseudopods contain multiple secretory granules measuring from 800 to 1700 Å. The granules have an electron-dense core separated from a surrounding limiting membrane by a thin electron-translucent halo. These resemble the granules found in the argentaffin cells of the intestines, the clear cells of the thyroid, pancreatic islet cells, and cells of the adrenal medulla and autonomic nerves. Similar granules are found abundantly in bronchial carcinoids. K-type cells occasionally appear, on EM, to have a close association with nerve processes. It is speculated that these specialized cells are possibly neuroectodermal in origin, have endocrine or chemoreceptor functions, and are capable of secreting and/or releasing acetylcholine, kinin activators, serotonin, and other amine groups. Terzakis [64] is of the opinion that these cells may also serve as an accessory source of goblet cells, since he has demonstrated neurosecretorylike granules in the cytoplasm of maturing goblet cells. Cutz and Conen [14] have recently identified similar granules in the bronchial mucosa of human fetal lungs.

Columnar and cuboidal cells throughout the bronchopulmonary tree are characterized by a relative abundance of cellular organelles, including free ribosomes, rough endoplasmic reticulum, mitochondria, and Golgi complexes. Numerous microvilli project from the free or luminal surfaces of the cells. Some columnar cells contain parallel ciliary basal bodies from which cilia arise and project into the lumina. Goblet cells contain numerous secretory vacuoles filled with globular material.

Bronchioles are lined by low columnar ciliated epithelial cells and pale vacuolated cuboidal cells (so-called clara cells), which possibly elaborate glycogen. Mucin-producing cells are not normally present. Over 90% of the alveolar walls are covered by Type I pneumocytes; the remaining alveolar surface is covered by Type II pneumocytes. Desmosomes (dense cytoplasmic membrane attachment plaques) are present between epithelial cells to assure integrity of the alveolar membrane.

Mature squamous cells, by EM, have uniform rounded nuclei, moderate numbers of organelles, and abundant cytoplasm. Cytoplasmic membranes are roughened by intercellular microvillous processes, which meet at desmosomes and form the intercellular bridges of light microscopy. The desmosomes serve to mechanically bind adjoining cells to each other [17]. Tonofibrils, osmiophilic parallel filaments or bundles, are found in perinuclear regions or may abut tangentially or parallel to the desmosomes. Keratohyaline granules, dense lamellar cytoplasmic structures, aggregate to form large round or angular bodies measuring up to 1000 Å which become enmeshed in the interstices of the tonofibrils.

IV. PATHOGENESIS

Bronchogenic carcinomas probably arise most commonly in segmental and subsegmental bronchi in response to repetitive carcinogenic stimuli, inflammation, and/or irritation [41, 43]. Particularly at the bifurcation of bronchial structures, the mucosal lining is most susceptible to injury. Ciliary mechanisms and superficial columnar lining cells tend to shed or become denuded, a process abetted by the physiologically altered air flows and reduced mucous flow rates at these sites. Carcinogenic agents are more likely to be deposited, absorbed, and retained in these zones. Basal (reserve) cells are stimulated to proliferate. Hyperplasia of mucin-secreting columnar epithelial cells is followed, in some instances, by an eventual replacement of the bronchial lining by an orderly arranged metaplastic stratified squamous epithelium. With progressive insult, the basal half of the metaplastic epithelium may become disorganized. Cells lose their usual polarity and individual cells develop atypical irregular hyperchromatic nuclei. Abnormal mitoses may be identified. The superficial layers of the mucosa retain a statified, flattened, but organized pattern. These changes have been termed "atypical metaplasia" or "dysplasia." Eventually, the entire thickness of the mucosa may be replaced by proliferating neoplastic cells (carcinoma-*in-situ*). Intraepithelial neoplasia may involve several centimeters of a bronchial mucosal lining or may be multicentric. Frankly infiltrating neoplasms may develop at some unpredictable future interval when the integrity of the basal membrane is lost. This mechanism particularly pertains to bronchial epidermoid malignancies in experimental animal models as well as in man [1, 2, 25, 26, 36]. Factors associated with these changes include smoking and occupational exposure to arsenic, uranium, chromium, and asbestos or other minerials [24].

The pathogenesis of small cell carcinoma remains an enigma. Its occurrence in smokers, particularly in miners who smoke [58], and the abnormal production of hormones by some of these tumors suggest that the small basal and granular cells are the progenitors [28]. The mechanism of chronic inflammation, additive irritation, and denudement of surface epithelium is implied in the development of this malignancy. Unlike epidermoid carcinomas, however, small cell tumors are rarely identified as arising from the bronchial mucosa. The mucosa may show foci of metaplasia, dysplasia, or basal cell hyperplasia, but it is usually separated from the underlying infiltrating malignancy by a thin but discrete lamina. Its origin from bronchial mucous glands has been suggested [28], but this is equally difficult to substantiate.

The pathogenesis of adenocarcinomas of the lung is also not clearly understood. A relatively small percentage of these tumors are bronchial in origin and may arise from the mucosal lining or from the submucosal bronchial mucous glands.

A significant number of lung tumors of all cell types arise in the periphery of the lung, unrelated to large or small bronchi except by contiguous growth [67]. Spencer states that at least three-quarters of adenocarcinomas, one-third of epidermoid carcinomas, and one-fifth of small cell carcinomas arise in peripheral locations [61]. Woolner [67] estimates that over three-quarters of large cell anaplastic malignancies originate in the periphery of the lung.

Exogenous and endogenous factors associated with adenocarcinomas are multiple and diverse. Implicated exogenous factors include pneumoconiotic dusts, asbestos, cadmium, chromium, beryllium, chemical gasses, mineral oils, viruses, and mycobacteria [8, 24, 43, 61]. Endogenous conditions that have been associated with these neoplasia include chronic interstitial pneumonitis and fibrosis, progressive systemic sclerosis (scleroderma), and scars associated with pulmonary infarctions. Bronchiectasis, chronic lung abscesses, and other necrotizing, destructive pulmonary diseases that terminate in fibrosis and/or local or diffuse honeycombing have also been implicated [3, 8–10, 43, 61].

Regardless of the factors associated, the basic lung pathology consists of progressive disruption and destruction of respiratory acini, fibrosis and inflammation of lung parenchyma, and hyperplasia and/or atypical metaplasia of bronchioloalveolar epithelium. In some instances, the epithelium may be converted to a metaplastic mucin-producing columnar epithelium that proliferates to line either preexisting alveoli or newly reorganized pulmonary spaces to form pseudoglandular or adenomatoid foci. Occasionally, the epithelium may be replaced by metaplastic squamous epithelium. In some cases, small basal-type cells proliferate to form so-called tumorlets, which are similar in arrangement and cell pattern to carcinoids. It is conceivable that these multiple variable metaplastic processes are responsible for the corresponding types of lung tumor found in peripheral locations. Tumors associated with scars, particularly healed infarcts and tuberculosis, tend to be located in the upper lobes. Tumors associated with diffuse interstitial fibrosis and honeycombing may be multicentric and bilateral. The pathogenesis of large cell carcinomas is possibly similar to the peripheral adenocarcinomas.

V. MORPHOLOGY

A. Epidermoid Carcinoma

1. GENERAL

Epidermoid carcinomas are tumors composed predominantly of flattened to polygonal-shaped neoplastic epithelial cells that tend to stratify, form intercellular bridges, and elaborate keratin on an individual cell basis or in the complex of an epithelial pearl. These tumors usually arise from the bronchial mucosa and are frequently associated with adjoining foci of intraepithelial malignancy or dysplasia. Such tumors are called squamous cell carcinoma when they arise from the skin. Many pathologists apply the term "squamous cell" carcinoma to stratifying or keratinizing malignancies arising from any site. Others use the synonymous term "epidermoid" carcinoma to designate a stratifying or keratinizing tumor arising from nonepidermal sources, such as the bronchus, esophagus, oral cavity, larynx, and cervix. The term "epidermoid" carcinoma will be used in this chapter.

Although epidermoid carcinomas probably arise in segmental or subsegmental bronchi, they frequently present as obstructing lesions in the lobar or main stem bronchi. Macholda relates this central growth of tumors to the more generous bronchial vascular bed available in the hilar zones. The tumors tend to be bulky, encroach upon bronchial lumina with the production of obstructing intraluminal granular or polypoid masses, and invade cartilage and adjoining lymph nodes. Symptoms relate to bronchial compromise and obstruction, with distal pneumonitis, atelectasis, bronchiectasis, or abscess formations. Cavitation of these tumors occurs in about 10% of the cases [19]. This may be related to the more peripheral location of some tumors, inadequate blood supply, and subsequent necrosis and liquefaction. Such tumors tend to be unusually well-differentiated and capable of elaborating an excess amount of keratin, which contributes to the central necrotic and caseous nature of the tumor.

2. LIGHT MICROSCOPY

Epidermoid carcinomas* (10) have been divided into three subtypes in the WP-L classification.

a. Well-Differentiated (11). These tumors are composed of proliferating polygonal-shaped to flattened epithelial cells that form sheets, stratifying pseudoductal structures with central zones of cornification and necrosis, and small nests. Individual cells have a "prickle" appearance because of regularly distributed intercellular bridges or may show evidence of intracellular keratinization. Epithelial pearl formation, a conglomeration of cornifying neoplastic cells that form small whorls or nests often devoid of nuclear detail, is frequent. Individual cells have enlarged irregular vesicular or hyperchromatic nuclei and moderate to abundant amounts of acidophilic cytoplasm. The cytoplasm of some cells may be abundant and clear. Nuclei may be giant and nucleoli may be prominent. Abnormal mitotic figures are present. Lymphatic invasion is usually identified if sufficient material is available for evaluation (Fig. 1). Pulmonary malignancies are rarely uniformly well-differentiated. To the contrary, the finding of a well-differentiated epidermoid carcinoma in a cervical lymph node or soft tissue suggests metastases from a primary oropharyngeal, laryngeal, or esophageal malignancy.

b. Moderately Differentiated (12). These tumors share the characteristics of well-differentiated malignancies, but show more nuclear atypism and less tendency to form epithelial pearls or to keratinize (Fig. 2).

c. Poorly Differentiated (13). These tumors are composed predominantly of anaplastic cells, frequently arranged in the classic pattern of

---

* Numbers in parentheses refer to WPL classification, see Table I.

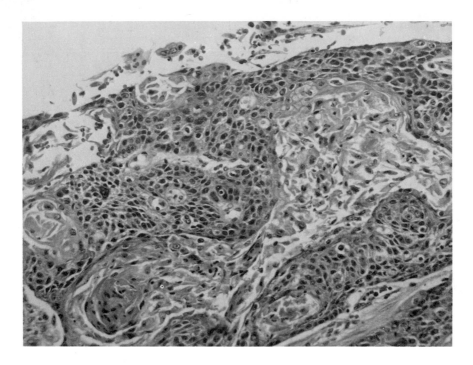

Fig. 1. Well-differentiated epidermoid carcinoma (11). Stratifying sheets of neoplastic cells, showing abundant keratinization and epithelial pearl formation. Hematoxylin and eosin; × 221.

stratifying sheets or pseudoductal structures. Much of the tumor may show little or no evidence of organization or maturation. Minimal but distinct evidence of individual cell keratinization and/or intercellular bridge formation are present. Cells may be loosely cohesive and infiltrate the stroma in small nests or isolated cell pattern. Individual cells have enlarged hyperchromatic or vesicular nuclei with prominent nucleoli. Giant nuclei and multinucleated forms may be present. The cytoplasm may be scant to moderate in amount and amphophilic to acidophilic in staining. (Fig. 3).

3. ELECTRON MICROSCOPY

Epidermoid malignancies share ultrastructural features of most epithelial neoplasms [23, 27, 48, 50, 54, 66]. Cells have distinct cytoplasmic membranes, enlarged nuclei with aberrant enfoldings of the nuclear membrane, prominent variable nucleoli, and dense congregations of nuclear chromosomal materials. Cytoplasmic organelles are not as abundant as in other varieties of tumors. Mitochondria tend to be swollen and irregular in size and shape. In moderately and well-differentiated tumors, numerous

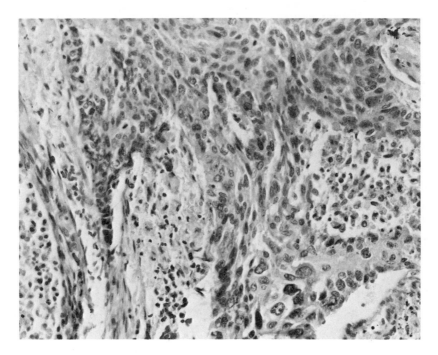

Fig. 2. Moderately differentiated epidermoid carcinoma (12). Stratifying sheets of neoplastic cells. Individual cells showed keratinization and intercellular bridge formation. Hematoxylin and eosin; × 221.

desmosomes and osmiophilic tonofilamentous structures may be identified. Villouslike cytoplasmic processes project from the surfaces of cells into adjoining intercellular spaces and meet at desmosomes. Hattori has described abundant glycogen granules in the vicinity of keratinized tonofibrils. Poorly differentiated tumors, in contrast, have no distinctive characteristics [27]. Desmosomes may be sparsely present. Cells are poorly cohesive.

4. COMMENT

Little difficulty exists in the diagnosis of moderately or well-differentiated epidermoid tumors. The predominantly anaplastic component of poorly differentiated tumors is responsible for discrepancies in diagnosis not only in cytology but also in diagnostic biopsies studied by light or electron microscopy. The inclusion of stratifying tumors that show no evidence of keratinization into this group of malignancies causes much of the discrepancies in diagnosis. A significant number of adenocarcinomas also stratify to form pseudoductal structures. Labeling such tumors undifferentiated epidermoid carcinomas appears to be a conflict in terms and is not

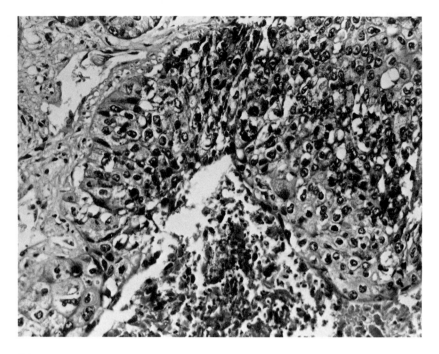

Fig. 3. Poorly differentiated epidermoid carcinoma (13). Stratifying sheets of neoplastic cells with small foci of intracellular keratinization and intercellular bridge formation. The majority of cells are anaplastic in nature. Hematoxylin and eosin; × 221.

always verifiable by EM. It would also seem hazardous to rely on a few ephemeral intercellular bridges, alone, to make a diagnosis of epidermoid malignancies, since their counterpart, the microvillous cytoplasmic processes, with or without desmosomes, are present in both squamous and glandular epithelial cells. It is possible that such poorly organized and differentiated tumors behave differently and should be studied separately in treatment plans that seek to treat and evaluate response to therapy of more differentiated epidermoid neoplasms.

B. Small Cell Carcinoma

1. GENERAL

Small cell (undifferentiated or anaplastic) carcinomas are composed of neoplastic cells with dark oval to round to spindled nuclei and scanty indistinct cytoplasm. These tumors may arise in any part of the tracheobronchial tree, tend to lift the mucosa slightly to form a velvety thickened lining, rapidly invade vascular channels, mediastinal lymph nodes, and soft tissue, and disseminate widely, often before pulmonary symptoms are recognized or provoked. Bronchial lumina may be stenosed circumferentially, but bulky intraluminal masses are rarely produced. The tumors frequently have a glossy, mucoid necrotic and/or hemorrhagic gross appearance. In a significant percentage of cases, the primary pulmonary lesion is obscure or may be overlooked at autopsy. Abnormal secretion of serotonin, antidiuretic hormone, adrenocorticotropic hormone and other similar substances may be associated with this tumor [21, 28].

2. Light Microscopy

Small cell carcinomas (20) have been subdivided into two subtypes in the WP-L classification.

a. Oat Cell (Lymphocytelike) (21). These tumors are composed of cells with round to oval nuclei that are almost twice the size of a lymphocyte. The cells tend to be arranged in ribbons, trabecular streams, cords, sheets, nests, or isolated cell patterns supported by a thin vascular fibrous stroma. Individual cells have darkly staining or vesicular nuclei with a delicate salt and pepper chromatin distribution. Nucleoli are usually indistinct. The cytoplasm is scanty and the majority of cells appear "naked" (Fig. 4). The cells tend to crush readily on biopsy, making interpretation difficult. Extensive areas of the tumor may be necrotic. Frequently within and adjacent to these necrotic foci, deposits of deep-blue staining material, resembling calcium, may be found within the necrotic tissues and in blood vessel walls. These deposits stain positive with Feulgen stains and probably represent excessive nucleic acid (DNA) released by necrotizing epithelial cells. Silver stains to identify neurosecretory granules are negative.

b. Intermediate Cell (22). The intermediate form is characterized by cells with somewhat larger more vesicular, fusiform or spindled nuclei. Nuclear chromatin retains a fine salt and pepper distribution, and nucleoli are indistinct. The cytoplasm is minimal or appears absent. Cells tend to be arranged in sheets, nests, pseudoductal, or individual cell patterns. On occasion, tubular or rosette patterns are formed. Smearing and crushing of neoplastic cells is a significant artifact. Syncytial giant cell formation may occur. In some portions of the tumors, cells may have a moderate amount of pale cytoplasm or appear polygonal in shape (Fig. 5). Silver stains are uniformly negative. DNA staining of necrotic tissues may be observed (Fig. 6).

3. Electron Microscopy

Small cell carcinomas are composed of multiple, variable-sized, small dark cells and clear cells. The clear cells have rounded nuclei and scanty condensed chromatin granules. The small dark cells have irregular molded nuclei and variable-sized, dense chromatin clumps. Nucleoli are small and indistinct. Cytoplasmic membranes are also indistinct. The cytoplasm con-

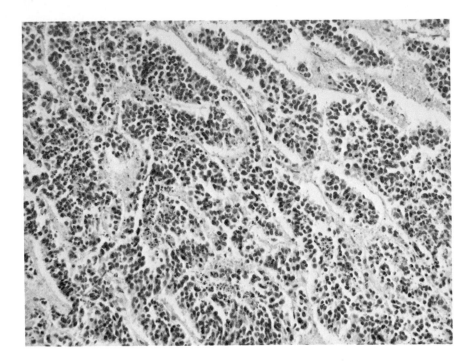

Fig. 4. Small cell carcinoma, lymphocytelike or oat cell type (21). Small round to oval dark cells, arranged in cords and nests separated by a thin vascular fibrous stroma. Hematoxylin and eosin; × 221.

tains a moderate number of organelles and forms pseudopodal structures. Some of the cells, particularly in the pseudopodal zones, contain neurosecretory granules similar to those described above in the K-type cells of the bronchial mucosa. The relative sparcity of these granules in the small cell tumors, in contrast to their abundance in bronchial carcinoid, probably explains their negative reaction to silver stains, in contrast to the relative positivity of the carcinoids. Hattori and co-workers [28] have pointed out that the granules of small cell tumors measure from 500 to 2000 Å, in contrast to granules in carcinoids, which measure from 1000 to 3000 Å. In 13 of 20 cases with small cell carcinoma, serum serotonin levels were elevated and correlated with the number of granules present in the tumors.

4. Comment

Diagnostic difficulties in small cell carcinoma are occasionally encountered in metastatic sites. The tubular or rosette pattern duplicated by this tumor is frequently exaggerated in sinusoidal organs, such as the liver, and

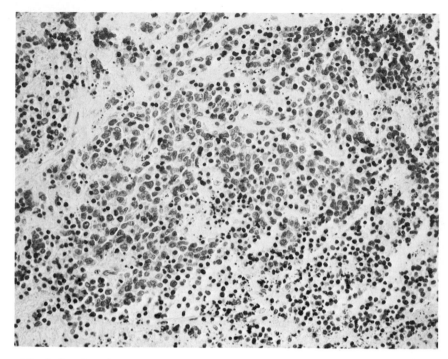

Fig. 5. Small cell carcinoma, intermediate type (22). Small dark necrotic cells in periphery cuff naked cells with larger more vesicular and fusiform nuclei. Hematoxylin and eosin; × 221.

may be misinterpreted as adenocarcinomas. The syncytial giant cell formation and polygonal appearance of some cells may be misinterpreted as large cell carcinomas. In rare instances, distinct but minute foci of keratin may be identified in the tumor, suggesting a poorly differentiated epidermoid malignancy. It is felt that the tubular pattern, giant cell formation, and/or rare foci of keratinization do not distinguish or specify this tumor but more likely express the inherent multipotentiality of the basal (reserve and/or granular) cells. The predominant cell pattern in primary and metastatic sites is inevitably the naked small cell. Electron microscopy is an invaluable aid in confirming the basic nature of this tumor.

C. Adenocarcinoma

1. General

Adenocarcinomas of the lung form acinar or granular structures, may have prominent intraluminal papillary processes and may be mucin-producing or provoke a desmoplastic stroma. Psammoma bodies, similar to

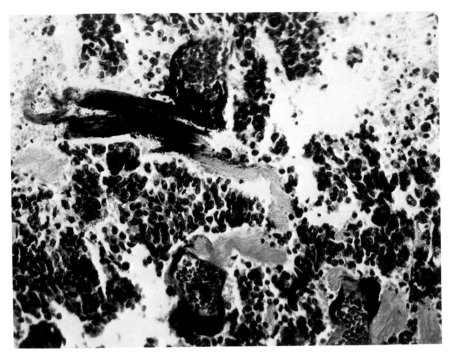

Fig. 6. Small cell carcinoma, intermediate type (22). DNA staining of stroma present in left upper half of figure. Hematoxylin and eosin; × 221.

those produced by neoplasms of the thyroid and ovary, may be found. A small percentage of adenocarcinomas of the lung may arise from the bronchial mucosal lining or underlying mucous glands [5, 11, 61]. These tumors tend to cuff and stenose the bronchial lumina and may be difficult to distinguish from neoplasms metastatic to the bronchi from other organ sites [38, 55, 57]. The majority of adenocarcinomas appear to originate in the periphery of the lung, not obviously related to any bronchus [8, 33, 39, 54, 61]. Such peripheral tumors are frequently circumscribed and subpleural with central pigmented fibrotic cores. Subpleural apical or subapical scars, frequently overlooked and not sampled at autopsy, may host a primary pulmonary malignancy. Over one-quarter of peripheral tumors are silent and may present as solitary distant metastases. In metastatic foci, in particular, it is difficult if not impossible to determine whether these malignancies originate from bronchial or bronchioloalveolar epithelium. Proof of the primary pulmonary nature of the tumor rests on the identification of preexisting pulmonary disease associated with bronchioloalveolar epithelial hyperplasia, metaplasia, or atypia [37].

Classical bronchioloalveolar carcinomas (so-called malignant pulmonary adenomatoses), whether single, multicentric, or lobar in type, tend to use existing alveolar septa as a framework for their growth. It is difficult, if not impossible, to distinguish these tumors from metastatic tumors to the lung, particularly from such organs as the colon, breast, and pancreas [16, 29, 30, 56]. There is a growing consensus of opinion that most adenocarcinomas of the lung are bronchiolar in origin and that the multicentric or lobar variety represents a variant of the disease [4].

2. LIGHT MICROSCOPY

Adencarcinomas (30) have been subdivided into well-, moderately, and poorly differentiated tumors and bronchiolopapillary malignancies in the WP-L classification.

a. *Well-Differentiated (3).* These tumors are composed of proliferating cuboidal to columnar epithelial cells that form distinct acinar or glandular structures. Intraluminal papillary processes, intracellular, or intraluminal mucin may be produced. Individual cells have moderately variable enlarged nuclei and moderate to abundant amounts of cytoplasm. Cytoplasm may be pink, granular, or replaced by mucicarmine positive vacuoles. Abnormal mitoses and psammoma bodies may be present (Fig. 7).

b. *Moderately Differentiated (32).* These tumors are composed of nests, sheets, cords, and isolated neoplastic cells that tend to form acinar, glandular, or complicated cribiform patterns. Individual cells are cuboidal to low columnar in type, have moderately pleomorphic nuclei, and prominent irregular nucleoli. Cytoplasm is moderately abundant and may contain mucin or secretory vacuoles. Intraluminal mucin may be produced (Fig. 8). The stroma is frequently desmoplastic.

c. *Poorly Differentiated (33).* These tumors are composed of anaplastic cells of variable size and shape. Individual cells may contain mucin or secretory vacuoles. Occasional cells have abundant clear cytoplasm. Nuclei may be enlarged or occasionally giant and multinucleated. Nucleoli are prominent, irregular and numerous. Cells may form small cords, nests, or stratifying sheets with central zones of necrosis. Distinct acinar formation is present. The stroma is frequently desmoplastic. The presence of mucin vacuoles per se is not sufficient to include a tumor in this category (Fig. 9).

d. *Bronchiolopapillary (34).* These tumors are predominantly well-differentiated and composed of proliferating cuboidal to columnar epithelial cells with uniform to pleomorphic nuclei, prominent nucleoli, and abundant pink or vacuolated cytoplasm. Cells tend to form relatively uniform large pseudoalveolar or glandular structures, may be arranged in single or

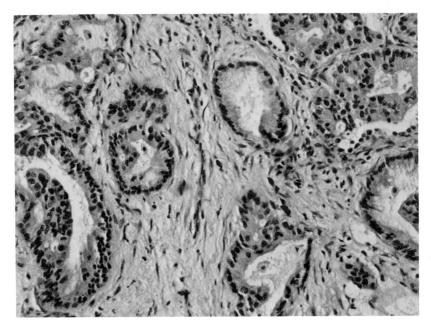

Fig. 7. Well-differentiated adenocarcinoma (31). Distinct neoplastic glands lined by single to several layers of columnar cells with basally located nuclei. Hematoxylin and eosin; × 221.

multiple layers, with basally located nuclei, and have mucicarmine-positive vacuoles in their cytoplasm. Atypical mitotic figures are present. Psammoma bodies may be found in 5–15% of the cases [65]. Individual cells proliferate to form glandular structures or may use the framework of the preexisting alveolar walls for their growth. Individual cells pile up to form small papillary structures that project into the lumina of glands or intra-alveolar spaces. In the majority of tumors, there is a central zone of fibrosis, with entrapped anthracotic pigment, infiltrated by a disorderly proliferation of neoplastic cells. The periphery of the tumor is usually more organized, and neoplastic cells may be identified migrating along preexisting alveolar walls or newly formed pulmonary spaces. Bronchiolar epithelial hyperplasia and atypia are commonly seen in the adjacent parenchyma (Fig. 10).

3. ELECTRON MICROSCOPY

Conspicuous features of adenocarcinoma of the lung include glandular arrangements of neoplastic cells, an abundance of microvilli that project in varying lengths and widths from cytoplasmic surfaces, occasional junctional

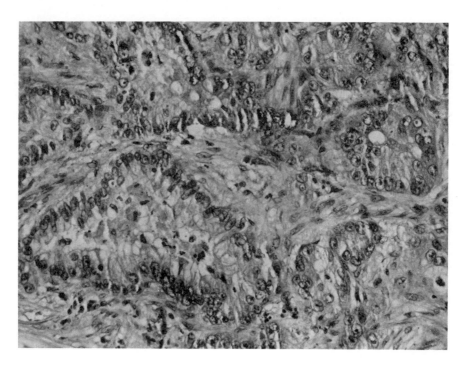

Fig. 8. Moderately differentiated adenocarcinoma (32). Multilayered neoplastic cells forming distinct glands and luminal spaces. Hematoxylin and eosin; × 221.

desmosomes, and terminal bars. Nuclei are enlarged, and nuclear membranes are irregularly enfolded. Chromatin clumps are prominent and eccentric. Nucleoli tend to be enlarged and variable in size and shape. Cytoplasmic structures that seem to appear within nuclei are an expression of abnormal nuclear membrane enfolding. Cytoplasmic organelles, including ribosomes, rough endoplasmic reticulum, and Golgi apparati, are abundant. Mitochondria are numerous, swollen, and atypical. Secretory vacuoles filled with loose globular material and ciliary bodies may be identified. Geller and Toker [20] have identified neurosecretorylike granules in some bronchiolar malignancies. Cells closely resembling the Type II pneumocyte, containing cytoplasmic lamellar osmiophilic inclusion bodies, have been described by other authors [12, 35, 49]. Filamentous intracytoplasmic particles, suggestive of viral inclusions, have also been described [62]. Nagaishi [48] experimentally induced "alveolar" cell carcinomas in mice by urethane administration. Columnar cells, on EM, contained cilia as well as osmiophilic lamellar bodies, suggesting the bronchiolar origin of these cells.

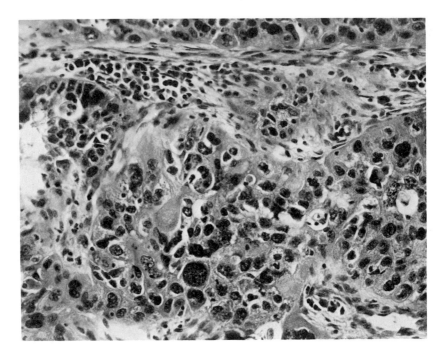

Fig. 9. Poorly differentiated adenocarcinoma (33). Left half of field is composed of anaplastic cells showing little or no evidence of differentiation. Small distinct acinus is formed in right half of field. Hematoxylin and eosin; × 221.

4. Comment

Embryologically and histogenetically, the epithelium of the tracheobronchial tree is entodermal in origin, columnar to cuboidal in type, and capable of producing mucin and cilia from the first trimester. One would anticipate, therefore, that the predominant tumor in the lung, as in the gastrointestinal tract, pancreas and biliary tree, would be an adenocarcinoma. It is not surprising that the features of glandular epithelium are identified by ultrastructural techniques in all varieties of adenocarcinomas and in some of the anaplastic tumors to be described below. The absence of mucin-secreting cells in normal bronchioles and the metaplastic capacity of these structures to form mucin in response to inflammation and/or injury suggest that the small bronchiolar basal cells, similar to their bronchial counterpart, retain the potential for producing globet cells. The presence of neurosecretorylike granules in mucin-producing tumors suggests that K-type cells may contribute to the production of these tumors. Whether such progenitors may be responsible for the production of gonad-

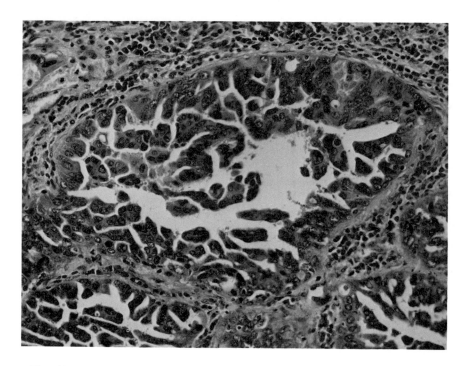

Fig. 10. Bronchiolopapillary adenocarcinoma (34). Cuboidal to columnar cells line or form pseudoalveolar structures and project in papillary pattern into lumina. Hematoxylin and eosin; × 221.

otropic or ACTH-like hormones in some of these tumors is a matter of speculation. The presence of ciliary bodies and mucin vacuoles in neoplastic cells supports the concept that adenocarcinomas are derived from bronchiolar rather than alveolar epithelium. The identification of lamellar osmiophilic bodies in some of these tumors suggest the innate ability of the bronchiolar "clara" cells to differentiate in this manner. The presence of ciliary bodies or processes and lamellar osmiophilic bodies tend to establish the primary pulmonary nature of the tumor.

C. Anaplastic Large Cell Carcinoma

1. GENERAL

The term "large cell carcinoma" is basically a wastebasket category that includes all tumors that show no evidence of maturation or differentiation. The tumors, in general, are composed of pleomorphic cells with variable enlarged nuclei, prominent nucleoli and nuclear inclusions, and abundant cytoplasm. Occasional cells may have giant nuclei or may be multinucleated. Intracellular mucin vacuoles may occasionally be identified. The tumors tend to form large bulky, somewhat circumscribed and necrotic masses, are frequently subpleural or peripheral in origin, invade locally, and disseminate widely [19, 32, 52]. In spite of the highly malignant and undifferentiated nature of these tumors, a surprisingly high 5-year cure rate can be obtained with curative surgical resections [19].

2. Light Microscopy

In the WP-L classification, large cell carcinomas (40) have been subdivided according to whether the tumors stratify, form mucin, giant cells, or clear cells. The tumors, in general, are composed of large cells with angular, oval to spindle configurations, with pleomorphic enlarged irregular vesicular or hyperchromatic nuclei and prominent irregular nucleoli. Cytoplasm is abundant and variable in staining characteristics. Hyaline droplets, mucin vacuoles, and intranuclear inclusions may be present. Cells may be arranged in small loose clusters, stratifying sheets, nests, strands, or isolated cell patterns. Hemorrhage and necrosis may be prominent features of the tumor. Tumors that tend to stratify but show no evidence of keratinization or intercellular bridge formation are classified as 40/10 (41), to permit comparability of data with those studies that diagnose these tumors as poorly differentiated or undifferentiated epidermoid carcinomas (Fig. 11). Tumors that elaborate intracellular mucin but show no evidence of acinar formation are classified as 40/30 (43), to permit comparability of data with those groups that diagnose such tumors as poorly differentiated or undifferentiated adenocarcinomas (Fig. 12). Such designations will permit retrieval of these anaplastic lesions for future study to evaluate behavior and response to therapy without obscuring the response of better differentiated tumors to therapy.

a. Giant Cell (42). These tumors are considered a variant of anaplastic large cell carcinomas and are similar to the tumors described above, with the exception that over one-third of the cell population is composed of cells with bizarre giant nuclei. Cells also show multinucleation and bizarre mitoses and have abundant cytoplasm. Neoplastic cells frequently phagocytize leukocytes, nuclear debris, and pigment granules. Mucin vacuoles may be present within the cytoplasm (Fig. 13).

b. Clear Cell (42). These tumors, in addition to the anaplastic features described above, tend to form nests, clusters, and sheets of neoplastic cells with large vesicular nuclei and abundant, almost clear cytoplasm (Fig. 14).

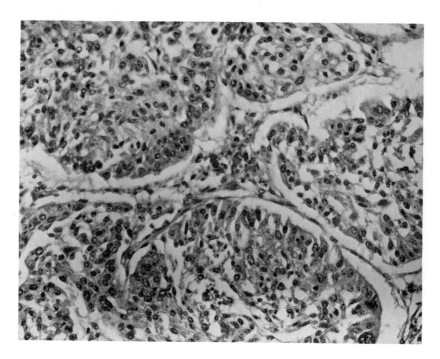

Fig. 11. Large cell carcinoma (41). Stratifying sheets and nests of polygonal-shaped neoplastic cells. No evidence of keratinization or intercellular bridge formation. Hematoxylin and eosin; × 221.

3. ELECTRON MICROSCOPY

A number of authors have stressed the fact that some anaplastic large cell tumors have no specific distinguishing features but appear to share common properties with poorly differentiated epidermoid malignancies and adenocarcinoma [27, 48, 54, 63]. The neoplastic cells are enlarged, have irregular or indistinct cell borders, and are loosely or poorly cohesive. Nuclei are enlarged and irregular; nuclear membranes are tortuous and enfolded. Nucleoli are prominent and irregular. The cytoplasm frequently contains an admixture of ribosomes, atypical mitochrondria, occasional desmosomes, and/or tonofilaments. Microvillous processes may be identified projecting into intercellular spaces.

Giant cell carcinomas, to the contrary, not infrequently contain prominent microvilli and abundant cytoplasmic organelles, including rough endoplasmic reticulum, Golgi, and secretory vacuoles filled with globular material. Nuclei are giant in size and grossly distorted in shape [18, 53]. Membrane-limited intranuclear vacuoles have been described which appear

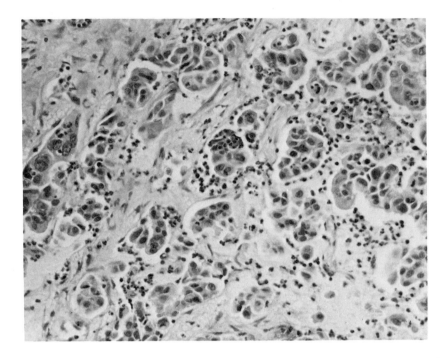

Fig. 12. Large cell carcinoma (43). Small nests and clusters of neoplastic epithelial cells. A few cells contained mucicarmine positive secretory vacuoles. Hematoxylin and eosin; × 221.

to be cytoplasmic artifacts due to an exaggerated nuclear membrane enfolding and polyploidy. Similar intranuclear cytoplasmic structures have also been found in poorly differentiated adenocarcinomas, as noted above.

No electron microscopic data of clear cell tumors has been found.

4. Comment

The cytoplasmic features, suggestive of both epidermoid and glandular malignancies on EM, emphasize the potential of large cell tumors to mature in either direction, in spite of the lack of differentiation seen by light microscopy. Although giant cell tumors contain cytoplasmic organelles of glandular epithelium, their bizarre pattern and behavior support the need for their retention in a separate classification, even when obvious glandular patterns may be identified by light microscopy in one or two isolated organs. The relatively benignant behavior of a small percentage of these anaplastic tumors is neither understood nor predictable at the present time. Stratifying mucin-producing tumors (so-called adenosquamous cell car-

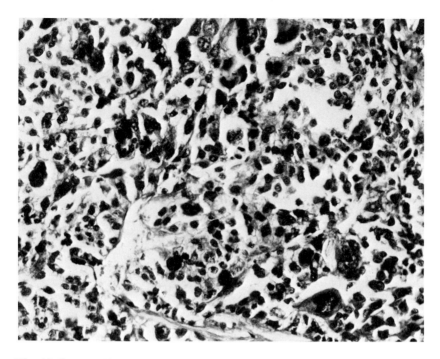

Fig. 13. Large cell carcinoma, giant cell variant (42). Prominent giant and multi-nucleated neoplastic cells, admixed with anaplastic cell clusters and supported by a thin vascular stroma. Rare giant cells in this tumor contained mucicarmine-positive vacuoles. Hematoxylin and eosin; × 221.

cinomas) tend to have this propensity. On the other hand, many pathologists, clinicians, and radiotherapists have anecdotedly encountered patients with anaplastic carcinoma of the lung, with or without adequate therapy and possibly lost to follow-up, who return in 8–10 years with progression of the disease. Such enigmas may hold the key to a better understanding of the disease, host resistance, and response to therapy.

VI. BEHAVIOR OF LUNG TUMORS AND RELATED PROBLEMS

A. General

The basic format of the WHO-oriented WP-L lung cancer classification has been in existence over 48 months. It seemed worthwhile to use this classification, prior to its activation and use by multiple pathologists, in a retrospective study of patients with lung cancer autopsied at the Veterans

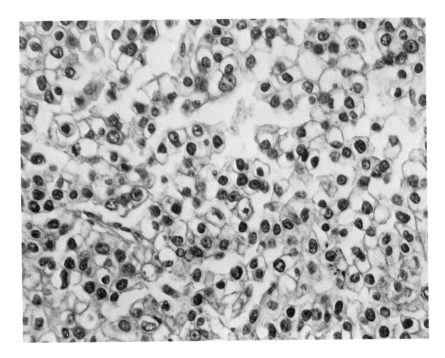

Fig. 14. Large cell carcinoma, clear cell variant (44). Cords, clusters, and nests of anaplastic cells with distinct cell membrane, somewhat uniform nuclei and abundant cytoplasm, clear and almost devoid of content. Hematoxylin and eosin; × 221.

Administration Hospital (VAH), Washington, D.C., over the past 10 years. It was hoped that such a review would identify problems that might be encountered with the classification and give some insight into whether, in fact, the pleomorphic patterns of lung tumors could be diagnosed consistently by participating pathologists. Retrospective evaluation of these cell types has raised questions that must be resolved in future clinical and pathological studies.

Autopsies, during the 10 year period, were performed on 418 patients with lung cancer, limited to the four main cell types. Patients with obvious combined adenosquamous carcinomas, carcinoids, or mesotheliomas were excluded from the study. One hundred and thirteen (113) of these patients were on chemotherapeutic and/or radiotherapeutic protocols, directed by the NCI-VA Medical Oncology Service (VAH), Washington, D.C., since late 1969. Less than 1% of the patients had received a curative or palliative pneumonectomy or lobectomy. The remaining patients received random variable chemotherapeutic, radiotherapeutic, or supportive measures. Rarely, pulmonary tumors were identified at autopsy that were incidental and unrelated to the cause of death.

Autopsy records and slides were reviewed on all patients. Approximately 25 slides, with several organs per slide, were available in the majority of cases. Approximately 50 slides, with several organs or sections per slide, were available on the protocol cases. All sections were stained by routine hematoxylin and eosin. Mucicarmine stains were available in a number of cases. No attempt was made to obtain this stain on all cases. Each case was reviewed and diagnosed according to the WP-L classification, regardless of its prior diagnosis or its protocol cell-type designation.

An attempt was made to evaluate each lung tumor in its primary and metastatic loci, and to place the tumor in one subtype, i.e., well-differentiated, moderately differentiated, poorly differentiated, or single subtypes of the small and large cell carcinomas. This was rarely possible. Relatively well-differentiated primary tumors were moderately or evenly poorly differentiated in some metastatic sites. On occasion, anaplastic tumors in the lung assumed identifiable characteristics of glandular (rarely keratinizing) malignancies in isolated distant foci, usually the adrenal, liver, brain, bone, or lymph nodes. Such discrepancies and inconsistencies of lung tumors are well known to pathologists and add to the problem of classification. Tumors were, therefore, frequently given double designations within a type (11/12 implying a well-differentiated to moderately differentiated tumor; and on occasion, 13/40/42, implying a poorly differentiated epidermoid carcinoma that had a marked anaplastic and giant cell component; 12/13 implying a moderately to poorly differentiated tumor). All organs involved in the metastases were recorded. Metastatic tumors identified grossly but not verified microscopically were excluded. Documented premortem metastases to long bones were included in this survey.

A summary of this retrospective study, according to cell type, follows. The survey of 418 autopsies was used to determine the difficulties that may be encountered in future studies with this classification. The 113 protocol patients were examined more closely to evaluate the behavior of the tumors according to cell subtype. In each cell type, tabulations are made comparing the incidence of metastases in both groups. Significant discrepancies in the percentage of metastases in the two groups may be explained by the larger number of sections studied and the somewhat greater attention paid to the protocol patients at autopsy. It is felt that these figures do not represent the true scope of metastatic disease and should be regarded as a minimal percentage. Approximately 90% of autopsies had brain permits; no attempt was made to correct the proportion of central nervous system metastases. All but four patients were male, reflecting the bias of the VAH population.

B. Epidermoid Carcinoma

Of the 418 patients autopsied over the 10-year period, 126 (30%) had epidermoid carcinoma. Of the 113 protocol patients, 35 (31%) had epidermoid malignancies. Table II compares the incidence and percentage of metastases of both groups.

Table IIA would appear to confirm the locally invasive nature of epidermoid malignancies. There is a striking parallel of incidence and percentage of metastases in the two series, particularly in involvement of the hilar or mediastinal lymph nodes, the pleura, the diaphragm, the alternate lung, the cardiovascular system (including the myocardium, parietal and visceral pericardium), the adrenals, bone, and central nervous system. Fifty-eight (46%) of the patients had no evidence of extension of tumor beyond the thorax. Local invasion of mediastinal lymph nodes, pleura, chest wall, rib, diaphragm, alternate lung, and/or pericardium was noted in these cases. Patients with myocardial, cervical, or thoracic vertebral involvement were excluded from this percentage. Metastases to extrathoracic sites, including the liver, adrenals, kidney, and bone, occurred in 20–25% of the cases.

Three patients had no identifiable tumor at autopsy. One of these patients had been treated by radiotherapy alone; one received radiotherapy prior to pneumonectomy and one received a pneumonectomy, only. All three tumors were well to moderately differentiated in biopsy or pneumonectomy specimens. One tumor metastasized to a parathyroid adenoma. Of the 126 total cases, 12 (10%) had cavitary lesions. Five of these were located in the left upper lobe; 2 in the right upper lobe; 3 in the left lower lobe; and 2 in the right lower lobe. Five well-differentiated tumors, in addition, showed extensive calcification of the primary tumor. Six of the patients had remote resections for carcinoma of the colon or rectum (3), tongue (1), floor of mouth (1) and larynx (1). Three had concomitant malignancies in other sites (2 in the prostate and 1 in the urinary bladder).

Table IIB examines the subtypes of the 35 protocol patients with epidermoid carcinoma. Twenty-nine tumors showed a well to moderately differentiated or a moderately to poorly differentiated pattern in primary and metastatic foci, with evidence of keratinization in all cases. Six tumors showed slight evidence of individual cell keratinization or intercellular bridging formation, stratification, and a predominance of anaplastic nondiagnostic malignant cells. Three of these, in addition, had a prominent giant cell component. Although the numbers are few, a striking pattern seems to emerge. The epidermoid carcinomas, showing moderate differentiation, appear to be locally invasive tumors involving predominantly regional lymph nodes, pleura, chest, and esophageal wall with some tendency

TABLE II

Epidermoid Carcinoma

Site of metastasis	A. Metastatic patterns of patients with epidermoid carcinoma — Total pts 126/418 (30%)	A. Protocol pts 35/113 (31%)	B. Metastatic patterns of protocol patients, according to subtype — Moderately differentiated 29/35 pts	B. Poorly differentiated 6/35 pts
Hilar/Med. lymph nodes	95 (77%)	28 (80%)	22 (75%)	6 (100%)
Pleura	43 (34%)	13 (37%)	8 (28%)	5 (83%)
Chest wall	23 (20%)	11 (31%)	7 (24%)	4 (67%)
Diaphragm	11 (9%)	3 (8.5%)	1 (3%)	2 (35%)
Alternate lung	27 (21%)	8 (23%)	4 (13%)	4 (67%)
Cardiovascular system (total)	27 (21%)	7 (20%)	4 (13%)	3 (50%)
Pericardium	23 (20%)	5 (14%)	3 (10%)	2 (33%)
Heart	10 (8%)	5 (14%)	2 (7%)	3 (50%)
Limited to thorax	58 (46%)	15 (43%)	15 (52%)	0 (0%)
Liver	31 (25%)	12 (34%)	6 (21%)	6 (100%)
Adrenals	29 (23%)	8 (23%)	3 (10%)	5 (83%)
Bone	20 (20%)	8 (23%)	4 (13%)	4 (67%)
Kidney	27 (21%)	10 (29%)	6 (21%)	4 (67%)
GI tract	22 (17.5%)	5 (14%)	3 (10%)	2 (33%)
Esophagus	15 (12%)	8 (23%)	3 (10%)	5 (83%)
Pancreas	17 (13%)	6 (17%)	5 (17%)	1 (17%)
Thyroid	6 (4%)	3 (8.5%)	—	3 (50%)
Spleen	6 (4%)	4 (11%)	1 (3%)	3 (50%)
Parathyroid	5 (3%)	2 (6%)	—	2 (33%)
Pituitary	1 (.8%)	1 (3%)	1 (3%)	—
Brain	2 (1.6%)	—	—	—
Abdominal lymph nodes	13 (10%)	6 (17%)	2 (7%)	4 (67%)

(21%) to metastasize to the liver and kidney (ipsilateral or bilateral). Fifty-two percent of these cases had disease limited to the thorax. The six poorly differentiated and anaplastic malignancies shared the locally agressive and metastatic potential of the better differentiated group, but, in contrast, appeared to metastasize more frequently to the alternate lung, cardiovascular system, adrenals, bone, thyroid, and gastrointestinal tract. Five of the six tumors metastasized to the mucosa or submucosa of the gastrointestinal tract, particularly the small bowel. None of the six patients had disease limited to the thorax. It is apparent that this observation is based on a small number of cases, but such a behavioral characteristic is worth evaluating closely in future studies. Response of these poorly differentiated tumors to therapy cannot be predicted at present.

C. Small Cell Carcinoma

Of the 418 patients in the overall series, 102 (24%) had small cell carcinomas; of the 113 protocol patients, 27 (25%) had small cell tumors. Table III compares the incidence and percentages of metastases of both groups. An attempt was made to evaluate both groups according to subtype to determine differences in behavior between the lymphocyte-type and the intermediate fusiform, spindle, or polygonal variety. No distinction could be made.

The predisposition of small cell tumors to metastasize to regional and abdominal lymph nodes, the alternate lung, liver, adrenals, bone, and central nervous system is apparent. Possibly one of the most perplexing aspects of this tumor is its propensity to metastasize to the pancreas (41% of the total 102 patients; 48% of the 27 protocol cases). Almost inevitably in these cases, metastases were also identified in abdominal lymph nodes. In small early undoubted pancreatic metastases, lymphatics were distended with neoplastic cells or peripheral lobules adjacent to neoplastic lymph nodes were invaded by tumor. In 11 cases, however, the pancreas was so massively involved that questions were raised concerning the primary site of the tumor. Almost all patients with pancreatic metastases had an associated focal acute pancreatitis with fat necrosis. Three had massive hemorrhagic pancreatitis. Pancreatic enzymes were rarely ordered on these patients prior to death. The clinical correlation and significance of these findings must await further studies.

Another interesting finding was the marked osteoblastic activity and new bone formation noted in 8 of 37 patients with bony metastases. The bony reaction was identical to that associated with metastases from prostatic and breast malignancies. Four of the 8 patients were on protocol. The mechanism of this bone formation is not understood. It may be an inherent but little recognized property of the tumor. It has been suggested that the

TABLE III

Small Cell Carcinoma

Sites of Metastasis	Metastatic patterns of patients with small cell carcinoma	
	Total pts 102/418 (24%)	Protocol pts 27/113 (25%)
Hilar/Med. lymph nodes	96 (96%)	23 (85%)
Pleura	34 (34%)	7 (26%)
Chest wall	13 (13%)	5 (18%)
Diaphragm	14 (14%)	1 (4%)
Alternate lung	34 (34%)	12 (44%)
Cardiovascular system (total)	21 (21%)	7 (26%)
Pericardium	18 (18%)	5 (18%)
Heart	14 (14%)	2 (7.4%)
Limited to thorax	4 (4%)	2 (7.4%)
Liver	74 (74%)	18 (66%)
Adrenals	55 (55%)	18 (66%)
Bone	37 (37%) (8 osteoblastic)	15 (55%) (4 osteoblastic)
Kidney	22 (22%)	6 (22%)
CNS	29 (29%)	8 (29%)
Meninges	3 (3%)	1 (3.7%)
Dura	1 (1%)	
GI tract	14 (14%)	2 (7.4%)
Esophagus	9 (14%)	2 (7.4%)
Pancreas	41 (41%)	13 (48%)
Thyroid	18 (18%)	5 (15%)
Spleen	10 (10%)	3 (11%)
Parathyroid	1 (1%)	—
Pituitary	15 (15%)	3 (11%)
Testes	7 (7%)	3 (11%)
Abdominal lymph nodes	52 (52%)	14 (52%)

bony reaction may be secondary to therapy or prolongation of life because of therapy [47].

The affinity of this tumor for endocrine organs is striking. The pancreas has already been mentioned. In addition, in the 102 patients, 18 tumors metastasized to the thyroid, 15 to the pituitary, 7 to the testes, and 1 to the parathyroid. Two tumors metastasized to pituitary adenomas, one metastasized to a thyroid adenoma, and one metastasized to a parathyroid adenoma. The presence of these adenomata causes as much speculation as the metastases in view of the possible "paracrine" or "endocrine" anlage nature of the small cell tumor.

Four patients had no identifiable tumor in the lung at autopsy. One of

these patients had been treated by radiotherapy and no tumor was identified at any site; two others treated by radiotherapy and chemotherapy had
residual disease in lymph nodes and liver. A fourth patient treated with
radiotherapy had no residual tumor in the lung but had multiple distant
metastases. Four patients (4%) had disease localized to the thorax.

Two patients had concomitant carcinoma of the prostate; one had a carcinoma of the colon; and one patient had a small localized carcinoid tumor
in the gastric mucosa. One patient had a cavitary moderately differentiated
epidermoid carcinoma in the lung immediately adjacent to a small cell
carcinoma. Metastases in the mediastinal lymph nodes, liver, and gastrointestinal tract were of a small cell (intermediate) type. Another patient had
a moderately differentiated epidermoid carcinoma identified in the lung,
but metastases in lymph nodes, liver, and bone were a combined lymphocytic and fusiform type of small cell carcinoma. A more diligent search
may have identified a small cell tumor of the lung. Whether this case
represents one or two primary tumors cannot be answered.

Since questions have been raised concerning the primary site of some of
these tumors, particularly those with massive pancreatic involvement, it
should be noted that small cell tumors, believed to be primary in the pancreas, have light and electron microscopic features identifical to their
pulmonary counterparts [51]. It is possible that a protocol designed for
bronchogenic small cell tumors would be equally effective for pancreatic
small cell carcinomas. Evaluation of the pancreas by biochemical and
radiologic techniques seems important in the staging of this disease. Consideration might be given to include upper abdominal lymph nodes in
the field of prophylactic irradiation to reduce the potential of pancreatic
metastases.

D. Adenocarcinoma

Of the 418 patients in the 10-year series, 110 (26%) had adenocarcinoma. Of the 113 protocol patients, 33 (30%) had adenocarcinoma.
Table IV compares the incidence and percentages of metastases of both
groups.

In Table IVA, there is a relative comparability of the incidence and
percentage of metastases in the two groups, particularly in involvement of
the opposite lung, central nervous system, chest wall and diaphragm.
Organs most frequently involved by invasion or metastases include regional
lymph nodes, pleura, adrenals, liver, central nervous system, bone and
cardiovascular system. Twenty cases (18%) had no evidence of extension
of disease beyond the thorax. Twelve of these were bronchiolopapillary
tumors, seven of which were associated with subpleural scars or sclerosing

TABLE IV Adenocarcinoma

Sites of metastasis	A. Metastatic patterns of patients with adenocarcinoma		B. Metastatic patterns of protocol patients, according to subtype	
	Total pts 110/418 (26%)	Protocol pts 33/113 (30%)	Moderately differentiated 23/33	Poorly differentiated 10/33
Hilar/Med. lymph nodes	88 (80%)	24 (73%)	16 (70%)	8 (80%)
Pleura	65 (60%)	23 (70%)	14 (61%)	9 (90%)
Chest wall	22 (20%)	6 (18%)	5 (21%)	1 (10%)
Diaphragm	12 (11%)	5 (15%)	3 (13%)	2 (20%)
Alternate lung	44 (60%)	12 (36%)	5 (21%)	7 (70%)
Cardiovascular system (total)	29 (26%)	13 (39%)	7 (30%)	6 (60%)
Pericardium	28 (25%)	11 (33%)	7 (30%)	4 (40%)
Heart	12 (11%)	7 (21%)	4 (17%)	3 (30%)
Limited to thorax	20 (18%)	3 (11%)	2 (9%)	1 (10%)
Liver	45 (41%)	17 (51%)	10 (43%)	7 (70%)
Adrenals	55 (50%)	20 (60%)	14 (61%)	6 (60%)
Bone	40 (36%)	15 (45%)	9 (39%)	6 (60%)
Kidney	25 (23%)	11 (33%)	8 (35%)	3 (30%)
CNS	41 (37%)	13 (39%)	7 (30%)	6 (60%)
Meninges	10 (10%)	4 (12%)	3 (13%)	1 (10%)
Dura	6 (5.3%)	1 (3%)	—	1 (10%)
GI tract	5 (4.5%)	4 (12%)	2 (9%)	2 (20%)
Esophagus	9 (8%)	5 (15%)	3 (13%)	2 (20%)
Pancreas	14 (12%)	4 (12%)	3 (13%)	1 (10%)
Thyroid	2 (2%)	1 (3%)	—	1 (10%)
Spleen	7 (6.3%)	—	—	—
Pituitary	5 (4.5%)	3 (9%)	1 (4%)	2 (20%)
Abdominal lymph nodes	26 (23%)	8 (24%)	5 (21%)	3 (30%)

tumors. In 9 cases (8%), psammoma bodies were prominent features of the tumor. Eight of the 9 were bronchiolopapillary malignancies. Only two of the nine cases had disease localized to the thorax. Three poorly differentiated tumors had a prominent clear cell component in primary and metastatic foci.

Twelve of 40 tumors that metastasized to bone showed prominent osteoblastic activity and new bone formation. Four of these tumors had an associated osteolytic and destructive bony component. Three of the 40 patients showed fibrosing and lytic changes compatible with the vanishing bone syndrome.

Diffuse microscopic meningeal metastases were identified in 10 cases. The meninges of the pituitary and spinal cord were involved in two of these cases.

One patient had no tumor identified at autopsy. He had received a prior pneumonectomy and was on a chemotherapy protocol. Three patients had microscopic foci of prostatic carcinoma at autopsy; one had a locally invasive prostatic malignancy and another had a history of prostatic carcinoma although no residual disease was identified in the prostate at autopsy. Two of these five patients had distinct bronchiolopapillary malignancies. The remaining three had poorly differentiated adenocarcinomas with prominent anaplastic or giant cell component. One patient had a coexistent chronic lymphocytic leukemia. One patient who had received radiotherapy for carcinoma of the lung had residual tumor in the lung, invasion of hilar lymph nodes and pleura, and partial replacement of the pancreas by an adenocarcinoma. Whether these represent two primaries, a primary pancreatic tumor with pulmonary metastases, or vice versa, is difficult to establish.

Table IVB examines the subtypes of the 33 protocol patients. Twenty-three had well to moderately differentiated tumors and/or bronchiolopapillary patterns. Ten tumors were poorly differentiated with prominent anaplastic, giant cell, or clear cell component. The propensity of the well-differentiated tumors to invade the pleura, involve the opposite lung and to spread by lymphohematogenous routes to regional lymph nodes, adrenals, liver, bone, cardiovascular and central nervous systems appear greatly exaggerated in the poorly differentiated group.

E. Anaplastic Large Cell Carcinoma

Of the 418 patients in the 10-year series, 80 (19%) were classified as large cell anaplastic carcinoma. Eighteen (16%) of the 113 protocol patients were similarly classified. Table V compares the incidence and percentages of both groups. Although less comparability of percentages

TABLE V Large Cell Carcinoma

Sites of metastasis	A. Metastatic patterns of patients with large cell cancer		B. Metastatic patterns of protocol patients according to subtype	
	Total pts 80/418 (19%)	Protocol pts 18/113 (16%)	Nongiant cell 7/18	Giant cell 11/18
Hilar/Med. lymph nodes	67 (84%)	17 (94%)	6 (86%)	11 (100%)
Pleura	54 (67%)	15 (83%)	6 (86%)	9 (81%)
Chest wall	15 (20%)	5 (28%)	3 (43%)	2 (18%)
Diaphragm	12 (15%)	7 (39%)	4 (57%)	3 (27%)
Alternate lung	27 (34%)	8 (44%)	3 (43%)	5 (45%)
Cardiovascular system (total)	26 (33%)	10 (55%)	3 (43%)	7 (63%)
Pericardium	20 (25%)	9 (50%)	3 (43%)	6 (54%)
Heart	12 (20%)	9 (50%)	3 (43%)	6 (54%)
Limited to thorax	11 (14%)	—	—	—
Liver	38 (48%)	11 (60%)	5 (71%)	6 (54%)
Adrenals	47 (59%)	14 (66%)	5 (71%)	9 (81%)
Bone	24 (30%)	10 (55%)	6 (86%)	4 (36%)
Kidney	22 (28%)	6 (33%)	2 (29%)	4 (36%)
CNS	20 (25%)	4 (22%)	2 (29%)	2 (18%)
Meninges	7 (9%)	2 (11%)	1 (14%)	1 (9%)
Dura	7 (9%)	2 (11%)	1 (14%)	1 (9%)
GI tract	16 (20%)	9 (50%)	1 (14%)	8 (72%)
Esophagus	2 (3%)	1 (6%)	1 (14%)	—
Pancreas	18 (22%)	4 (22%)	1 (14%)	3 (27%)
Thyroid	5 (6%)	3 (17%)	1 (14%)	2 (18%)
Spleen	10 (13%)	1 (6%)		1 (9%)
Pituitary	2 (3%)	2 (11%)	1 (14%)	1 (9%)
Abdominal lymph nodes	24 (30%)	7 (39%)	3 (43%)	4 (36%)
Skin	5 (6%)	4 (22%)	2 (29%)	2 (18%)
Gallbladder bed	3 (4%)	2 (11%)	1 (14%)	1 (14%)

appears to exist in these two groups, the predilection for involvement of mediastinal lymph nodes, pleura, liver, adrenals, cardiovascular and central nervous systems, and bone is strikingly similar to the adenocarcinoma series.

Eleven patients (14%) had no evidence of extrathoracic metastases. In three of these cases, the tumors were cavitary with superimposed abscess formation in one. One of the 11 cases was associated with an apical scar. Four patients had associated carcinomas of the prostate. One had a previous resection for a carcinoma of the larynx. One patient had a subpleural anaplastic large cell carcinoma in the left upper lobe and a well-differentiated epidermoid carcinoma in the left lower lobe bronchus. All metastases in this latter case were of the large cell anaplastic type.

Table VB examines subtypes of the 18 protocol patients with large cell carcinoma. Seven tumors were large cell types, with varying degrees of stratification, mucin vacuole formation, and/or clear cell patterns. Eleven tumors, in addition, contained prominent giant cells that comprised from 10 to 30% of the neoplastic cell population. Involvement of the regional lymph nodes, pleura, cardiovascular system, liver, adrenals, and bone are reminiscent of the behavior of poorly differentiated adenocarcinomas. The mucosal and submucosal gastrointestinal spread of tumors with giant cell component is striking and recalls the behavior of the poorly differentiated epidermoid group. The numbers in this group are too few to draw any conclusions. However, close attention should be paid to the intestinal tract, particularly the small bowel, in future studies.

Fourteen of the 80 tumors showed evidence of differentiation in one, rarely two, metastatic sites. In 12 cases, the differentiation was glandular in type. This occurred most frequently in the adrenals (4), bone (2), brain (2), lymph nodes (2), liver (1), and small bowel mucosa (1). Small cell carcinoma patterns were identified in the mediastinal lymph nodes of one patient and in the kidney and pancreatic metastases of another case. These foci were not representative of the tumor as a whole. It has seemed worthwhile to retain these cases in the large cell category for purposes of consistency and because of the likelihood that prognosis and behavior of such tumors may be predicted on the basis of predominant components. Prediction of response of these tumors to therapy is not justified at this time.

VII. PROBLEMS IN CYTODIAGNOSIS OF PULMONARY MALIGNANCIES

Cytologic examination of sputa, bronchial washings, and/or brushings, in experienced hands, is a highly reliable and effective mechanism of diagnosing pulmonary malignancies. The percentage of false positives is negligible. The percentage of false negatives can be reduced significantly by proper collection techniques, by examination of three to five serial sputum specimens per patient, and by fiberoptic bronchial washings and/or brushings [44].

If cytologic typing of lung cancer were to approach the accuracy and consistency of histologic typing, it would not only be feasible but mandatory that this mode of diagnosis become acceptable as a substitute for tissue diagnosis in some cases. Staging procedures and appropriate surgical, radiotherapeutic, and/or chemotherapeutic protocols could be initiated in an earlier and relatively more salvageable stage of the disease.

Members of the Pathology Committee of the WP-L, cognizant of this problem, devised both a retrospective and a prospective study to evaluate the consistency and reliability of cytologic typing. Lukeman [40] reevaluated 103 cases of known lung cancer at the M.D. Anderson Hospital, Houston, Texas, in which both cytologic and histologic specimens were available for analysis. Cytology slides were examined and classified according to cell types. These diagnoses were compared with histologic diagnoses, which at the time did not conform to the WP-L Lung Cancer Classification. In 77 of the 103 cases, cytologic diagnoses were consistent with the histologic diagnoses. Discrepancies occurred in 24 cases. Twenty-two cases were diagnosed histologically as poorly differentiated adenocarcinoma. Sixteen of these were diagnosed cytologically as poorly differentiated epidermoid carcinoma, five were considered unclassifiable, and one was classified as an undifferentiated small cell carcinoma.

Kanhouwa and Matthews [31] undertook a prospective study to evaluate the accuracy of cytologic typing of lung cancer, as compared to the histologic diagnoses, utilizing the WP-L classification. One hundred and thirty-eight (138) cases of lung cancer were diagnosed at the VAH, Washington, D.C., over a 13 month period, in which both cytologic and histologic specimens were submitted for study. All cytology specimens were classified according to cell type. There was one false positive (0.6%) and ten (7.2%) false negatives. Consistent diagnoses were reached in 77% of the cases. Fifty moderately and well-differentiated epidermoid carcinomas were diagnosed accurately; 14 moderately and well-differentiated adenocarcinomas were diagnosed correctly; 17 of 19 small cell tumors were diagnosed accurately; and 5 of 6 large cell carcinomas had consistent diagnoses. In 25 cases (22.5%), cytologic diagnoses were at variance with histologic diagnoses. Of 18 cases classified as large cell anaplastic carcinoma, cytologically, 13 proved to be poorly differentiated adenocarcinoma and 5 proved to be poorly differentiated epidermoid carcinoma. The remaining discrepancies involved poorly differentiated and anaplastic malignancies.

It is considered that the reliability and consistency of cytologic diagnoses of moderately and well-differentiated tumors and small cell carcinomas are equivalent to the accuracy of tissue diagnoses. The WP-L Pathology Committee has, therefore, recommended that the cytologic diagnoses of these groups of tumors be acceptable for entry of patients into various cell-type oriented protocols, particularly when tissue diagnoses are unobtainable. Secondary and tertiary reviews of positive material have assured consistency and accuracy in these cases.

The studies cited above reaffirm the difficulty encountered in recognizing poorly differentiated and anaplastic tumors by light and/or electron microscopy. This does not preclude the possibility that accuracy and reliability of identifying these tumors will improve in future studies, which utilize a uniform histologic classification.

VIII. SUMMARY

The pleomorphism and multiplicity of cell types of lung tumors are basically responsible for the discrepancies and lack of consistency encountered in diagnosing these neoplasms. Tumors that have matured sufficiently to form readily identifiable markers (e.g., keratin and gland formation) appear to have a less aggressive nature. A striking difference in behavior is recognized between epidermoid and adenocarcinomas. The former tend to be localized to the thorax (46%) and metastasize to the liver and kidneys in less than a quarter of the cases. Metastases to other organ sites are even less frequent. Adenocarcinomas, to the contrary, metastasize frequently and predictably to the adrenals, liver, bone, kidney, and central nervous system.

Anaplastic tumors, including large and small cell types, and poorly differentiated tumors with predominantly anaplastic and/or giant cell components, metastasize widely and to unlikely sites. The majority of small cell tumors, metastasize to multiple distant organs, notably to the liver, adrenals, bone, central nervous system, pancreas, and endocrine organs. Anaplastic large cell tumors metastasize in a pattern reminscent of adenocarcinomas. Poorly differentiated epidermoid tumors, and tumors with prominent giant cell component, in addition, metastasize with exceptional frequency to the mucosa and submucosa of the gastrointestinal tract.

Further studies are required to validate these impressions. These findings will have some significance if some measurable difference in response to therapy and survival can be identified in the different cell subtypes.

REFERENCES

1. Auerbach, O., Gere, J. B., Pawlowski, J. M., Muehsam, G. E., Smolin, H. S., and Stout, A. P. *J. Thorac. Surg.* **34,** 298–307 (1957).
2. Auerbach, O., Stout, A. P., Hammond, E. G., and Garfinkel, L., *N. Engl. J. Med.* **265,** 253–269 (1961).

3. Batsakis, J. G., and Johnson, H. A., *AMA Arch. Pathol.* **69**, 633–638, (1960).
4. Bennett, D. D., and Sasser, W. F., *Cancer* **24**, 876–885 (1969).
5. Bennett, D. D., Sasser, W. F., and Ferguson, T. B., *Cancer* **23**, 431–439 (1969).
6. Bensch, K. G., Gordon, G. B., and Miller, L. R., *Cancer* **18**, 592–602 (1965).
7. Bensch, K. G., Gordon, G. B., and Miller, L. R., *J. Ultrastruct. Res.* **12**, 668–686 (1965).
8. Berkheiser, S. W., *Cancer* **12**, 449–508 (1959).
9. Berkheiser, S. W., *Cancer* **16**, 205–211 (1963).
10. Berkheiser, S. W., *Cancer* **18**, 516–521 (1965).
11. Campobasso, O., *Brit. J. Cancer* **22**, 655–662 (1969).
12. Coalson, J. J., Mohr, J. A., Pirtle, J. K., Dee, A. L., and Rhoades, E. R., *Amer. Rev. Resp. Dis.* **101**, 181–197 (1970).
13. Conen, P. E., and Balis, J. O., *in* "Anatomy of the Developing Lung" (J. Emery, ed.), Chapter 3, pp. 18–48. Heinemann, London, 1969.
14. Cutz, E., and Conen, P. E., *Anat. Rec.* **173**, 115–122 (1972).
15. De Haller, R., *in* "Anatomy of the Developing Lung" (J. Emery, ed.), Chapter 6, p. 94. Heinemann, London, 1969.
16. Delarue, N. C., Anderson, W., Sanders, D., and Starr, J., *Cancer* **29**, 90–97 (1972).
17. Ebe, T., and Kobayashi, S., *in* "Fine Structures of Human Cells and Tissues," (T. Ebe, ed.), pp. 242–243. Wiley, New York, 1972.
18. Friedberg, E. C., *Cancer* **18**, 259–264 (1965).
19. Galofre, M., Payne, W. S., Woolner, L. B., Clagett, O. T., and Gage, R. P., *Surg., Gynecol. Obstet.* **119**, 51–61 (1964).
20. Geller, S. A., and Toker, C., *Arch. Pathol.* **88**, 148–154 (1969).
21. George, J. M., Capen, C. C., and Phillips, A. S., *J. Clin. Invest.* **51**, 141–148 (1972).
22. Gmelich, J. T., Bensch, K. G., and Liebow, A. A., *Lab. Invest.* **17**, 88–98 (1967).
23. Greene, J. G., Brown, A. L., and Divertie, M. B., *Mayo Clin. Proc.* **44**, 85–95 (1969).
24. Harris, C. C., *Cancer Chemother. Rep.* **4**, 59–62 (1973).
25. Harris, C. C., Kaufman, D. G., Sporn, M. B., and Saffiotti, U., *Cancer Chemother. Rep.* **4**, 43–54 (1973).
26. Harris, C. C., Sporn, M. B., Kaufman, D. G., Smith, J. M., Baker, M. S., and Saffiotti, U., *Cancer Res.* **31**, 1977–1989 (1971).
27. Hattori, S., Matsuda, M., Tateishi, R., and Terozawa, T., *Gann* **58**, 283–290 (1967).
28. Hattori, S., Matsuda, M., Tateishi, R., Nishihara, H., and Horai, T., *Cancer* **30**, 1014–1024 (1972).
29. Herbut, P. A., *Arch. Pathol.* **41**, 175–184 (1946).
30. Hewer, T. F., *J. Pathol. Bacteriol.* **81**, 323–330 (1961).
31. Kanhouwa, S., and Matthews, M. J., *Acta Cytol.* (in press).
32. Kirklin, J. W., McDonald, J. R., Clagett, O. T., Moersch, H. J., and Gage, R. P., *Surg., Gynecol. Obstet.* **100**, 429–438 (1955).
33. Knudson, R. J., Hatch, H. B., Mitchell, W. T., Jr., *et al., Dis. Chest* **48**, 514–516 (1965).
34. Kreyberg, L., "Histological Typing of Lung Tumors." World Health Organ., Geneva, 1967.
35. Kuhn, C., *Cancer* **30**, 1107–1118 (1972).
36. Kuschner, M., *Amer. Rev. Resp. Dis.* **98**, 573–590 (1968).
37. Liebow, A. A., *Advan. Intern. Med.* **10**, 329–358 (1960).

38. Lisa, J. R., Trinidad, S., and Rosenblatt, M. B., *Cancer* **17**, 395–401 (1964).
39. Lisa, J. R., Trinidad, S., and Rosenblatt, M. B., *Amer. J. Clin. Pathol.* **44**, 375–384 (1965).
40. Lukeman J. M., *Cancer Chemother. Rep.* **4**, 79–93 (1973).
41. Macholda, F., *Acta Univ. Carol., Med. Monogr.* **39**, 62 (1970).
42. Matthews, M. J., *Cancer Chemother. Rep.* **4**, 229–302 (1973).
43. Meyer, E. C., and Liebow, A. A., *Cancer* **18**, 322–350 (1965).
44. Meyer, J. A., and Umiker, W. O., *Med. Clin. N. Amer.* **41**, 1233–1244 (1961).
45. Moersch, H. J., and McDonald, J. R., *Dis. Chest* **23**, 621–633 (1963).
46. Moore, K. L., *in* "The Developing Human," (K. L. Moore, ed.), pp. 167–173. Saunders, Philadelphia, Pennsylvania, 1973.
47. Muggia, F. M., and Hansen, H. H., *Cancer* **30**, 801–805 (1972).
48. Nagaishi, C., Okada, Y., Genka, E., Ikeda, S., and Kitano, M., *Exp. Med. Surg.* **23**, 177–202 (1965).
49. Nash, K. G., Langliniais, P. C., and Greenawald, K. A., *Cancer* **29**, 322–326 (1972).
50. Obiditsch, M. I., and Breitfellner, G., *Cancer* **21**, 945–951 (1968).
51. Patchefsky, A. S., Solit, R., Phillips, L. D., Craddock, N., Harrer, W. V., Cohn, H. E., and Kowlessar, O. D., *Intern. Med.* **77**, 53–61 (1972).
52. Patton, M. M., McDonald, J. R., and Moersch, H. J., *J. Thorac. Surg.* **22**, 88–93 (1951).
53. Razzuk, M. A., Lynn, J. A., Kingsley, W. B., Race, G. J., Urschel, H. C., and Paulson, D. L., *J. Thorac. Cardio. Surg.* **59**, 574–580 (1970).
54. Razzuk, M. A., Martin, J. A., and Paulson, D. L., *J. Thorac. Cardiov. Surg.* **59**, 581–587 (1970).
55. Rosenblatt, M. B., Lisa, J. R., and Collier, F., *Dis. Chest* **51**, 587–595 (1967).
56. Rosenblatt, M. B., Lisa, J. R., and Collier, F., *Dis. Chest* **52**, 147–152 (1967).
57. Rosenblatt, M. B., Lisa, J. R., and Trinidad, S., *Dis. Chest* **49**, 396–404 (1966).
58. Saccomanno, G., Archer, V. E., Auerbach, O., Kuschner, M., Saunders, R. P., and Klein, M. G., *Cancer* **27**, 515–523 (1973).
59. Selawry, O. S., and Hansen, H. H., *in* "Cancer Medicine" (J. Holland and E. Frei, eds.), pp. 1473–1518. Lea & Febiger, Philadelphia, Pennsylvania, 1973.
60. Soroken, S. P., *in* "Histology" (R. D. Greeg and L. Weiss, eds.), pp. 675–712. McGraw-Hill, New York, 1973.
61. Spencer, H., "Pathology of the Lung," 2nd ed., pp. 778–863. Pergamon, Oxford, 1968.
62. Stinson, J. C., Leibovitz, A., Brindley, G. V., Hayward, R. H., Turner, R. A., and McCombs, W. B., *J. Nat. Cancer Inst.* **49**, 1483–1493 (1972).
63. Stoebner, P., Cussac, Y., Porter, A., and Legal, Y., *Cancer* **20**, 286–294 (1967).
64. Terzakis, J. A., Sommers, S. C., and Anderson, B., *Lab. Invest.* **26**, 127–132 (1972).
65. Unterman, D. H., and Reingold, I. M., *Amer. J. Clin. Pathol.* **57**, 297–302 (1972).
66. Watson, J. H., Bryant, V., and Brinkman, G. L., *Proc. Int. Cong. Electron Microsc., 6th, 1966* pp. 759–760 (1966).
67. Woolner, L. B., "Atlas of Peripheral Lung Tumors." Amer Soc. Clin. Pathol., Chicago, Illinois, 1969.
68. Yesner, R., *Cancer Chemother. Rep.* **4**, 55–57 (1973).
69. Yesner, R., Gerstl, B., and Auerbach, O., *Ann. Thorac. Surg.* **1**, 33–49 (1965).

Chapter 3

Rates and Patterns of Growth of Lung Cancer

A. Philippe Chahinian and Lucien Israel

There are many reasons, both technical and ethical, for the paucity of accurate data on the growth of solid tumors in man [15]. The lung is a privileged site for the study of tumor growth because of the possibility of measuring the tumor on successive chest X-rays. This is possible only for tumors with clearly defined contours and simple geometric shape, namely, spherical. Although the majority of pulmonary metastases fit this description, only a small proportion of primary bronchogenic tumors (evaluated at 8 to 30% of all primary bronchogenic tumors depending on the statistical series considered and the recruitment [1]) meet these requirements.

I. THE EXPONENTIAL MODEL IN MAN

Collins *et al.* [13] in 1956 were the first to establish this model in man through roentgenographic study of the growth of 24 cases of pulmonary metastases. Using Mottram's experimental investigations [41] as a basis, these authors remarked that tumor growth followed an exponential pattern throughout the entire macroscopic, clinical course. In this model, growth becomes linear when semilogarithmic coordinates are used, and the doubling time in terms of volume (DT) remains constant. These authors used a simple graphic method for measuring the DT (see Section VI), which they found to be between 11 and 164 days with a mean of 62 days. Schematically speaking, if a tumor is considered to arise from a single cell likened to a spere 10 μm in diameter, it takes $20DT$ to produce 10^6 cells, which represent a tumor 1 mm in diameter, and $30DT$ to produce 10^9 cells, which constitute a tumor 1 cm in diameter, this being the usual threshold of roentgenographic diagnosis [13]. Ten DT later, i.e., when the tumor has doubled its volume 40 times, its diameter is 10 cm and it weighs approximately 1 kg. This corresponds to the mortality zone.

Since these initial investigations, numerous studies involving over 700 cases [27] have confirmed the constancy of the DT and the validity of this exponential model with the exception of a few cases, which will be discussed later. These studies have been performed both on primary lung tumors (summarized in Table I) and on pulmonary metastases of various origins [6, 7, 9, 10, 12, 14, 22, 42, 47, 51, 52, 60, 61]. Moreover, the lung was not the only organ investigated—the DT has also been measured in colonic carcinoma [62], breast cancer [3, 26, 43], lymph node metastases

TABLE I
Growth Rates of Different Pathologic Groups of Human Tumors[a]

Pathologic type	DT (geometric mean in days)	95% confidence interval	Median DT (days)
Lung metastases from squamous cell carcinoma	58.0	47.8–70.3	56
Primary squamous cell carcinoma	81.8	69.2–95.5	80
Lung metastases from adenocarcinoma	82.7	71.9–95.5	89
Primary adenocarcinoma	166.3	122.5–225.7	207

[a] Adapted from Charbit *et al.* [12].

[36], and osteogenic sarcoma [48]. In a cumulative study involving 530 cases of solid tumors, the mean geometric *DT* was calculated to be 58 days [12]. With regard to primary lung cancers, the following data have been established.

A. *DT* Distribution

The distribution of *DT* values is of the log-normal type [10, 12, 52]. This finding is fundamental for statistical calculations that must use the logarithm of the *DT*. Nathan *et al.* [42] collected 177 cases of measurable primary or secondary lung tumors that they used to assess the maximum *DT* range, which proved to be from 7 to 465 days. This range defines the "malignant zone." If the doubling time of a lung nodule is between these values, a malignant tumor should be suspected (with a probability greater than 0.95). In contrast, a *DT* of less than 7 days suggests an infectious or inflammatory lesion, while a *DT* exceeding 465 days is highly suggestive of a benign tumor.

B. Histologic Type and *DT*

As a rule, the slowest doubling time is that of adenocarcinomas, while the fastest is that of undifferentiated tumors, epidermoid tumors being intermediate [22, 51, 60]. However, considerable overlap of *DT* values occurs between the different histologic types, and the histology of a tumor cannot be deduced from its *DT* [6].

C. Doubling Times of the Primary Tumor and of Its Metastases

The rate of tumor growth varies according to the organ or tissue bed. This is the so-called "zone effect" [52]. In breast cancer, for example, *DT* was slowest for the primary tumor and progressively faster for pulmonary metastases, lymph node metastases, and local metastases [30]. Growth rates of different pulmonary metastases in the same individual may vary [30]. The growth rate of metastases from adenocarcinomas and squamous cell carcinomas exceeds that of the primary tumor [12] (Table I). Pulmonary metastases can be considered as autologous transplants that often show a faster growth rate than the primary tumor in experimental situations [12].

II. ANALYSIS OF *DT*

It is striking to compare the *DT* of a tumor, expressed in weeks or months, to the cell cycle, expressed in days, in various experimental systems or in humans [9]. Tumor volume is made up of two parts, namely, the cancer cells themselves and the stroma.

A. Cancer Cells

Three factors are involved in tumor growth. These are the duration of the cell cycle (*CC*), the growth fraction (*GF*), and the cell loss (*CL*). Tumor growth is conditioned by the algebraic sum of these three factors.

1. CELL CYCLE (*CC*)

Only in rare instances, such as L 1210 leukemia, for example, is the *DT* equal to the duration of the *CC* [57]. In solid tumors, the *CC* is extremely variable [2], but it is usually longer than that of normal cells from the same tissue [4, 18].

2. GROWTH FRACTION (*GF*)

A tumor is composed of dividing and nondividing cells. There is some experimental evidence to suggest that a certain number of cells within a tumor are in the G^0 phase [29, 40, 58]. The potential *DT* of a tumor (DT_{pot}) is the *DT* that would be observed in the absence of cell loss. It is based on thymidine labeling indices [18]. The mean DT_{pot} can be calculated using the relationship [54]

$$DT_{pot} = \lambda \, (Ts/LI)$$

where *Ts* is the duration of the S phase, *LI* the mean labeling index, and λ a constant factor.

The growth fraction can be calculated using the equation

$$GF = LI \, (Tc/Ts)$$

where *Tc* is the duration of the cell cycle [38]. Mendelsohn estimated this growth fraction to be 40% of the tumor volume on the average [40].

3. CELL LOSS (*CL*)

Since the potential *DT* is, in fact, much shorter than the *DT* observed, the third factor, cell loss, must be taken into account. The reality of this factor is evident when one considers the possibility of local cell necrosis,

TABLE II

**Tumor and Cell Kinetics in Human Squamous Cell
Carcinoma and Adenocarcinoma[a, b]**

Pathologic type	Mean actual DT (days)	LI (%)	DT_{pot} (days)	Estimated GF (%)	CL (%)	Rate of CL (per 10^9 cells per day)
Squamous cell carcinoma	58	8.3	6.0	25	90	111×10^6
Adenocarcinoma	83	2.1	23.8	6	71	21×10^6

[a] Adapted from Malaise et al. [38].
[b] LI, labeling index; DT_{pot}, potential doubling time; GF, growth factor; CL, cell loss.

cell desquamation, and dissemination via blood and lymphatics [54]. Direct measurement of CL is impossible at the present time, but its value (ϕ) may be deduced from the following formula [54]:

$$\phi = 1 - (DT_{pot}/DT)$$

Cell loss has been estimated to be between 50 and 90% [37, 54]. Thus the rate of cell loss (L) appears to be considerable. It measures the number of cells lost daily per 10^9 cells. This value is equal to $10^9 \phi [\exp(kt) - 1]$, where $k = \log 2/DT_{pot} = 0.69/DT_{pot}$ and $t = 1$ day [38].

A few values for these various parameters have been evaluated by Malaise et al. [38] and are summarized in Table II.

These authors have come to the following conclusions.

a. As a rule, the differences in DT of various tumors cannot be accounted for by differences in cell loss.

b. Cell loss is conditioned by the rate of cell proliferation, i.e., the higher this rate the greater the cell loss.

c. The GF varies considerably between various histologic types and shows the closest correlation with growth rate.

B. Stroma

The stroma is not a static tumor component. It may constitute up to 50% of the tumor volume [22]. It has often been suggested that this tissue is perpetually changing, adapting to tumor growth itself. New vascular tissue is formed at approximately the same rate as cell growth, and it thus makes up a nearly constant fraction of the total tumor volume [16] through proliferation and even formation of new capillaries [46]. Folkman *et al.* [20] demonstrated the existence of a tumor angiogenesis factor that stimulates mitosis in endothelial cells and leads to the rapid formation of new capillaries.

III. IS THE *DT* CONSTANT?

To answer this question, two aspects of tumor growth must be considered: growth during the macroscopic phase, when the tumor is visible and measurable, and microscopic growth starting from the very first cell, which is largely invisible.

A. Macroscopic Growth

If the definition of measurable tumors is strictly adhered to [9, 10] and if tumors with an indistinct geometric configuration or lymphangitic spread are discarded [52], the *DT* is usually constant. According to Spratt *et al.* [53], the log-normal distribution of the diameters of randomly observed tumors supports the concept that growth is exponential.

However, periodic variations in growth rate may occur, probably because of inadequate nutrition and space for the growing mass or because of other factors involved in the tumor–host relationship [52]. Two exceptions to exponential growth have been reported: spontaneous regression and linear nonexponential growth. The incidence of these exceptions is low and varies according to different investigators: 7 cases out of 77 according to Breur [6], 3 cases out of 15 according to Spratt *et al.* [51], 3 cases out of 11 according to Steele and Buell [56], and 3 cases out of 6 according to Weiss [59].

One of the major causes of nonexponential growth appears to be the occurrence of *tumor necrosis* [6, 51, 56]. When active cell division is confined to a sheath of cells on the surface of the tumor while necrosis occurs at its core, the growth curve is downwardly concave when plotted on a semilogarithmic graph [51]. This linear growth was described by Mayneord [39] as early as 1932. Such tumors should not, therefore, be used for the calculation of doubling times, but this type of necrosis may appear secondarily and may remain invisible on X-rays. Most atypical curves appear to be accounted for by this factor, at least for peripheral primary bronchogenic carcinoma.

As for pulmonary metastases, Breur [6] pointed out that other factors may be involved. The first appears to be of a hormonal nature and would explain the longer *DT* of pulmonary metastases from breast cancer at the onset of menopause. Another factor appears to be immunologic and would account for spontaneous regression of pulmonary metastases from placental choriocarcinoma, for example. Other causes of error are discussed in Section VI.

B. Microscopic Growth—Birth of Tumors

Mottram, who established the exponential model experimentally, suggested that this law could be validly applied to the early microscopic phase of tumor growth, since there was a close relationship between the length of the latent period and the DT of tar-induced skin tumors in mice [41]. He concluded that this invisible microscopic phase constituted two-thirds or three-fourths of the natural history of the tumor. Hoffman reported similar findings [24]. Using this data as a basis, Collins et al. [13] calculated that, starting from a single cell, it takes a tumor 5 years to reach a diameter of 1 cm ($30DT$) if the DT is 60 days and 8 years if the DT is 100 days. The mean length of this microscopic phase is 10.8 years for squamous cell bronchogenic carcinomas and 18.6 years for adenocarcinomas according to Garland et al. [22].

In fact, this evaluation is debatable in the light of experimental investigations. In small animals, the tumor growth curve is not linear, when plotted on a semilogarithmic graph, but convex upward [55]. This growth model has been adjusted to the Gompertzian function mainly by Laird [31, 32] and MacCredie et al. [35].

$$V = V_o \exp \{(A/a) [1 - \exp (-at)]\}$$

where V is the tumor volume at time t, V_0 the initial volume, A the growth rate, and a the deceleration rate.

In this model, the DT increases uniformly with time. However, when a is small, the curve is very nearly exponential. The reasons for this slowing of growth rate are complex. Cell kinetic studies using tritiated thymidine have shown a drop in the cell proliferation coefficient [21], sometimes associated with a longer cell cycle [33]. The precise role of cell loss, which is assessed indirectly at the present time, cannot be defined.

MacCredie and Inch [34] showed that the growth of mammary adenocarcinomas in mice is almost exponential when the tumors arise spontaneously, while it is Gompertzian-like for transplanted tumors. This is largely due to tumor necrosis and a relative decrease in blood supply.

In multicell spheroid tumors, grown in soft agar, Folkman and Hochberg [19] observed a phase of exponential growth preceding the onset of central necrosis. When the latter appeared growth became linear until the tumor reached a critical diameter beyond which no further expansion occurred.

These experimental models imply that growth is exponential in the absence of cell necrosis, while it is Gompertzian when cell necrosis occurs [8]. Using transplantation of Lewis lung carcinoma in mice, DeWys [17] demonstrated a synchronous slowing of growth rate of the implanted tumor and its renal and pulmonary metastases after an initial period of exponential growth. The total cell load appeared to determine tumor growth rate. This author rejected the role of immunologic factors and suggested that systemic factors, such as nutritional deficiency (or competition for nutrients) and growth-inhibiting tumor by-products, were a more likely explanation for the findings reported.

Extrapolating these experimental results to man has its drawbacks. Small laboratory animals show a remarkable tolerance to metastases, particularly to tumor grafts of enormous size in relation to body weight [14]. Taking into account the ratio of tumor weight to host body weight, Gompertzian curves differ significantly from the exponential pattern only when this ratio exceeds 10^{-2}. In man, this corresponds to a tumor 10 cm in diameter, i.e., the terminal phase of disease [7].* It may be said, nevertheless, that in man, even if tumor growth follows a Gompertzian-like pattern, the error associated with considering the growth pattern as exponential is in fact negligible, at least during the clinical macroscopic period (Fig. 1). On the other hand, long-term extrapolation and calculation of the "date of birth" of the tumor would be overestimated and is not justified at the present time.

IV. PERSONAL DATA

We have collected 150 cases that fit the definition of measurable lung tumors as previously outlined [10]. The tumors included were all either spherical or slightly elliptical and their entire contour was visible. The diameter considered was the mean of two perpendicular diameters. All measurements were taken from either anteroposterior or lateral chest X-rays. Tomograms, which show a slightly larger diameter, were not used. Under these conditions, correction for magnification was not done since the error would not exceed 5% [22] and had no influence on the slope of the curve. At least three successive measurements were required. Of the 150 cases studied, 73 involved primary lung tumors (48 squamous cell carcinomas, 16 adenocarcinomas, and 9 undifferentiated or oat cell carcinomas) and 77 involved pulmonary metastases of various origins.

The DT was calculated by means of a Wang 720 computer using the method of least squares. The advantage of this method over Collins'

---

* By studying 256 cases of radiation-induced osteosarcomas in adult beagles, Thurman et al. [56a] found also an exponential tumor growth in these animals.

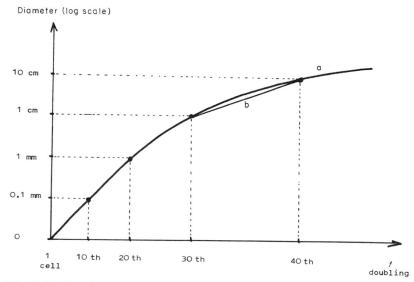

Fig. 1. During the clinical period from the thirtieth to the fortieth doubling, the difference between the Gompertzian curve and the exponential curve is minimal. (a) Gompertzian curve, (b) exponential curve.

graphic procedure [13] is that it is possible to determine the probability of the points being aligned when plotted on semilogarithmic axes. The mean geometric DT was 55.3 days for primary lung tumors (95% range, 12–248 days) and 51.2 days for pulmonary metastases (95% range, 8–311 days) (Table III). Spontaneous growth was observed for an average length of time of $1.7DT$ in primary lung cancer and $2DT$ in pulmonary metastases.

The statistical test performed using the method of least squares showed that for $p < 0.05$ the curve obtained could indeed be considered a straight line in 129 cases. Thus, according to these statistical criteria 21 cases (14%) did not fit the exponential model. These cases did not differ significantly from the overall group in the distribution of primary versus metastatic lesions, in the length of observation of spontaneous growth, or in the DT range. We may thus conclude from this work that 86% of lung tumors studied showed a constant DT during the period of observation.

V. PRACTICAL CONSEQUENCES AND NATURAL HISTORY OF SOLID TUMORS

Lung tumors do not suddenly begin to grow more rapidly during their final stages. This is simply an optical illusion easily explained by the shape of the exponential curve. In fact, growth rate remains constant. It takes the

TABLE III
Rates of Growth of Lung Cancer[a]

Type of Cancer	No. of cases	Doubling time[b]				Exponential growth constant (b)[c] equivalent to doubling time	
		Mean (ln)	Standard deviation (ln)	Mean (days)	95% range (days)	Mean	95% range
Primary	73	4.0134	0.7499	55.3	12–248	0.0125	0.0028–0.0577
Metastases	77	3.9358	0.9026	51.2	8–311	0.0135	0.0022–0.0866

[a] Personal data.

[b] Computer calculated using the method of least squares.

[c] $b = (\log 2 \text{ or } 0.69315)/\text{doubling time (days)}$, b is the growth constant in $V = V_0 \exp(bt)$, the equation for exponential volume increase.

same time for a tumor to increase in size from 1 to 2 cm as it does to increase from 4 to 8 cm [6, 9, 13, 28, 41, 47, 49].

Similarly, the term "acute progressive bout" is incorrect, at least for non-hormone-dependent tumors. All that can be said is that there are fast-growing tumors (DT between 10 and 40 days), tumors of moderate growth rate (DT of 40 to 80 days), and slow-growing tumors (DT > 80 days). The growth curve remains a straight line when semilogarithmic coordinates are used, at least during the macroscopic clinical phase.

Metastases occur more frequently and appear earlier in fast-growing tumors (see Chapter 5). Conversely, there is no logical basis for the concept of "dormant" metastases to explain their appearance years after the removal of the primary tumor. Since the majority of metastases arise when the primary tumor itself is in its microscopic phase [25, 47, 50] and since they are not detected before they have reached a diameter of 2 to 3 cm, it appears logical to assess their presence from a probability viewpoint based on the DT of the primary tumor, rather than from the clinical work-up.

The preclinical microscopic phase accounts for two-thirds or three-fourths of the natural history of exponentially growing tumors [13, 41]. However, although the monocellular or paucicellular origin of cancer is generally recognized [22, 41], the validity of the exponential growth pattern during the microscopic phase has not been conclusively demonstrated. Assuming growth to be Gompertzian (Fig. 1) extrapolation back to the first cell would markedly differ from the exponential model. It is probable, however, that the preclinical phase lasts several years [44, 45].

Adopting an exponential model, at least during the macroscopic phase, enables short-term extrapolation, which is of considerable usefulness in determining therapeutic strategy and assessing the prognosis [11].

VI. APPENDIX: MEASUREMENT OF DOUBLING TIME

The tumor is usually measured on successive chest roentgenograms. Two methods can be used: either direct measurement of tumor volume or measurement of one or several diameters of the tumor.

A. Direct Measurement of Tumor Volume

If the tumor volume V is known at two or several different dates, the DT can be easily calculated. Several formulas can be used. For perfect spheres

$$V = (\pi/6)d^3 = 0.52d^3$$

where d is the diameter of the tumor. For slightly nonspherical tumors [26, 47]

$$V = [(4/3)\pi^{1/2}]\,A^{3/2}$$

where A is the area of the largest cross section, i.e., the roentgenographic picture. This formula can be simplified to

$$V = \tfrac{3}{4}\,A^{3/2}$$

Other formulas have been suggested:

$$V = (\pi/6)d_1d_2^{2} \qquad \text{and} \qquad V = d_1d_2^{3/2}$$

where d_1 and d_2 are two diameters of the tumor [4].

$$V = (\tfrac{4}{3})\,\pi abc$$

for an elliptic tumor where a, b, and c are the three diameters.

B. Graphic Method for Measuring Diameters [13]

This is by far the most convenient and most widely used method. In the exponential model the growth equation is

$$V = V_0\exp(bt) \qquad \text{or} \qquad d = d_0\exp[(b/3)t]$$

and for spheres

$$V/V_0 = (d/d_0)^3$$

If $V = 2V_0$, $t = DT$, which gives the following values for b:

$$b = \log 2/DT = 0.69315/DT$$

by using natural or Napierian logarithm. The exponential regression coefficient or growth constant b determines the slope of the exponential growth curve [51]. If the cells contained in a malignant tumor are considered as units of volume, b expresses the relative rate of cell replication. Multiplied by 10^3, this then represents relative growth expressed in terms of the number of new cells per 10^3 cells per day [51].

The fraction $1/b$ is equal to the mean life-span of a cell [51]. Mean values for b in primary lung cancer have been evaluated by Spratt and Spratt [52] (Table IV). Our personal data are summarized in Table III.

When the diameter of a tumor d doubles, the volume is multiplied by 2^3. When the volume V doubles, the diameter is multiplied by only $2^{1/3}$,

TABLE IV

**Mean Value and 95% Range for b (Exponential Growth Constant) in
Primary Lung Cancer[a]**

		b	
Type of cancer	No. of cases	Mean	95% range
Adenocarcinoma	8	0.0055	0.0006–0.0533
Epidermoid	13	0.0099	0.0028–0.0330
Undifferentiated	13	0.0075	0.0019–0.0289
TOTAL	34	0.0079	0.0015–0.0385

[a] From Spratt and Spratt [52].

i.e., 1.26. From the above equations it is apparent that the doubling time
expressed in terms of diameter is three times as long as the *DT* expressed
in terms of volume.

Figure 2 illustrates the method of graphic measurement. Semilogarithmic paper is used. Diameters are plotted on the *y* axis (logarithmic scale)
and time is plotted on the *x* axis (arithmetic scale). One-third of the *DT*
expressed in terms of diameter equals one volume *DT* [13].

C. Use of Nomogram for Measurement

Gerstenberg [23] has suggested using a nomogram, or an ingenious
graduated ruler, which makes direct reading of *DT* possible.

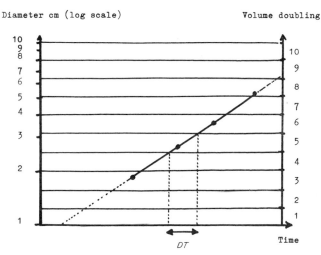

Fig. 2. Graphic measurement of doubling time (*DT*) 1*DT* in terms of volume
equals one-third of the *DT* expressed in terms of diameter.

D. Criticism and Causes of Error of the Graphic Method

The main criticism that may be directed against this method stems from the fact that the tumors measured are not always strictly spherical. In this case the diameter used is either the mean of two perpendicular diameters or, if the tumor grows concentrically, the longest diameter [61]. In effect the *DT* reflects volume variations and a constant error does not change the slope of the graph.

The dimensions measured are, in fact, projections of the tumor on a roentgenographic film. It is, therefore, essential that films are made under identical technical conditions. In practice, this means using standard chest X-rays. Correction for magnification is thus not necessary since the error does not exceed 5% [22] and does not change the slope of the curve. Under these conditions the causes of absolute errors are obvious and include variations in technical characteristics of roentgenographic equipment, poor quality films, and indistinct or poorly defined tumor margins. Otherwise, the error in measurement itself is slight, on the order of 1 or 2 mm [6, 7, 14].

Relative error has been estimated at approximately 7 to 10% [7, 14, 42]. In fact, in this case the error depends on the type of distribution of the different points as calculated by Brenner *et al.* [5]. A minimum of three adequately spaced points must be obtained for correct determination of *DT*.

The main objection concerning the graphic method is that personal judgment, rather than statistical calculation, is used in fitting a straight line to the points. To override this objection, it appears preferable to use the method of least squares to calculate the slope of the curve statistically and to determine the probability with which the growth curve can be likened to a straight line (Table III).

REFERENCES

1. Bariéty, M., Delarue, J., Paillas, J., and Rullière, R., "Les Carcinomes Bronchiques Primitifs." Masson, Paris, 1967.
2. Baserga, R., The relationship of the cell cycle to tumor growth and control of cell division. *Cancer Res.* **25**, 581 (1965).
3. Berger, S., Ingleby, H., and Gershon-Cohen, J., Roentgenography and biopsy in mammary cancer. *Radiology* **73**, 891 (1959).
4. Bertalanffy, F., and Lau, C., Rates of cell division of transplantable malignant rat tumors. *Cancer Res.* **22**, 627 (1962).
5. Brenner, M., Holsti, L., and Pertalla, Y., The study by graphical analysis of the growth of human tumors and metastases of the lung. *Brit. J. Cancer* **21**, 1 (1967).

6. Breur, K., Growth rate and radiosensitivity of human tumours. I. Growth rate of human tumours. *Eur. J. Cancer* **2**, 157 (1966).
7. Bru, A., Combes, P. F., Douchez, J., and Regis, H., Etude des variations du temps de doublement des métastases pulmonaires des cancers rectocoliques traités par le fluoro-5-uracile. *Bull. Cancer* **55**, 63 (1968).
8. Burton, A., Rate of growth of solid tumors as a problem of diffusion. *Growth* **30**, 157 (1966).
9. Chahinian, P., "Le temps de doublement des cancers broncho-pulmonaires. Problèmes posés par la croissance des tumeurs humaines (à propos de 50 cas)," No. 355. Thesis of Medicine. University of Paris, 1969.
10. Chahinian, P., Relationship between tumor doubling time and anatomoclinical features in 50 measurable pulmonary cancers. *Chest* **61**, 340 (1972).
11. Chahinian, P., and Israel, L., Survival gain and volume gain. Mathematical tools in evaluating treatments. *Eur. J. Cancer* **5**, 625 (1969).
12. Charbit, A., Malaise, E. P., and Tubiana, M., Relation between the pathological nature and the growth rate of human tumors. *Eur. J. Cancer* **7**, 307 (1971).
13. Collins, V. P., Loeffler, R. K., and Tivey, H., Observations on growth rates of human tumors. *Amer. J. Roentgenol., Radium Ther. Nucl. Med.* [N.S.] **76**, 988 (1956).
14. Combes, P. F., Douchez, J., Carton, M., and Naja, A., Etude de la croissance des métastases pulmonaires humaines comme argument objectif d'évaluation du pronostic et des effets thérapeutiques. *J. Radiol.* **49**, 893 (1968).
15. Cooper, E. H., Cell kinetics and the growth of solid tumors in man. *In* "The Design of Clinical Trials in Cancer Therapy" (M. Staquet, ed.), p. 156. Editions Scientifiques Européennes, Brussels, 1972.
16. Day, E. D., Vascular relationships of tumor and host. *Progr. Exp. Tumor Res.* **4**, 57 (1964).
17. DeWys, W. D., Studies correlating the growth rate of a tumor and its metastases and providing evidence for tumor-related systemic growth-retarding factors. *Cancer Res.* **32**, 374 (1972).
18. Fabrikant, J. I., Vitak, M. J., and Wisseman, C. L., The kinetics of cellular proliferation in normal and malignant tissues. Nucleic acid metabolism in relation to the cell cycle in human tissues. *Growth* **36**, 173 (1972).
19. Folkman, J., and Hochberg, M., Self-regulation of growth in three dimensions. *J. Exp. Med.* **138**, 745 (1973).
20. Folkman, J., Merler, E., Abernathy, C., and Williams, G., Isolation of a tumor factor responsible for angiogenesis. *J. Exp. Med.* **133**, 275 (1971).
21. Frindel, E., Malaise, E., Alpen, E., and Tubiana, M., Kinetics of cell proliferation of an experimental tumor. *Cancer Res.* **27**, 1122 (1967).
22. Garland, L., Coulson, W., and Wollin, E., The rate of growth and apparent duration of untreated primary bronchial carcinoma. *Cancer* **16**, 694 (1963).
23. Gerstenberg, E., Die Tumorverdopplungszeit, ihre röntgenologishe Bestimmung und ihre Bedeutung für die Röntgendiagnostik. *Fortschr. Roentgenstr.,* **101**, 39 (1964).
24. Hoffman, J., Goltz, H., Reinhard, M., and Warner, S., Quantitative determination of the growth of a transplantable mouse adenocarcinoma. *Cancer Res.* **3**, 237 (1943).
25. Igot, J., and Legal, Y., Age des adénopathies métastatiques dans le cancer mammaire. *Ann. Anat. Pathol.* **13**, 449 (1968).
26. Ingleby, H., Moore, L., and Gershon-Cohen, J., A roentgenographic study of the growth rate of 6 "early" cancers of the breast. *Cancer* **11**, 72 6(1958).

27. Israel, L., L'évaluation de traitements anticancéreux par l'étude des tumeurs mesurables. *In* "The Design of Clinical Trials in Cancer Therapy" (M. Staquet, ed.), p. 190. Editions Scientifiques Européennes, Brussels, 1972.

28. Israel, L., and Chahinian, P., Le temps de doublement des cancers bronchiques. *Rev. Fr. Etud. Clin. Biol.* **14**, 703 (1969).

29. Israel, L., Duchatellier, M., and Chahinian, P., Les tumeurs mesurables broncho-pulmonaires comme moyen d'évaluation de la chimio-résistance et du coefficient de prolifération cellulaire. Conséquences thérapeutiques. *Presse Med.* **78**, 1137 (1970).

30. Kusama, S., Spratt, J. S., Donegan, W. L., Watson, F. R., and Cunningham, C., The gross rates of growth of human mammary carcinoma. *Cancer* **30**, 594 (1972).

31. Laird, A. K., Dynamics of tumor growth. *Brit. J. Cancer* **18**, 490 (1964).

32. Laird, A. K., Dynamics of tumor growth: Comparison of growth rates and extrapolation of growth to one cell. *Brit. J. Cancer* **19**, 278 (1965).

33. Lala, P., and Patt, H., Cytokinetics analysis of tumor growth, *Proc. Nat. Acad. Sci. U.S.* **56**, 1735 (1966).

34. McCredie, J. A., and Inch, W. R., Variations tissulaires au cours de la croissance du carcinome mammaire de la souris. *Laval Med.* **39**, 684 (1968).

35. McCredie, J. A., Inch, W. R., Kruuv, J., and Watson, T. A., The rate of tumor growth in animals. *Growth* **29**, 331 (1965).

36. McDonald, J. S., Laugier, A., and Schlienger, M., Observations on the growth of tumors in lymph nodes changing from normal to abnormal while remaining apacified after lymphography. *Clin. Radiol.* **19**, 120 (1968).

37. Malaise, E., Données actuelles sur la cinétique des tumeurs humaines. *Rev. Fr. Etud. Clin. Biol.* **14**, 11 (1969).

38. Malaise, E. P., Chavaudra, N., and Tubiana, M., The relationship between growth rate, labelling index and histological type of human solid tumours. *Eur. J. Cancer* **9**, 305 (1973).

39. Mayneord, M. W., On law of growth of Jensen's rat sarcoma. *Amer. J. Cancer* **16**, 841 (1932).

40. Mendelsohn, M. L., Autoradiographic analysis of cell proliferation in spontaneous breast cancer of C_3H mouse. III. The growth fraction. *J. Nat. Cancer Inst.* **28**, 1015 (1962).

41. Mottram, J. C., On origin of tar tumors in mice, whether from single cells or many cells. *J. Pathol. Bacteriol.* **40**, 407 (1935).

42. Nathan, M. H., Collins, V. P., and Adams, R. A., Differentiation of benign and malignant pulmonary nodules by growth rate. *Radiology* **79**, 221 (1962).

43. Philippe, E., and Legal, Y., Growth of seventy-eight recurrent mammary cancers. *Cancer* **21**, 461 (1968).

44. Rigler, L. G., O'Longhlin, B., and Tucker, R., The duration of carcinoma of the lung. *Dis. Chest* **23**, 50 (1953).

45. Rigler, L. G., A roentgen study of the evolution of carcinoma of the lung. *J. Thorac. Surg.* **34**, 283 (1957).

46. Rubin, P., and Casarett, G., Microcirculation of tumors. Part I. Anatomy, function and necrosis. *Clin. Radiol.* **17**, 220 (1966).

47. Schwartz, M., A biomathematical approach to clinical tumor growth. *Cancer* **14**, 1272 (1961).

48. Spratt, J. S., The rates of growth of skeletal sarcomas. *Cancer* **18**, 14 (1965).

49. Spratt, J. S., The rates and patterns of growth of neoplasms of the large intestine and rectum. *Surg. Clin. N. Amer.* **45**, 1103 (1965).
50. Spratt, J. S., and Ackerman, L. V., Small primary adenocarcinomas of the colon and rectum. *J. Amer. Med. Ass.* **179**, 337 (1962).
51. Spratt, J. S., Spjut, H. J., and Roper, C. L., The frequency distribution of the rates of growth and the estimated duration of primary pulmonary carcinomas. *Cancer* **16**, 687 (1963).
52. Spratt, J. S., and Spratt, T. L., Rates of growth of pulmonary metastases and host survival. *Ann. Surg.* **159**, 161 (1964).
53. Spratt, J. S., Ter Pogossian, M., and Long, R., The detection and growth of intrathoracic neoplasms. *Arch. Surg. (Chicago)* **86**, 283 (1963).
54. Steel, G., Cell loss as a factor in the growth rate of human tumours. *Eur. J. Cancer* **3**, 381 (1967).
55. Steel, G., and Lamerton, L., The growth rate of human tumours. *Brit. J. Cancer* **20**, 74 (1966).
56. Steele, J. D., and Buell, P., Asymptomatic solitary pulmonary nodules. Host survival, tumor size, and growth rate. *J. Thorac. Cardiov. Surg.* **65**, 140 (1973).
56a. Thurman, G. B., Mays, C. W., Taylor, G. N., Christensen, W. R., Rehfeld, C. E., and Dougherty, T. F., Growth dynamics of Beagle osteosarcomas. *Growth* **35**, 119 (1971).
57. Tubiana, M., La cinétique des populations de cellules. *Ann. Biol. Clin. (Paris)* **26**, 793 (1968).
58. Valleron, A. J., and Frindel, E., Computer stimulation of growing cell populations. *Cell Tissue Kinet.* **6**, 69 (1973).
59. Weiss, W., The growth rate of bronchogenic carcinoma: Is it constant? *Cancer* **32**, 167 (1973).
60. Weiss, W., Boucot, K., and Cooper, D., Growth rate in the detection and prognosis of bronchogenic carcinoma. *J. Amer. Med. Ass.* **198**, 1246 (1966).
61. Weiss, W., Boucot, K., and Cooper, D., The survival of men with measurable proved lung cancer in relation to growth rate. *Amer. J. Roentgenol. Radium Ther. Nucl. Med.* [N.S.] 98, 404 (1966).
62. Welin, S., Youker, J., and Spratt, J., The rates and patterns of growth of 375 tumors of the large intestine and rectum observed serially by double contraste enema study. *Amer. J. Roentgenol., Radium Ther. Nucl. Med.* [N.S.] **90**, 673 (1963).

Chapter 4

Tumor Antigens Associated with Lung Cancer

Paul Lo Gerfo

The hypotheses that neoplastic tissue can be distinguished from normal tissues by properties that are unique to tumor cells is not a new one. At the turn of the century investigators had shown that transplantable animal tumors could be rejected by the recipient, and this stimulated a great deal of interest in an area now known as tumor immunology. It did not become apparent until the late twenties, however, that this rejection of tumor tissue was governed by the genetics of the histocompatibility antigens rather than tumor-specific antigens (TSA). This problem of distinguishing genetically controlled antigenic differences between animals from those antigens related to neoplastic transformation could not be resolved until genetically identical laboratory animals became available for investigation. Even today this fundamental problem plagues studies on tumor specific antigens, and investigations in this area were not looked upon with favor by the scientific community until the last few decades [30].

In retrospect the first identification of a tumor-specific antigen can probably be attributed to Gross (1943), but because of a limited study and an inadequate number of controls his work was largely ignored by his peers. A new interest was stimulated in this area mainly as a result of research carried out by Foley in 1953 [7] using methylcholanthrene-in-

duced mouse tumors, but doubt about the existence of tumor-specific antigens was prevalent until 1957 when Prehn and Main conclusively demonstrated their presence using a similar methycholanthrene-induced mouse
sarcoma [35]. These tumor antigens were relatively weak at inducing immunity in animals when compared to normal histocompatability antigen
and the immunity induced could easily be overcome by giving a large
challenging dose of tumor cells.

In the last decade intensive studies on animal tumors have revealed that
the agent responsible for malignant transformation has a major influence
on the nature of antigens produced by the tumor. At the present time tumor antigens can be classified into one of three general categories and
these will be discussed individually.

I. CHEMICALLY OR PHYSICALLY INDUCED
TUMOR ANTIGENS

Antigens found in chemically induced tumors are *unique* in each tumor
and *do not share common antigenic properties*, even though the tumors in
which they are found may appear histologically identical or may have been
induced by the same carcinogen [34]. Even two separate tumors induced
in the same host at the same time by the same carcinogen are antigenically
different. The reason for this is unclear, since in theory it would seem
plausible that the carcinogen might behave as a haptene and some degree
of cross-reactivity would be expected. It is of interest that some of these
chemically induced antigens show cross-reactivity with fetal antigens from
the same species. These antigens that show cross-reactivity with fetal tissues may not be specifically related to a carcinogen but rather represent a
form of antigence regression found in many tissues undergoing malignant
transformation.

Carcinogen-induced tumor-specific antigens differ in their ability to elect
an immune response in a host, and this response is poor when compared
to normal transplantation antigen [34]. In general, methylcholanthrene-induced tumor antigens incite a relatively strong host immune response compared to antigens induced by other carcinogens. The strength of the chemically induced antigens can be predicted in part by the latent period that
occurs between carcinogen exposure and tumor development, the longer
the latent periods being associated with weaker antigens.

Chemically induced pulmonary neoplasms in animals can be produced
using a number of carcinogens. The ability of these carcinogens to induce
tumors, however, can be modified by a wide variety of factors. These factors include genetic makeup, infection, bacterial flora, and vitamin A [6,

36, 39]. Some of these same factors appear to play a role in human lung cancer [45]. Whether any of these chemically induced animal pulmonary cancers are associated with tumor-specific antigen is unknown at present. Some information, however, is available on carcinogen-induced pulmonary adenomas in mice. Prehn reported that one of eight urethane-induced adenomas had detectable tumor antigens but that these were very weak [34]. Recently it has been shown that the antigenicity of chemically induced tumors can be increased by using immunodepression, and with this technique a high percentage of these pulmonary adenoma in mice contain tumor-specific antigen (TSA) [3, 14].

Lung cancer in man appears to be related to carcinogens found in cigarette smoke and in some instances to environmental carcinogens associated with certain occupations [40, 45]. The induction period for these tumors is very long, and if experience with chemically induced tumor in animals can be applied to man it is apparent that chemically induced tumor-specific antigens in lung cancer, if present, are very weak. The rapid demise of patients with this form of cancer would suggest that if an immune response to these antigens occurs, it is poor at best or that it takes the form of a blocking factor. Unfortunately we have little to support the concept that chemically related tumor-specific antigens exist in man and most antigens described to date can be attributed to unmasking of repressed fetal genetic information.

II. VIRAL-INDUCED TUMOR ANTIGENS

There are a large number of RNA and DNA viruses that are capable of inducing cancer in animals, and some of these oncogenic animal viruses are members of the adenovirus group commonly found in humans. Although there is no definitive proof to show that any human cancer is caused by a virus, there is considerable evidence that points to an association of some human cancers with viruses that have oncogenic potential. In animal models these oncogenic viruses can be transmitted by the gametes of the parents, via the milk, or by direct contact depending on the virus system involved. The transfer of some viruses via the normal reproductive genetic apparatus has led to a speculation about the role of such "oncogenes" in human cancer [13]. The mechanism of tumor inductions of these viruses cannot be discussed here, but it is of interest that the antigens found in these tumors include both the viral antigens themselves and new antigens induced by the virus.

The tumor-specific antigens found in virally transformed cells, unlike carcinogen-induced antigens, are *similar* in all tumors induced by the same virus regardless of the morphological appearance of the tumor [38]. For example, all tumors induced by the mammary tumor virus share *common* tumor-specific antigens, but these antigens are not shared with tumors produced by other viruses, even though they may be histologically similar. There are some viruses that do share common antigenic properties, but this is unusual. The production of these induced tumor-specific antigens is controlled by the viral genome rather than the cellular genome except in some cases where these antigens may represent an unmasking of genes controlling the production of embryonic antigens.

Tumors induced by viruses are much more susceptible to immunological therapy because the antigens produced are relatively good immunizing agents. In fact, it is difficult to infect adult animals with these viruses since they usually can mount a good immune response against the virus. This, however, is an extremely complex problem since it involves the genetic makeup of the exposed animals, which may in part be controlled by a viral oncogene [13]. In general, however, some exposure to intact viruses or viral antigens in fetal or neonatal period is necessary for viral infection to take place in the adult animal. Even if this has occurred, it is possible to alter the effect of the oncogenic virus by immunization with chemically treated virus. This immunization may result in a temporary delay in tumor growth or completely protect the animal against tumor development. Some of these effects might be related to the production of interferon, since active virus infection seems more effective in prevention of tumor growth.

Electron microscopy studies on animal pulmonary neoplasia have revealed the presence of intracisternal A particles and C type viruses [1, 2, 18]. The latter are generally considered to have oncogenic potential, but the A type particles have never been conclusively shown to possess biological activity and are ubiquitous in both normal and neoplastic tissue. Since these tumors are usually chemically induced, the role of the virus in the pathogenesis of these lesions is unclear, but there is no doubt that these C particles are associated with tumor-induced antigens specifically related to the virus [1]. This would imply that if the animals could be immunized against these viral antigens and if the viral antigens were necessary to maintain neoplastic growth, immunization might protect the animal against tumor development. This is obviously pure speculation, but it is important to understand the concept that the etiological role of the virus may not be important when using immunotherapy against the tumor.

Lung carcinoma in sheep (jagsiekte) has been studied extensively and appears to be transmitted by a virus [44]. Virus particles morphologically similar to other feline and rodent oncogenic virus have been observed in these tumors using electron microscopy [33]. These tumors appear to have some antigenicity that elects a cellular immune response associated with a hyperglobulenemia and occasional myeloma-like serum spikes [12]. In addition, a small percentage of animals appears to have humoral antibodies against the tumor. Whether the immune responses in these animals are directed against virus-induced antigens remains to be determined.

The analogy between alveolar cell carcinoma in humans and the pulmonary neoplasms seen in sheep has been discussed by others [40]. Attempts, however, to document viral particles in human alveolar cell carcinoma have been unsuccessful, and the antigenicity of these tumors has not been studied but such studies would be of considerable interest [20]. There is some evidence that tumor-specific antigens are present in oat cell carcinoma of the lung. These antigens appear to be a common or cross-reacting antigen, suggesting that a virus may play a role in antigen production, but there is no evidence to support the hypothesis that viruses play a significant part in the etiology of this form of human lung cancer [32]. Hopefully viral antigens may be of value in immunotherapy or prevention of some forms of lung cancer, but at the present time this seems unlikely.

III. FETAL ANTIGENS

These probably represent the great majority of human tumor antigens described to date, and they may account for a significant number of common tumor antigens previously attributed to chemical carcinogens or oncogenic viruses. It has been postulated that a multipotential embryonic cell matures to assume its life's role by suppression of certain genomes. In fetal tissue some of these genomes are expressed as unique substances in the cell and are detectable by immunological techniques, hence the term "fetal antigens." As the fetal cell matures, the genomes are suppressed and the fetal antigens disappear. When these cells undergo malignant transformation, a derepression of some of these genomes occurs and the fetal antigens reappear in the malignant cell. This process has been referred to as "antigenic regression" and has been described in detail [9]. Such fetal antigens would be expected to occur in a wide variety of human neoplasms, since in theory at least all cells would have the suppressed genetic information. The presence of fetal antigens in essence represents a regression to a more embryonic state and does not necessarily imply that malignant transformation has taken place. For instance fetal antigens have been found in rapidly regenerating tissues, tumors produced by chemical carcinogens, in tumors produced by oncogenic viruses.

It is apparent from many studies that fetal antigens never entirely disappear from the adult cell but are present in such low levels that they cannot be detected except with sensitive immunological techniques [6, 7]. This is important from a clinical standpoint, since they do not represent substances that are foreign to the host, and it would be difficult to imagine a significant number of cancer patients developing an immune response to a normal tissue antigen. Reports of antibody to fetal antigens can be found, but have never been documented by other authors despite many attempts [8, 21]. The function of these fetal antigens is unknown but may in some way be important in protecting the cell from the normal immunologic surveillance mechanism.

IV. CARCINOEMBRYONIC ANTIGEN (CEA)

This antigen is characterized as a glycoprotein with a molecular weight of approximately 200,000 and appears to be related to the blood group substances [19]. Described by Gold and Freedman in 1965 it was originally thought to be specific for endodermally derived gastrointestinal tract neoplasms and fetal gastrointestinal tissue [10]. Initial studies using radioimmunoassay techniques demonstrated that the antigen could be detected only in the serum of patients with gastrointestinal neoplasms [42]. This specificity has never been confirmed by others, and Gold's laboratory in a double blind study was unable to support its original findings [11, 21, 23, 28, 47]. The wide discrepancy between Gold's initial results and those of others led some authors to believe they were studying a closely related but antigenically distinct antigen [22–25]. Since this antigen was referred to as tumor-associated antigen some confusion in terminology has resulted. It is now apparent that CEA is associated with many types of neoplasms and some benign diseases. Slightly elevated serum levels of CEA are not uncommon in some apparently healthy individuals, especially those who are heavy smokers [11] and all evidence supports the concept that CEA and tumor-associated antigen are identical [23]. The distribution of this antigen in the plasma of individuals is shown in Tables I and II. These tables are based on a large collaborative study carried out by Hoffman La Roche using an assay for CEA that will soon be commercially available, and a detailed report of these results can be found elsewhere [11]. It is obvious that there is considerable overlap in the plasma CEA values obtained from patients with and without malignant disease. In general, high levels of CEA are associated with malignancy, and in patients with colon carcinoma the incidence of elevated CEA values correlates with the stage of the disease. On the basis of many reports it is questionable if this assay will be of value as a screening procedure except in selected patient populations.

Small amounts of CEA have been detected in normal lung tissue from

TABLE I

CEA Titers in Selected Groups of Subjects

	Number	Percent with CEA levels of			
		0.0–2.5 ng/ml	2.6–5.0 ng/ml	5.1–10.0 ng/ml	>10.0 ng/ml
Nonsmokers	892	97.0	2.8	0.2	0
Presently smoking	620	80.4	15.0	3.6	1.0
Former smokers	235	93.4	4.6	1.0	1.0
Bronchitis	61	67.0	25.0	7.0	1.0
Pulmonary emphysema	49	43.0	37.0	16.0	4.0
Alcoholic cirrhosis	120	30.0	44.0	24.0	2.0
Ulcerative colitis	146	69.0	18.0	8.0	5.0
Regional ileitis	97	60.0	27.0	11.0	2.0
Granulomatous colitis	59	53.0	27.0	15.0	5.0
Gastric ulcer	94	55.0	29.0	15.0	1.0
Duodenal ulcer	166	70.0	22.0	6.0	2.0
Rectal polyps	90	81.0	15.0	3.0	1.0

TABLE II

CEA Titers in Patients with Clinically Suspected Malignancy

Histologically proven site	Subjects	Percent with CEA levels of			
		0.0–2.5 ng/ml	2.6–5.0 ng/ml	5.1–10.0 ng/ml	>10.0 ng/ml
Lung	181	24	25	25	26
Colorectal	544	28	23	14	35
Pancreas	55	9	31	25	35
Stomach	79	39	32	10	19
Breast	125	53	20	13	14
Other[a]	343	51	28	12	9

[a] Prostate, head and neck, ovary, cervix, etc.

adult patients who died with nonmalignant disease, but attempts to demonstrate CEA in fetal lung have been unsuccessful [25]. The presence of CEA in adult lung tissue might indicate that some early premalignant changes may have taken place in these tissues since most of these individuals were smokers. This CEA in lung tissue could account for the high percentage of heavy smokers who have elevated plasma CEA values. If the plasma CEA levels reflect the lung tissue levels of CEA it might serve as a marker for individuals who are at risk to develop lung cancer, and be useful in selecting patients requiring close observation. Long-term follow-up studies on smokers with serial plasma CEA levels and autopsy specimens from smokers and nonsmokers would provide some answers to these questions.

The presence of CEA in extracts of lung cancer has recently been reported and is consistent with the previous findings of high CEA levels in the plasma of patients with this disease [37]. There are several studies dealing with the value of CEA determinations in patients with lung cancer [16, 25, 43]. The standards used by Lo Gerfo in an early study were slightly different from those employed by others and the table has been corrected to account for this (Table III). Sixty percent of the patients in these series had CEA levels greater than 5 ng/ml, and over 70% had levels greater than 2.5 ng/ml. The distribution of those who had levels over 5 ng/ml on basis of cell type is shown in Table IV. All cell types were associated with a significant number of elevated CEA values, and these results are similar to those obtained by Vincent.

There is some correlation between the stage of the disease and the level of CEA in all series to date. CEA levels greater than 10 are usually associated with disseminated disease, but even some individuals with localized disease have plasma CEA values in this range (Table V). Whether the preoperative CEA values are of prognostic significance in patients with lung carcinoma remains to be determined, but in patients with colon car-

TABLE III

CEA Levels in Patients with Lung Carcinoma

Number of patients	Percent with CEA levels (ng/ml) of			
	0–2.5	2.5–5.0	5.0–10	>10
61	17	17	20	24
38	8	5	4	8
117	27	13	37	41

TABLE IV

**Incidence of Elevated CEA Levels in Patients with
Various Types of Lung Carcinomas**

Types of lung Carcinomas	Number of patients studied	Number of patients with elevated levels of CEA
Squamous cell	38	30
Oat cell	10	7
Adenocarcinoma	9	5
Undifferentiated type	4	2

cinoma on a stage for stage basis high CEA levels are associated with a poorer prognosis. It is intriguing that in the postoperative period CEA levels have been shown to increase markedly and remain so for considerable periods in patients who have had curative pulmonary resection [43]. This would indicate that CEA was still being produced elsewhere or that its excretion mechanism was blocked. Further clinical studies may provide some insight into this phenomenon, which is probably of prognostic significance.

V. GAMMA FETAL PROTEIN (GFP)

This antigen was first described by Edynak and is antigenically distant from CEA and can be found in many tumors, including sarcomas and leukemias. GFP is present in fetal tissues from several animal species but like CEA quantitative rather than qualitative similarities exist between benign and malignant tissues. Using microimmunodiffusion techniques, GFP can be demonstrated in human lung cancer extracts [4]. Early results using a radioimmunoassay procedure to detect GFP in human serum indicate that this assay may be of value as a screening test for neoplastic disease

TABLE V

CEA Levels in Patients with Localized Disease

Level of CEA/ml	Number of patients	Percentage undergoing thoracotomy
Less than 10 ng	21	50
Greater than 10 ng	25	20

[5]. In patients with malignant disease, the serum levels of GFP are usually greater than 20 ng/ml, the highest levels being found in patients with sarcomas. Experience with lung carcinoma is limited, but 5 of 9 such patients had levels of GFP greater than 20 ng/ml. An extensive clinical evaluation of this assay for GFP needs to be carried out.

VI. REGAN ISOENZYME ALKALINE PHOSPHATASE (RI)

This enzyme was first identified in the serum of a patient with lung carcinoma and represents an embryonic isoenzyme of adult alkaline phosphatase. It is not detectable with the usual chemical methods in adult serum and is biochemically and immunologically identical to placental alkaline phosphatase [41]. Approximately 14% of all cancer patients and 13% of lung cancer patients have detectable levels of this enzyme [31]. The highest incidence of RI occurs in germ cell tumors followed by carcinomas of lung, breast, pancreas, and cervix. Benign conditions occasionally associated with serum RI include ulcerative colitis, cirrhosis, some vascular diseases, and pregnancy.

VII. OTHER FETAL ANTIGENS ASSOCIATED WITH LUNG CARCINOMA

Yacki has identified at least one fetal cross-reacting antigen in extracts of lung carcinoma, but follow-up studies of this have not been reported [46]. In addition there has been one report in the literature where a patient with lung carcinoma metastatic to the liver had increased levels of α-fetoprotein in his serum. The latter is extremely rare and probably only occurs in patients with liver metastases.

REFERENCES

1. Buccinarelli, E., and Ribacchi, R., C Type particles in primary and transplanted lung tumors induced in BALB/c mice by hydrazine sulfate: Electron microscopy and immunodiffusion studies. *J. Nat. Cancer Inst.* **49,** 673 (1972).
2. Calafat, J., den Engelse, L., and Emmelot, P., Studies on lung tumors: Morphological alterations induced by dimethyl nitrosamine in mouse lung and liver and their relevance to tumorigenesis. *Chem.-Biol. Interact.* **2,** 309 (1970).
3. Colnaghi, M. I., Menard, S., and Della-Porta, G., Demonstration of cellular immunity against urethane-induced lung ademomas of mice. *J. Nat. Cancer Inst.* **17,** 1325 (1971).

4. Edynak, E. M., Lardis, M. P., and Pizzaia, L. M., "Mammary Cancer in Experimental Animals and Man," 8th Meet., p. 55. U.S. Dept. of Health, Education and Welfare, Washington, D.C., 1973.
5. Edynak, E. M., Old, L. J., Vrana, M., and Lardis, M. P., A fetal antigen associated with human neoplasia. *N. Engl. J. Med.* **286**, 1178 (1972).
6. Flaks, A., Pulmonary tumor induction *in vitro* genetic influence. *Eur. J. Cancer* **6**, 259 (1970).
7. Foley, E. J., Antigenic properties of methylchexanthrene induced tumors in mice of the strian of origin. *Cancer Res.* **13**, 835 (1953).
8. Gold, P., Circulating antibodies against carcinoembryonic antigens of colonic tumors. *Cancer Res.* **20**, 1663 (1967).
9. Gold, P., Antigenic reversion in human cancer. *Annu. Rev. Med.* **22**, 85 (1971).
10. Gold, P., and Freedman, S. O., Specific carcinoembryonic antigens of the human digestive system. *J. Exp. Med.* **122**, 467 (1965).
11. Hansen, H. J., Schnieder, J. J., Miller, E., Vandevoorde, J. P., Miller, O. M., Henz, L. R., and Burns, J. J., Carcinoembryonic antigen assay: Lab adjunct in diagnosis and management of cancer. *J. Hum. Pathol.* **5**, 139 (1974).
12. Hod, I., Perk, K., Nobel, T. A., and Klopfer, U., Lung carcinoma of sheep (jaagsievite): Lymph node, blood, and immunoglobulin. *J. Nat. Cancer Inst.* **48**, 451 (1972).
13. Huebner, R. J., and Todaro, G. J., Oncogenes of RNA tumor viruses as determinants of cancer. *Proc. Nat. Acad. Sci. U.S.* **64**, 1087 (1900).
14. Johnson, S., The effect of thymectomy and of dose of 3-methylcholanthrene on the induction and antigenic properties of sarcoma in C57BL mice. *Brit. J. Cancer* **22**, 93 (1968).
15. Kaplan, M. M., Alkaline phosphatase. *N. Engl. J. Med.* **286**, 200 (1972).
16. Kashmiri, R., Hunter, L., Clapp, W., and Griffin, W. O., Clinical evaluation of carcinoembryonic antigen test. *Arch. Surg. (Chicago)* **107**, 266 (1973).
17. Kellermann, G., Shaw, C. R., and Loyten-Kellerman, M., Aryl hydrocarbon hydroxylase inducibility and bronchogenic carcinoma. *N. Engl. J. Med.* **289**, 934 (1973).
18. Kimura, I., Miyake, T., Ishimato, A., and Ito, Y., Intracisternal A type and C type particles observed in pulmonary tumors in mice. *Gann* **63**, 563 (1972).
19. Krupey, J., Gold, P., and Freedman, S. O., Purification and characterization of carcinoembryonic antigens of the human digestive system. *Nature (London)* **215**, 67 (1967).
20. Kuhn, C., Fine structure of bronchoalveolar cell carcinoma. *Cancer* **30**, 1107 (1972).
21. Laurence, D. J., Stevens, V., Bettelheim, R., Darcey, D., Leese, C., Tuberville, C., Alexander, C., Johns, E. W., and Munroeville, A., Role of plasma carcinoembryonic antigen in diagnosis of gastrointestinal, mammary and bronchial carcinoma. *Brit. Med. J.* **9**, 605 (1972).
22. Lo Gerfo, P., Bennett, S., and Herter, F. P., Absence of circulating antibodies to carcinoembryonic antigen in patients with gastrointestinal malignancies. *Int. J. Cancer* **9**, 344 (1972).
23. Lo Gerfo, P., Hansen, H. J., and Krupey, J., Demonstration of an antigen common to several varieties of neoplasia. *N. Engl. J. Med.* **285**, 138–143 (1971).
24. Lo Gerfo, P., Herter, F. P., and Bennett, S., Studies on tumor associated antigen. *J. Surg. Res.* **15**, 290 (1973).
25. Lo Gerfo, P., Herter, F. P., Braun, J., and Hansen, H. J., Tumor associated antigen with pulmonary neoplasms. *Ann. Surg.* **175**, 495–500 (1972).

26. Lo Gerfo, P., Herter, F. P., and Hansen, H. J., Tumor associated antigen in normal lung and colon. *J. Surg. Oncol.* **4,** 1–7 (1972).
27. Martin, F., and Martin, F. S., Radioimmunoassay of carcinembryonic antigen in extracts of human colon and stomach. *Int. J. Cancer* **9,** 642–647 (1972).
28. Martin, F., Martin, F. S., Bordes, M., and Bourgeaux, C., The specificity of carcino-foetal antigens of the human digestive tract tumors. *Eur. J. Cancer* **8,** 315–321 (1972).
29. Miller, A. B., A collaborative study of a test for carcinoembryonic antigen in the sera of patients with carcinoma of the colon and rectum. A joint National Cancer Institute of Canada/American Cancer Society Investigation. *Can. Med. Ass. J.* **107,** 25 (1972).
30. Morton, D. L., and Wells, S. A., "Textbook of Surgery." Saunders, Philadelphia, Pennsylvania, 1972.
31. Nathanson, L., and Fishman, W. H., New observations on the regan isoenzyme of alkaline phosphatase in cancer patients. *Cancer* **27,** 1390 (1971).
32. Oboshi, S., Seido, T., and Tsugawa, S., Antibody in sera of pulmonary cancer patients against specific surface antigen of oat cells. *Gann* **62,** 515 (1971).
33. Perk, K., Hod, I., and Nobel, T. A., Pulmonary adenomatosis of sheep (jaagsievite) ultrastructure of the tumor. *J. Nat. Cancer Inst.* **46,** 525 (1971).
34. Prehn, R. T., Specific isoantigenicites among chemically induced tumors. *Ann. N.Y. Acad. Sci.* **101,** 107 (1962).
35. Prehn, R. T., and Main, J. M., Immunity to methylcholanthrene-induced sarcomas. *J. Nat. Cancer Inst.* **18,** 769 (1957).
36. Schreiber, H., Nettesheim, P., Lijinsky, W., Richter, C. B., and Walberg, H. E., Induction of lung cancer in germfree specific-pathogen free, and infected rats by *N*-nitrosoheptamelthyeneimine: Enhancement by respiratory infection. *J. Nat. Cancer Inst.* **49,** 1107 (1972).
37. Sizaret, P., and Martin, F., Carcinoembryonic antigen in extracts of pulmonary cancers. *J. Nat. Cancer Inst.* **50,** 807 (1973).
38. Sjögren, H. O., Hellström, I., and Klein, G., Transplantation of polyoma virus induced tumor antigens in mice. *Cancer Res.* **21,** 329 (1961).
39. Smith, W. E., Yazdi, E., and Miller, L., Carcinogenesis in pulmonary epithelia in mice on different levels of vitamin A. *Environ. Res.* **5,** 152 (1972).
40. Spencer, H., "Pathology of the Lung," pp. 778–844. Pergamon, Oxford, 1969.
41. Stolbach, L. L., Krant, M. J., and Fishman, W. H., Ectopic production of an alkaline phophatase isoenzyme in patients with cancer. *N. Engl. J. Med.* **281,** 757 (1969).
42. Thomson, D. M., Krupey, J., Freedman, S. O., and Gold, P., The radio immunoassay of circulating carcinoembryonic antigen of the human digestive system. *Proc. Nat. Acad. Sci. U.S.* **64,** 161.
43. Vincent, R. G., and Chu, T. M., Carcinoembryonic antigen in patients with lung carcinoma. *J. Thorac. Cardiov. Surg.* **66,** 320 (1973).
44. Wandera, J. G., Sheep pulmonary adenomatosis. *Advan. Vet. Sci. Comp. Med.* **15,** 251 (1971).
45. Wynder, E. L., Etiology of lung cancer. *Cancer* **30,** 1332 (1972).
46. Yachi, A., Matsuura, Y., Carpenter, C. M., and Hyde, L., Immunochemical studies on human lung cancer antigens soluble in 50% saturated ammonium sulfate. *J. Nat. Cancer Inst.* **40,** 663 (1968).
47. Zamcheck, N., Moore, T. L., Dhar, P., and Kupchik, H. Z., Immunological diagnosis and prognosis of human digestive tract cancer: Carcinoembryonic antigens. *N. Engl. J. Med.* **286,** 83 (1972).

Chapter 5

Prognostic Value of Doubling Time and Related Factors in Lung Cancer

A. Philippe Chahinian and Lucien Israel

The doubling time (*DT*) is the only presently available dynamic parameter of a tumor. By measuring tumor growth itself its prognostic implications are entirely unique.

I. *DT* AND POSTOPERATIVE SURVIVAL

This correlation makes it possible to assess the prognostic value of the *DT*. The degree of this correlation has been invariably substantiated in all investigations comparing the *DT* of a tumor to survival after surgical excision. Thus, in 57 cases of measurable peripheral lung cancer, Steele and Buell [30] reported a 21% 5-year survival rate in the group whose *DT* was less than 120 days as against a 39% survival rate in the group whose *DT* exceeded 135 days. The difference remained significant from the first to the seventh year following excision. Similarly, in 19 cases of lung cancer of which 13 underwent surgery, Weiss *et al.* [35] found a correlation coefficient of 0.61 between *DT* and survival (measured from the time the cancer was 1 cm in diameter). This figure is highly significant ($t = 3.16$, $p < 0.01$). Median survival in the groups with a rapid *DT* (1.8 to 3.9 months), moderate *DT* (4.0 to 6.6 months), and slow *DT* (6.7 to 10.0 months) was 26, 40, and 54 months, respectively. Meyer [23] reached a similar conclusion and stated that the growth rate of operable primary bronchogenic carcinomas appeared to be a determinant of the probability of surgical cure—the slower the *DT*, the longer the survival.

These data, derived from primary lung tumors, have also been shown to apply to surgically excised pulmonary metastases of various origins [11, 16] and metastases from breast cancer [19].

One of the most plausible explanations for the prognostic value of the *DT* is undoubtedly the correlation between it and the invasive and metastatic potential of the tumor. Bronchogenic carcinomas that are inoperable from the onset are usually tumors with a rapid *DT* [23]. Martinez *et al.* [21] showed experimentally that production of lung metastases from a transplantable mouse adenocarcinoma was related to the growth rate of the primary tumor. In tumors with a rapid *DT*, metastases occurred earlier and more frequently [21]. Similarly, in man, the metastatic potential of primary bronchogenic carcinomas appears to be directly related to the *DT* [35]. This is a fundamental point that should be emphasized when considering the indication for surgery, as we have already pointed out [12]. Indeed, it appears likely that the 40% death rate during the 12 months following adequate local excision of lung cancer is largely due to tumors with rapid *DT* which are associated with microscopic metastases already present at the time of intervention. This point has been demonstrated for colonic cancers [8, 27]. The primary tumor appears to give rise to metastases before it becomes detectable (1 cm) by usual investigative methods. In breast cancer, the peak number of occurrence of lymph node metastases presumably appears when the primary tumor is approximately 3 mm in diameter [10].

II. CORRELATION BETWEEN *DT* AND VARIOUS PARAMETERS

The *DT* is a reliable and convenient parameter for prognostic assessment [34]. However, in contrast to pulmonary metastases, the number of measurable primary lung cancers is small, ranging from 8 to 31% according to various statistics and depending on the recruitment of each particular center [1].

In an attempt to extend the prognostic information of the *DT* to all types of primary bronchogenic carcinoma, whether measurable or not, it appears necessary to develop some correlations between the *DT* and various parameters.

A. *DT* and Histological Characteristics

1. CELL DIFFERENTIATION

It is generally recognized that the higher the degree of differentiation of a tumor, the better the prognosis, particularly in cases of squamous cell carcinoma. In a personal series of 45 measurable squamous cell bronchogenic carcinomas, we attempted, retrospectively, to establish a correlation between *DT* and the degree of cell differentiation [13], assessed according to Matthews' criteria [22]. As shown in Table I, we found no significant difference between the geometric mean of the *DT* of well-differentiated (10 cases, mean *DT* = 54.2 days), moderately differentiated (9 cases, mean *DT* = 43.6 days), and poorly differentiated epidermoid carcinomas (26 cases, mean *DT* = 56.4 days). Moreover, there was a considerable overlap between the 3 distributions as shown by the range of the *DT*'s.

It is evident that this result should be accepted with some reservation because of the small number of cases and especially because of the heterogeneous histological material. Indeed, in most cases, histological diagnosis was made through bronchial biopsy and aspiration material obtained by bronchoscopy, and such specimens cannot claim to reflect the true histological characteristics of the entire tumor. Indeed, the degree of differentiation may vary appreciably from one area of the tumor to another [18].

TABLE I

Growth Rates and Cell Differentiation of Bronchial Squamous Cell Carcinomas

Differentiation	No. cases	Doubling time				
		Mean (ln)	Standard deviation (ln)	Mean (days)	95% range (days)	Median (days)
Poorly differentiated	10	3.9927	0.9411	54.2	8–356	53
Moderately differentiated	9	3.7762	0.7875	43.6	9–211	51
Well-differentiated	26	4.0318	0.9440	56.4	8–372	46
Total	45	3.9719	0.9003	53.1	9–321	51

Last, the criteria of differentiation are difficult to assess, and there is considerable variation between the interpretations of various pathologists. Weiss *et al.* [35] tried to establish a correlation between *DT* and degree of keratinization of epidermoid bronchogenic carcinomas, but they had to give up this study because of the disagreement between pathologists. Different specimens examined by two groups of pathologists are similarly interpreted in less than half the cases (Table II) [36].

Surprisingly enough, Table II shows that over half the lung tumors initially classified as squamous cell were later considered to be adenocarcinomas, undifferentiated small cell, or large cell carcinomas by a second group of pathologists. Moreover, it is edifying to remark that the classification of the World Health Organization has been criticized by its very author [18].

Although we do not wish to question the prognostic value of cell differentiation, it is unfortunate that its assessment is purely qualitative. There is no information available regarding the relative volumes of differentiated and undifferentiated zones within the tumor. The need has now arisen for a quantitative and objective assessment of the histologic, cytologic, and

TABLE II

Correspondence of Diagnostic Groups in Old and New Cellular Readings for Epidermoid Lung Cancer[a]

	Original reading	
Subsequent reading	Well-differentiated epidermoid (180 cases)	Poorly differentiated epidermoid (31 cases)
Well-differentiated epidermoid	73 (41%)	2
Poorly differentiated epidermoid	59	8 (26%)
Well-differentiated adenocarcinoma	17	3
Poorly differentiated adenocarcinoma	14	3
Undifferentiated small cell	4	3
Undifferentiated large cell	13	12

[a] Adapted from Yesner *et al.* [36].

kinetic characteristics of tumors in order to draw more accurate prognostic implications.*

2. CELL NECROSIS

In primary bronchogenic carcinoma, microscopic cell necrosis appears to be more intense and more frequent for tumors of short DT [18, 28, 35]. This factor warrants investigation and should be mentioned in all pathologic reports.

3. MITOTIC INDEX (MI)

Weiss et al. [35] were able to estimate the mitotic activity in 17 cases of measurable bronchogenic carcinoma by counting the *number of mitoses* per 50 microscopic fields under oil immersion ($\times 970$). Although the number of mitoses was difficult to count, and in spite of substantial variations from one slide to another, a significant negative correlation was established with the DT: the longer the DT, the smaller the number of mitoses [35].

The routine application of this method entails serious difficulties. The number of microscopic fields examined must be large in order to minimize variations from one tumor specimen to another. Moreover, the evaluation of the number of mitoses is subject to some criticism and error. It constitutes a static evaluation of a dynamic parameter. In fact, all things being equal, the number of mitoses at a given time depends on the duration of mitosis and also on the cell size. Since it is measured per unit area, the number of mitoses is greater when cells are smaller or when the stroma is less abundant [35].

To overcome some of these problems, Weiss [33] studied more recently the mitotic index or number of mitoses per 1000 cells. In a total of 37 cases of bronchogenic carcinoma, there was no significant correlation between MI and survival from the time of tumor detection [33]. In a subgroup of 12 cases with measurable tumor, the relationship between MI and survival was not linear on arithmetic coordinates, and the MI reflected growth rate only in the most rapidly growing cancers. The Spearman correlation coefficient between MI and DT was -0.69, significant with $p < 0.02$. It should be mentioned, however, that Weiss used arithmetic co-

---

* An effort toward morphometric studies in lung cancer has been accomplished by Gerstl et al. [9a].

ordinates. It is well established that *DT* is a log-normal parameter. Therefore, we repeated this calculation using log *DT* instead of *DT*.* The
correlation with *MI* was much closer, and the correlation coefficient was
-0.78, significant with $p < 0.01$. Further investigations appear necessary,
but other experimental and clinical studies have stressed the usefulness of
MI as a prognostic indicator.

For chemically induced tumors in mice, the percentage of cells undergoing mitosis was 0.96% for fast-growing tumors and 0.70% for slow-
growing tumors [6]. In man, Breur [5] found a relationship between
mitotic frequency of fibrosarcomas and *DT* of their pulmonary metastases.
The mean number of mitoses in the primary tumor with metastases having
a *DT* between 80 and 160 days was approximately half that of tumors
with metastases having a *DT* between 20 and 80 days. A significant correlation has similarly been demonstrated between prognosis and mitotic
frequency in cases of fibrosarcomas [32] and breast cancer [3].

4. LABELING INDEX WITH TRITIATED THYMIDINE

Intravenously injected tritiated thymidine (^{3}HT) disappears from the
blood a few minutes after injection and turns up in cell nuclei, thus labeling
only cells in S phase (DNA synthesis). This will undoubtedly be an accurate and convenient method for studying cell kinetics in human tumors.
This method has already been applied to man by injection of ^{3}HT a few
hours before surgical excision of a tumor. This method makes it possible
to define the number of cells in the S phase at a given time, to make an
approximate assessment of the duration of the G_2 phase, and to count the
number of labeled mitoses.

A few trials involving glioblastoma [14], breast cancer [15], and colonic
and gastric carcinomas [17] demonstrated a correlation between the number of labeled mitoses and the prognosis.

This method could well be applied to operable cases of lung cancer.
Straus [31] has determined that the radioactive exposure from this method
is less hazardous than previously thought. Serial bronchoscopies may yield
adequate cells in each biopsy sample for complete kinetic analysis [31].
Malaise *et al.* [20] found a significant negative correlation between *DT* and
mean labeling index *in vitro* for different histologic types of solid tumors.

In cases with easily accessible metastases, *intratumoral* rather than intravenous injection on ^{3}HT can be performed. By this method, labeled mitosis
curves have been obtained in patients with carcinoma of the breast and

---

* In collaboration with Dr. Harry Smith, Jr., Department of Biostatistics, Mount
Sinai School of Medicine, New York.

malignant melanoma [37]. Muggia employed intratumoral injections of ³HT into subcutaneous nodules, metastatic lymph nodes, and bone marrow metastases from lung cancer [24]. He demonstrated in 28 patients that the labeling index (LI) was highest in cases of small cell carcinoma (mean LI = 15.0 ± 6.1), followed by large cell undifferentiated carcinoma (mean LI = 10.3 ± 5.9). Patients with adenocarcinoma and epidermoid carcinoma had the lowest LI (mean 3.6 ± 1.1 and 3.6 ± 3.2, respectively). These data are in accordance with the actual tumor doubling time of these various histologic types. Such information is of great value in order to assess the natural history, prognosis, and therapeutic response of lung cancer.

B. *DT* and Symptomatic Pattern

The prognostic value of the nature and duration of symptoms in primary bronchogenic carcinoma was emphasized by Feinstein with regard to 678 cases [9] and confirmed by Senior *et al.* in 646 cases [25]. In an earlier investigation [7], we sought a correlation between the DT in 19 measurable primary bronchogenic carcinomas (14 squamous cell, 3 small cell, 2 adenocarcinomas) and the clinical spectrum according to Feinstein's classification, which includes 5 subgroups of symptoms: (a) asymptomatic; (b) long primary (pulmonary symptoms only, for six months or longer); (c) short primary (pulmonary symptoms only, for less than six months; (d) systemic (anorexia, finger clubbing, endocrine effects, etc.); and (e) metastatic (thoracic and/or extrathoracic). These five subgroups were consolidated into three main groups according to Feinstein [9]: indolent, (a) and/or (b); obtrusive, (c) and/or (d); deleterious, (e) in any combination.

The regression equation of $y(\log DT)$ in relation to x (three classes of symptoms mentioned above) was

$$y = 5.128 - 0.654x$$

Figure 1 shows the scatter diagram of corresponding points, the mean value of log DT for each class of x, and the standard deviation for each class of symptoms. The regression coefficient was highly significant (t = 2.87, $p < 0.01$). This test showed the close relationship between the classification of symptoms and the DT [7].

This method can only be used if an accurate and reliable medical history is available and if there are no other concomitant but unrelated diseases or other bronchopulmonary diseases. With these exceptions, its major advan-

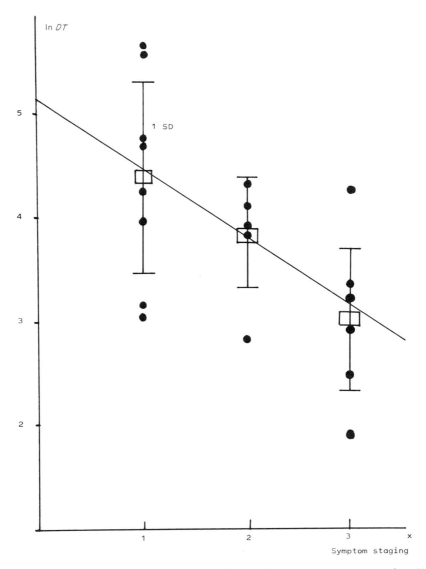

Fig. 1. Regression equation between ln DT and Feinstein's symptom staging (1, indolent; 2, obtrusive; 3, deleterious) for 19 primary lung cancers. The square points represent the mean value for each class, with the standard deviation (SD) (adapted from Chahinian [7], and reproduced with permission of the publishers of *Chest*).

tage lies in the fact that it may be used in all cases of primary bronchogenic carcinoma, whether measurable or not. Moreover, it also bears a relationship with the stage of the disease, which is of prime prognostic importance [26].

III. *DT* AND OTHER PARAMETERS

A. Age

Measurable primary bronchogenic carcinomas in young patients are too rare to allow statistical analysis. However, age does not appear to be a very reliable prognostic determinant. Thus, for pulmonary metastases of various origins, fast-growing tumors are common in young patients, but in old patients both fast-growing and slow-growing tumors are encountered [7].

B. Sex

The number of measurable primary bronchogenic carcinomas in women is still too small in our series. For pulmonary metastases, there was no significant difference in *DT* between sexes [7]. In primary bronchogenic carcinomas considered as a whole, the prognosis in women does not appear to differ significantly from that in men, although this point still remains controversial [2].

C. Sedimentation Rate

It is common knowledge that a normal erythrocyte sedimentation rate does not rule out the possibility of cancer [1]. In patients with primary bronchogenic carcinoma (excluding those with anemia or an infectious syndrome), no significant correlation was found between *DT* and sedimentation rate [7].

D. Tumor Size on the First Roentgenogram

Tumor size on the first roentgenogram (*T*1) is a "puzzling factor" [26]. Some reports have indicated a better prognosis when *T*1 is small while others have found no relationship with postoperative survival [26]. As *T*1 follows a log-normal distribution [29], we attempted to demonstrate a correlation between log *T*1 and log *DT* in 27 cases of measurable primary lung cancer [7]. This calculation showed an *r* value (correlation coefficient) of 0.34 with 25 degrees of freedom This value was just below the level of significance ($r = 0.38$) for $p = 0.05$. Thus, the borderline result of this test of significance did not permit us to reach a definite conclusion. The correlation between log *T*1 and log *DT* appears to be poor. One possible explanation might be that the faster a tumor grows, the earlier the symptoms occur and vice versa. This factor thus minimizes the relationship between *DT* and tumor size on the first roentgenogram. For an identical

$T1$, a slow-growing tumor would have a longer latency than a fast-growing tumor.

E. DT and Immune Status

In a previous work [7] no correlation was found between DT and response to tuberculin skin test in 15 patients. However, in view of the small number of patients investigated and the necessity of applying more elaborate tests, both *in vivo* and *in vitro*, to assess the immune status, one cannot rule out the possibility of a correlation. In 40 patients with carcinoma of the rectum, Bone and Camplejohn [4] found no relationship between skin response to dinitrochlorobenzene and proliferation rate or potential doubling time of the tumor.

IV. CONCLUSION

The possibility remains that certain parameters (such as age, tumor size, immune status) may be of individual prognostic significance. However, their significance appears to be independent of that of the DT. Present histologic criteria seem too qualitative and too subjective and their reliability is often open to question. Histologic methods for objective and quantitative assessment should be developed. In contrast, there is a close correlation between DT and symptom classification. This provides the clinician with a useful tool that makes it possible, within the limits of its application, to extend the prognostic implications derived from the study of the DT to cases of nonmeasurable bronchogenic carcinoma.

REFERENCES

1. Bariéty, M., Delarue, J., Paillas, J., and Rullière, R., "Les Carcinomes Bronchiques Primitifs." Masson, Paris, 1967.
2. Bignall, J. R., and Martin, M., Survival experience of women with bronchial carcinoma. *Lancet* **2**, 60 (1972).
3. Bloom, H. J., Prognosis in carcinoma of the breast. *Brit. J. Cancer* **4**, 259 (1950).
4. Bone, G., and Camplejohn, R., The role of cellular immunity in control of neoplasia. *Brit. J. Surg.* **60**, 824 (1973).
5. Breur, K., Growth rate and radiosensitivity of human tumors. *Eur. J. Cancer* **2**, 157 (1966).
6. Brues, A. M., Weiner, A. E., and Andervont, H. B., Relation between latent period and growth rate in chemically induced tumors. *Proc. Soc. Exp. Biol. Med.* **42**, 374 (1939).
7. Chahinian, P., Relationship between tumor doubling time and anatomoclinical features in 50 measurable pulmonary cancers. *Chest* **61**, 340 (1972).

8. Collins, V. P., Time of occurrence of pulmonary metastasis from carcinoma of colon and rectum. *Cancer* **15**, 387 (1962).
9. Feinstein, A. R., A new staging system for cancer and reappraisal of "early" treatment and "cure" by radical surgery. *N. Engl. J. Med.* **279**, 747 (1968).
9a. Gerstl, B., Switzer, P., and Yesner, R., A morphometric study of pulmonary cancer. *Cancer Res.* **34**, 248 (1974).
10. Igot, J., Légal, Y., Age des adénopathies métastatiques dans le cancer mammaire. *Ann. Anat. Pathol.* **13**, 449 (1968).
11. Ishihara, T., Kikuchi, K., Ikeda, T., and Yamazaki, S., Metastatic pulmonary diseases: Biologic factors and modes of treatment. *Chest* **63**, 227 (1973).
12. Israel, L., and Chahinian, P., De l'impossibilité de guérir les cancers bronchiques par la chirurgie seule. Données statistiques. Raisons théoriques. Déductions thérapeutiques. *Presse Med.* **77**, 389 (1969).
13. Israel, L., and Chahinian, P., Absence de corrélation entre la vitesse de croissance et le degré de différenciation des cancers bronchiques. *Presse Med.* **79**, 1567 (1971).
14. Johnson, H. A., Haymaker, W. E., Rubini, J. R., Fliedner, T. M., Bond, V. P., Cronkite, E. P., and Hugues, W. L., A radioautographic study of a human brain and glioblastoma multiforme after the *in vivo* uptake of tritiated thymidine. *Cancer* **13**, 636 (1960).
15. Johnson, H. A., Rubini, J. R., Cronkite, E. P., and Bond, V. P., Labelling of human tumor cells *in vivo* by tritiated thymidine. *Lab. Invest.* **9**, 460 (1960).
16. Joseph, W. L., Morton, D. L., and Adkins, P. C., Prognostic significance of tumor doubling time in evaluating operability in pulmonary metastatic disease. *J. Thorac. Cardiov. Surg.* **61**, 23 (1971).
17. Kissel, P., Duprez, A., Schmitt, J., and Dollander, A., Autohistoradiographie des cancers digestifs humains *in vivo*. *C. R. Soc. Biol.* **159**, 1400 (1965).
18. Kreyberg, L., Comments on the histological typing of lung tumours. *Acta Pathol. Microbiol. Scand., Sect. A* **79**, 409 (1971).
19. Kusama, S., Spratt, J. S., Donegan, W. L., Watson, F. R., and Cunningham, C., The gross rates of growth of human mammary carcinoma. *Cancer* **30**, 594 (1972).
20. Malaise, E. P., Chavaudra, N., and Tubiana, M., The relationship between growth rate, labelling index and histological type of human solid tumours. *Eur. J. Cancer* **9**, 305 (1973).
21. Martinez, C., Miroff, G., and Bittner, J., Effect of size and/or rate of growth of a transplantable mouse adenocarcinoma on lung metastasis production. *Cancer Res.* **16**, 313 (1956).
22. Matthews, M. J., Morphologic classification of bronchogenic carcinoma. *Cancer Chemother. Rep., Part 3* **4**, 299 (1973).
23. Meyer, J. A., Growth rate versus prognosis in resected bronchogenic carcinomas. *Cancer* **31**, 1468 (1973).
24. Muggia, F. M., Cell kinetic studies in patients with lung cancer. *Oncology* **30**, 353 (1974).
25. Senior, R. M., and Adamson, J. S., Survival in patients with lung cancer. An appraisal of Feinstein's symptom classification. *Arch. Intern. Med.* **125**, 975 (1970).
26. Slack, N. H., Chamberlain, A., and Bross, I. D., Predicting survival following surgery for bronchogenic carcinoma. *Chest* **62**, 433 (1972).
27. Spratt, J. S., and Ackerman, L. V., Small primary adenocarcinomas of the colon and rectum. *J. Amer. Med. Ass.* **179**, 337 (1962).

28. Spratt, J. S., Spjut, H. J., and Roper, C. L., The frequency distribution of the rates of growth and the estimated duration of primary pulmonary carcinomas. *Cancer* **16,** 687 (1963).
29. Spratt, J. S., Ter-Pogossian, M., and Long, R. T. L., The detection and growth of intrathoracic neoplasms. *Arch. Surg. (Chicago)* **86,** 283 (1963).
30. Steele, J. D., and Buell, P., Asymptomatic solitary pulmonary nodules. Host survival, tumor size, and growth rate. *J. Thorac. Cardiov. Surg.* **65,** 140 (1973).
31. Straus, M. J., The growth characteristics of lung cancer and its application to treatment design. *Semin. Oncol.* **1,** 167 (1974).
32. Van der Werf-Messing, B., and Unnik, J. A., Fibrosarcoma of the soft tissues: A clinicopathologic study. *Cancer* **18,** 1113 (1965).
33. Weiss, W., The mitotic index in bronchogenic carcinoma. *Amer. Rev. Resp. Dis.* **104,** 536 (1971).
34. Weiss, W., Tumor doubling time and survival of men with bronchogenic carcinoma. *Chest* **65,** 3 (1974).
35. Weiss, W., Boucot, K., and Cooper, D., Survival of men with peripheral lung cancer in relation to histologic characteristics and growth rate. *Amer. Rev. Resp. Dis.* **98,** 75 (1968).
36. Yesner, R., Gelfman, N. A., and Feinstein, A. R., A reappraisal of histopathology in lung cancer and correlation of cell types with antecedent cigarette smoking. *Amer. Rev. Resp. Dis.* **107,** 790 (1973).
37. Young, R. C., and DeVita, V. T., Cell cycle characteristics of human solid tumors *in vivo*. *Cell Tissue Kinet.* **3,** 285 (1970).

Chapter 6

The Relationship of Prognosis to Morphology and the Anatomic Extent of Disease: Studies of a New Clinical Staging System

Clifton F. Mountain

Historically, lung cancer has been considered by most physicians as a single disease entity. The roles of surgery, radiotherapy, and chemotherapy, as unique modalities of treatment, were generally agreed upon, and their relative contributions to survival were regarded as established. Treatment was selected on a rank order basis; surgery, radiotherapy, chemotherapy, according to the estimated extent of disease at the time of initiating therapy. The extent of disease was conveniently designated as local, regional, or systemic. Thus each classification was easily identified with one of the three therapeutic modalities. This was a simple and attractive conceptual approach which served as an uncomplicated guide to the choice of treatment, and it became dogma among practitioners. Few critical questions were raised, and even fewer explanations offered, regarding the variability of results within each method of management.

In recent years, the problem of lung cancer has been the target of increasing critical attention by oncologists. This has measurably increased our understandings of the biological behavior of the disease. These understandings argue for a more sophisticated conceptual approach to management and bring into focus existing gaps in our knowledge. The rational development of new therapeutic approaches must, accordingly, take into account the morphology, any unique biologic characteristics, the extent of disease at onset of treatment, and the cell kill potential for each individual and combined modality approach. This requires identification of subsets of the total lung cancer population that exhibit generally similar behavioral patterns. In addition, some understanding of the dynamics of survival patterns and of the prognostic implications of the extent of disease at diagnosis seems of value. Finally, it is essential that a reliable and valid system for clinical staging, adaptable for international use, be employed for reporting of end results.

I. GENERAL CONSIDERATIONS IN STAGING

Staging is the process of classifying patients into comparatively homogenous groups with respect to the anatomic extent or biologic severity of their neoplastic disease. A coded designator, or index, is assigned each patient in accordance with an established set of rules. The salient feature of such an index should be that patients within any staged group, who survive equivalent treatment, will demonstrate a generally similar age-adjusted life expectancy. Clinical staging depends only on those evaluations of the disease's extent which are obtained from diagnostic and evaluative studies accomplished prior to any major exploratory surgery and before treatment is initiated. The classification of patients with respect to estimates of their prognosis, prior to the implementation of any therapy, is essential if different modalities of treatment are to be compared and if results of therapy are to be communicated in meaningful terms. [28].

The central problems in designating a useful staging system [20] are (1) to identify and give proportionate weight to those measurable factors that will reliably and validly predict survival and (2) to develop rules that, when applied to these factors, will permit assignment of an index of disease extent. The design should relate to both current and projected therapeutic strategies in order to aid in the selection of the most effective treatment, and it should be of assistance in determining prognosis. It should also be sufficiently uncomplicated in its basic form in order to be widely utilized in daily practice, and yet be flexible and adaptable in expanded forms to meet the more sophisticated needs of documentation required in clinical research. Such requirements must be met within the framework of a broadly acceptable and easily understood set of rules. Therefore, the system necessarily must be based on the evaluation of few but powerful predicting factors whose influence on prognosis is measurable. Such design proposals place an obvious restraint on any system of classification, but they also serve to narrow the focus to the development of a useful tool.

II. THE CLASSIFICATION OF NEOPLASTIC DISEASE EXTENT

Improvements in diagnostic and evaluative techniques and in the results of therapy have been accompanied by an increased awareness of the value of clinical staging. Through the years, numerous proposals for the classification of disease extent have been made by individual investigators for almost all neoplastic processes. Most of these have been based on topographical–anatomical criteria. The TNM classification principles, initially proposed by Denoix [6] and subsequently applied by the TNM Committee on Classification of the International Union Against Cancer (UICC) [11–13] represented the first systematic approach to the problem with common features applicable to a number of primary disease sites. In 1958 the UICC published its initial classification brochure on "Cancer of the Breast and Larynx." Twenty-two sites, including lung, classified by TNM rules were described in the 1969 booklet, "Livre de Poche" [12].

The TNM system utilizes a common language to provide a basis for categorizing the extent of disease. The letter "T," with appropriate number, describes the primary tumor. The letter "N," with its number, describes the extent of regional lymph node involvement. The letter "M," with its number, designates the absence or presence of disseminated metastatic spread. The nature and degree of tumor involvement is appropriately defined for each letter and number according to the primary tumor site.

The UICC recommendations for classification are limited to describing disease extent in terms of the TNM definitions with no provision for assigning the various TNM subsets to stage groups. The initial UICC definitions were judgmental, being derived by a panel of experts with provision for modification through the results of subsequent clinical trials. The American Joint Committee for Cancer Staging and End Results Reporting (AJC) organized in 1959, adopted the TNM principles of nomenclature in its independent approach to classification. Proposals of the AJC are initially derived from clinical investigations undertaken by various site-oriented task forces. Definitions of the various TNM factors are constructed by analyzing patterns of survival. Subsets of TNM combinations, which display generally similar survival, are grouped into "stages" of disease. Recommendations for staging of disease at ten primary sites have now been published. The AJC proposal for the clinical staging of lung cancer [1, 3, 5], based on a study of over 2000 patients with proven bronchogenic carcinoma [20], is presented in the present manuscript. The elements of this proposal have been jointly adopted and published by the UICC [14].

Since the first successful pneumonectomy by Evarts Graham in 1933, a number of proposals for the classification of lung cancer have been published [2, 4, 7, 8, 10, 16, 24, 25]. Several systems utilize the TNM concept of nomenclature [7, 12, 23]. Proposals based on two recent studies vary only in minor detail with our own recommendations [15, 17]. However, to date, no single system has achieved wide acceptance in terms of common usage. A number of probable reasons may be advanced to explain this situation. Some systems have been faulted due to their inadequate or, indeed, nonexistent data base. Other proposals have been found wanting when tested in clinical trials. In other instances, the proposed systems have apparently been found too complex. Perhaps most importantly, there has been a general lack of appreciation among physicians as to the inherent values and clinical usefulness of judging and recording disease extent utilizing some common language of expression adaptable for international usage.

III. THE NEW TNM SYSTEM FOR CLASSIFYING LUNG CANCER

In this system three capital letters are used to classify the primary lesion and the extent of involvement: T, primary tumor; N, regional lymph node metastasis; M, distant metastasis.

These designations are further expanded with appropriate subscripts. For the *T—primary tumor designation*—the subscripts describe increasing sizes of tumor involvement and/or the involvement by direct extension (T0, TX, T1, T2, T3). For the *N—regional lymph node involvement—* the subscripts specify and describe the absence of such involvement or increasing degrees of such involvement (N0, N1, N2, N3). For the letter *M, distant metastasis,* the subscripts describe the absence of such metastasis or the increasing degree of spread of the tumor (M0, M1). In each instance, the highest category of T, N, and M is utilized which best describes the full extent of disease.

T—Primary Tumors

T0

No evidence of primary tumor.

TX

Tumor proved by the presence of malignant cells in bronchopulmonary secretions but not visualized roentgenographically or bronchoscopically, or any tumor which is not evaluable.

TIS

Carcinoma *in situ*.

T1

A tumor that is 3.0 cm or less in greatest diameter, surrounded by lung or visceral pleura and without evidence of invasion proximal to a lobar bronchus at bronchoscopy (graphic representation shown in Fig. 1; survival pattern shown in Fig. 4).

T1

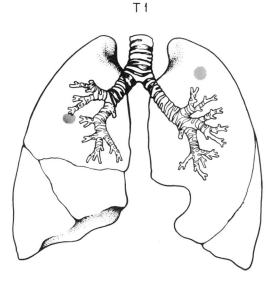

Fig. 1. A solitary tumor that is 3.0 cm or less in greatest diameter, surrounded by lung or visceral pleura and without evidence of invasion proximal to a lobar bronchus at bronchoscopy. Two examples of T1 lesions are shown.

T2

A tumor more than 3.0 cm in greatest diameter or a tumor of any size which invades the visceral pleura or with its associated atelectasis or obstructive pneumonitis, extends to the hilar region. At bronchoscopy the proximal extent of demonstrable tumor must be within a lobar bronchus or at least 2.0 cm distal to the carina. Any associated atelectasis or obstructive pneumonitis must involve less than an entire lung, and there must be no pleural effusion (graphic representation shown in Fig. 2, survival pattern shown in Fig. 4).

T3

A tumor of any size with direct extension into an adjacent structure such as the chest wall, the diaphragm, or the mediastinum and its contents; or demonstrable bronchoscopically to involve a main bronchus less than 2.0 cm distal to the carina; any tumor associated with atelectasis or obstructive pneumonitis of an entire lung or pleural effusion (graphic representation shown in Fig. 3; survival pattern shown in Fig. 4).

T 2

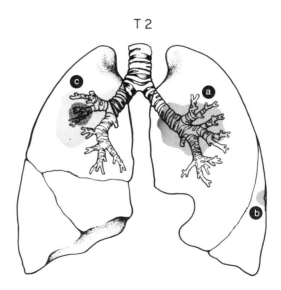

Fig. 2. The primary tumor is more than 3.0 cm in greatest diameter as depicted in (a), or a tumor of any size invading visceral pleura (b), or which, with its associated atelectasis or obstructive pneumonitis, extends to the hilar region (c). At bronchoscopy the proximal extent of demonstrable tumor must be within a lobar bronchus or at least 2.0 cm distal to the carina. Any associated atelectasis or obstructive pneumonitis must involve less than an entire lung and there must be no pleural effusion.

T 3

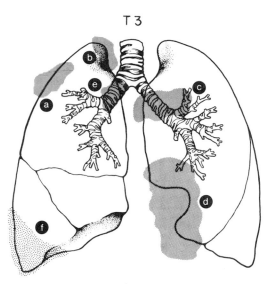

Fig. 3. A primary tumor of any size with direct extension into an adjacent structure such as chest wall (a) mediastinum and its contents (b) with direct invasion of the aorta, main pulmonary artery or veins, recurrent or phrenic nerves (c) or with invasion of the pericardium or diaphragm (d). *T3* lesions include tumors demonstrable bronchoscopically to involve a main bronchus less than 2.0 cm distal to the carina (e), and any tumor associated with a pleural effusion (f) or with atelectasis or obstructive pneumonitis of an entire lung.

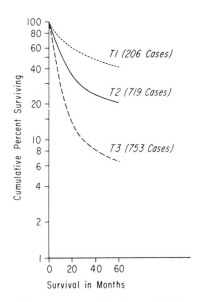

Fig. 4. Survival pattern of lung cancer patients stratified by *primary tumor classification*, T, anatomic extent of disease (semilog plot).

N—Regional Lymph Nodes

N0

No demonstrable metastasis to regional lymph nodes (survival pattern shown in Fig. 7).

N1

Metastasis to lymph nodes in the peribronchial and/or the ipsilateral hilar region (graphic representation shown in Fig. 5; survival pattern shown in Fig. 7).

N2

Metastasis to lymph nodes in the mediastinum (graphic representation shown in Fig. 6; survival pattern shown in Fig. 7).

M—Distant Metastasis

M0

No distant metastasis (survival pattern shown in Fig. 8).

N1

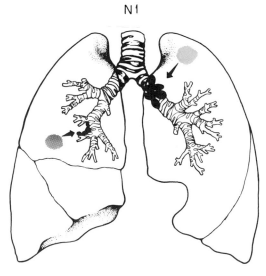

Fig. 5. Spread to lymph nodes in the peribronchial and/or ipsilateral hilar regions (including direct extension).

N 2

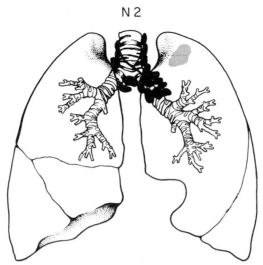

Fig. 6. Spread to mediastinal lymph nodes.

M1

Distant metastasis, such as in scalene, cervical or contralateral hilar lymph nodes, contralateral lung, brain, bones, liver (survival pattern shown in Fig. 8).

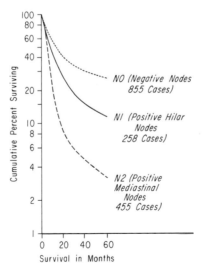

Fig. 7. Survival pattern of lung cancer patients stratified by presence or absence of regional node involvement and degree of involvement, *N classification* (semilog plot).

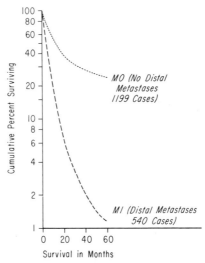

Fig. 8. Survival pattern of lung cancer patients stratified by presence or absence of distal metastasis, *M classification* (semilog plot).

IV. STAGE GROUPING OF TNM COMBINATIONS

The T, N, and M descriptors define those anatomic factors most highly predictive of survival. The various combinations and permutations of these descriptors are grouped into stages of disease such that each stage is substantially homogenous with respect to survival and so that the force of mortality is stage I < stage II < stage III.

Occult Carcinoma

TX N0 M0

An occult carcinoma with bronchopulmonary secretions containing malignant cells but without other evidence of the primary tumor or evidence of metastasis to the regional lymph nodes or distant metastasis.

Stage I

TIS N0 M0—Carcinoma *in situ*
T1 N0 M0
T1 N1 M0
T2 N0 M0

A tumor that can be classified T1 without any metastasis or with metastasis to the lymph nodes in the ipsilateral hilar region only, or a tumor that can be classified T2 without any metastasis to nodes or distant metastasis.

Note: TX N1 M0 and T0 N1 M0 are also theoretically possible, but such a clinical diagnosis would be difficult if not impossible to make. If such a diagnosis is made, it should be included in Stage I.

Stage II

T2 N1 M0

A tumor classified as T2 with metastasis to the lymph nodes in the ipsilateral hilar region only.

Stage III

T3 with any N or M
N2 with any T or M
M1 with any T or N

Any tumor more extensive than T2, or any tumor with metastasis to the lymph nodes in the mediastinum, or with distant metastasis.

Without regard to morphology, the dynamics of survival for these anatomically defined sets, as grouped into three stages, demonstrate a marked and statistically significant difference in the prognostic implications of each stage (Fig. 9). At 24 months there is an interstage cumulative survival difference of 19 percentage points between stage I and stage II disease; 37 percentage points between stage I and III disease; and 18 per-

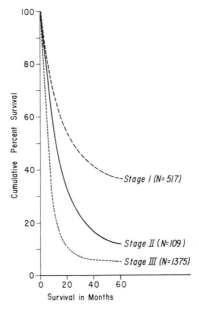

Fig. 9. Survival pattern of lung cancer patients stratified by *stage of disease,* TNM combinations.

centage points between stage II and stage III disease. At 60 months there differences are 24, 31, and 7%, respectively.

V. SURVIVAL PATTERNS OF ANATOMIC TNM SUBSETS

The survival dynamics for each anatomic stage grouping, stratified by TNM subsets is depicted in Figs. 10–14. Cases of undifferentiated small cell carcinoma have been excluded from the analysis of stage III disease as the bias of morphology, in this instance, tends to obscure some important aspects of intrastage variability. This point will be discussed more fully when the effects of morphology on survival are described.

Small primary tumors arising distally to a lobar orifice and completely contained within the anatomic boundaries of the lung have the best prognosis. The 5-year cumulative survival rate for this antaomic extent of disease (T1 N0 M0) is 40%. When such primary lesions, 3 cm or less in greatest diameter, clinically manifest metastatic hilar lymphadenopathy (T1 N1 M0) the 5-year survival rate decreases to approximately 34% if there is no clinical evidence of mediastinal lymph node involvement or of distal spread. More extensive primary tumors (T2) that are confined to the lung without evidence of extension to the hilar or mediastinal nodes (T2 N0 M0) have an

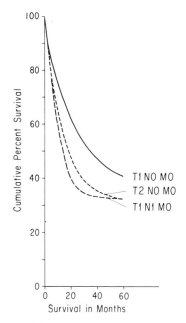

Fig. 10. Survival pattern of lung cancer patients; *stage I,* stratified by anatomic TNM subsets.

equivalent prognosis after 5 years but have an improved intermediate survival as evidenced by the slope of the survival curve (Fig. 10).

Stage II is defined in terms of a single subset (T2 N1 M0). This clinical extent of disease is found in approximately 5% of the patient population. The survival curve for this group (Fig. 11) indicates a markedly morbid effect of ipsilateral hilar lymph node metastases in the presence of a T2 primary lesion with a 5-year cumulative survival rate of 12%. Such cases should be technically resectable and theoretically curable almost to the same extent as stage I disease. This suggests a tendency to clinically underestimate the true anatomic extent of disease in this category more than in stage I. The initial number of number of cases studied with this estimated extent of disease (N = 109) was relatively small and further studies may alter the characteristics of the survival curve. In spite of this uncertainty, the survival of patients in this anatomic stage is clearly intermediate between stage I and stage III disease.

Within stage III the survival curves for the anatomic TNM subsets are reasonably well clustered (Figs. 12–14) with an average 5-year cumulative survival rate of 5%. There are two notable exceptions that are amplified by the exclusion of undifferentiated small cell carcinomas in this particular

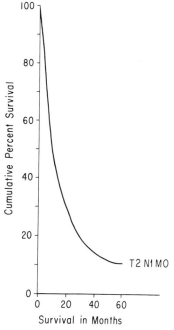

Fig. 11. Survival pattern of lung cancer patients, *stage II,* stratified by anatomic TNM subsets.

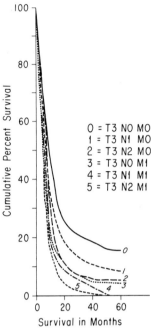

Fig. 12. Survival pattern of lung cancer patients, *stage III*, stratified by TNM subsets according to extent of any T3 primary tumor.

analysis. These exceptions are the subsets T3 N0 M0 and T3 N1 M0, which are composed almost exclusively of patients with superior sulcus tumors associated with either a painful apical syndrome or a true Pancoast's syndrome. For some time now it has been appreciated that such tumors enjoy a unique behavior with respect to the natural history of other bronchogenic carcinomas [22]. Compared to similarly invasive primary lesions elsewhere in the lung, superior sulcus tumors have a relatively more favorable biological potential and exhibit an appreciably better response to therapy. In these cases, the mediastinal lymph nodes are seldom involved, and evidence of distant metastatic disease is relatively uncommon. The cumulative 5-year survival rate is 18% for T3 N0 M0 lesions and 10% for T3 N1 M0 lesions. When cases of undifferentiated small cell carcinoma are included, the survival rate falls to 12% and 5%, respectively.

The subset T3 N2 M0 has a prognosis similar to the group of T3 lesions without mediastinal lymph node metastases but with clinical evidence of distal extension present (T3 N0 M1). There is little variability between TNM subsets, which share the common factor of mediastinal lymph node involvement regardless of the extent of the primary lesion. When the disease is manifest outside the hemithorax of origin (M1), all survival curves rapidly fall toward the 1% level at 5 years.

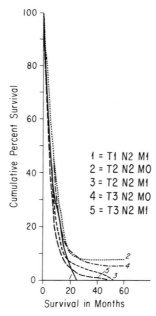

Fig. 13. Survival pattern of lung cancer patients, *stage III,* stratified by TNM subsets according to presence of any N2 mediastinal metastasis.

VI. THE EFFECT OF MORPHOLOGY ON ANATOMIC SURVIVAL PATTERNS

Within the universe of lung cancer, epidermoid (squamous) cell carcinoma occurs in about 50% of all patients, adenocarcinoma in 18%, undifferentiated large cell in 9%, and undifferentiated small cell (oat cell) carcinoma in 19%. Other miscellaneous cell types constitute the remaining 4%. In examining survival by major morphologic patterns of disease, regardless of any other tumor, host, or therapeutic influence, it becomes clear that lung cancer cannot be regarded as a single disease entity. With respect to histology alone, three explicit and statistically significant patterns of survival are evident (Fig. 15). As a group, patients with epidermoid carcinoma have the best prognosis. A remarkably similar intermediate survival is seen among patients with adenocarcinoma and undifferentiated large cell carcinoma. The survival of patients with undifferentiated small cell carcinoma is manifestly disastrous at the present time with only 5% surviving 18 months and less than 1% surviving beyond 42 months. This, and other evidence to be presented, indicates that each major cell type of tumor exhibits a unique spectrum of biologic behavior. It is imperative, therefore, that all lung cancer cases be stratified by cell type as well as by anatomic

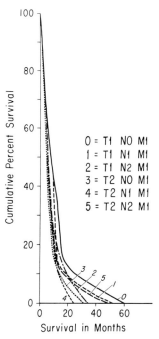

Fig. 14. Survival pattern of lung cancer patients, *stage III*, stratified by TNM sub-sets according to presence of any M1 distal metastasis.

extent of disease prior to any institution of therapy or any analysis of therapeutic results.

The relative influence of histology on the anatomic survival pattern of *T1* lesions, regardless of other parameters of disease extent is shown in Fig. 16. The cumulative percentage of patients surviving 5 years with squamous cell carcinoma is 46%, with adenocarcinoma it is 38%, and with large cell carcinoma it is 17% compared with an overall survival rate of about 39% for *T1* lesions (Fig. 4). Less than half as many patients survive 5 years in the *T2* category, (21%, Fig. 4); however, further analysis by cell type shows that for squamous cell carcinoma the 5-year survival is 28%, for large cell carcinoma it is 16%, and for adenocarcinoma it is 11% (Fig. 17). Seven percent of all patients with a primary tumor classification of *T3* survive 5 years (Fig. 4). Squamous cell and large cell carcinoma have a nearly identical prognosis for *T3* primary lesions (about 8% surviving 5 years) while 2% with adenocarcinoma (Fig. 18) and less than 1% with small cell carcinoma survive 5 years. Thus the greater extension of disease, more central location, and the widespread complications characterized in *T3* lesions have a more deleterious effect on survival in adenocarcinoma than in the other cell types. The size of the primary lesion in large cell carcinoma, however, is a relatively poor prognostic indicator.

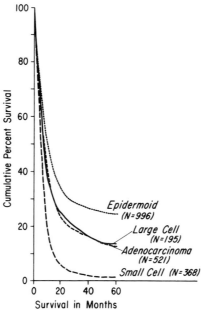

Fig. 15. Survival pattern of lung cancer patients stratified by histologic type of tumor.

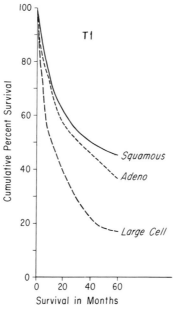

Fig. 16. Survival pattern of lung cancer patients, *primary tumor classification T1,* stratified by histologic type of tumor.

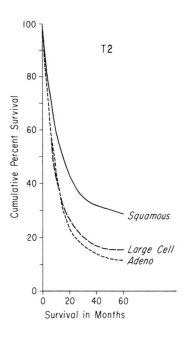

Fig. 17. Survival pattern of lung cancer patients, *primary tumor classification T2,* stratified by histologic type of tumor.

The influence of morphology on the anatomic survival patterns of the N classifications is similarly evident. As an isolated observation, the absence of lymph node involvement (N0) portends a superior prognosis for all cell types, excepting small cell carcinoma (Fig. 19). The survival in squamous cell carcinoma is 30%, for large cell carcinoma it is 20%, and for adenocarcinoma it is 18% compared to the overall rate for the N0 group, of 26% (Fig. 7). The relative influence of cell type on prognosis, in the presence of ipsilateral hilar lymph node metastasis, (N1 classification) is illustrated in Fig. 20. For squamous cell carcinoma the 5-year survival is 19%, while that for adenocarcinoma drops to about 7% and for undifferentiated large cell carcinoma to 5%.

The survival pattern in cases classified as N2 (extension to the mediastinal lymph nodes) is slightly influenced by the histology of the tumor. The prognosis for squamous cell carcinoma and adenocarcinoma is somewhat better than the overall rate of about $3\frac{1}{2}$% (Fig. 7). Figure 21 shows a similar survival pattern for three cell types up to about 40 months, at which point survival for large cell carcinoma plunges to zero. The 5-year survival for small cell carcinoma is less than 1% for all values of N.

The survival pattern of patients according to the M (distant metastasis

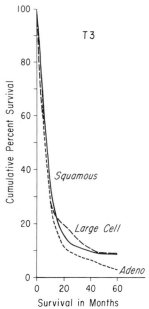

Fig. 18. Survival pattern of lung cancer patients, *primary tumor classification T3,* stratified by histologic type of tumor.

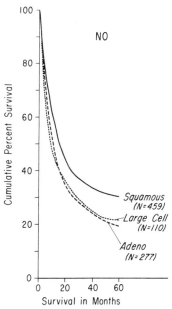

Fig. 19. Survival pattern of lung cancer patients, *regional node classification N0,* no involvement, stratified by histologic type of tumor.

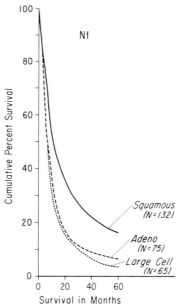

Fig. 20. Survival pattern of lung cancer patients, *regional node classification N1,* metastasis to lymph nodes in the ipsilateral hilar region (including direct extension) stratified by histologic type of tumor.

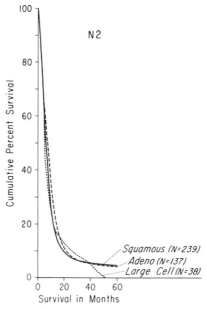

Fig. 21. Survival pattern of lung cancer patients, *regional node classification N2,* metastasis to lymph nodes in the mediastinum, stratified by cell type.

classification) is also modified with stratification by histologic type (Fig. 22). With no clinical evidence of distant metastatic spread, the 5-year survival rate is 26% for squamous cell carcinoma, 20% for adenocarcinoma, and 18% for large cell carcinoma as compared to 25% for all cases combined (Fig. 8). The effect of extrathoracic extension of disease (M1) is disastrous regardless of the cell type, as shown in Fig. 23, with the survival rate falling rapidly to nearly zero.

The combined bidirectional effects of morphology and overall disease extent on the force of mortality, according to stage definitions, is illustrated in Figs. 24–26. Patients with squamous cell carcinoma have a markedly better prognosis in each stage of disease. Forty percent of these patients with stage I disease survive 5 years; 17% with stage II disease survive 5 years; and 9% with stage III disease survive 5 years. If the primary tumor exceeds 3 cm, metastasis to hilar lymph nodes is predictive of a much poorer prognosis in adenocarcinoma and large cell carcinoma than in squamous cell carcinoma. In stage III disease the 5-year survival drops to 5% for large cell carcinoma and 3% for adenocarcinoma. In the population sampled, the survival experience in undifferentiated small cell carcinoma (N = 360) bears no relationship to the clinically recognized anatomic extent of disease (Fig. 27). For this reason such patients are not assigned to a stage group. However, in view of promising current investi-

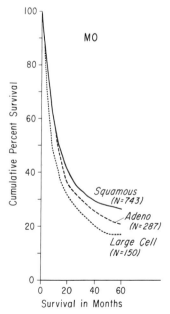

Fig. 22. Survival pattern of lung cancer patients, *distant metastasis classification M0,* no distal metastasis present, stratified by histologic type of tumor.

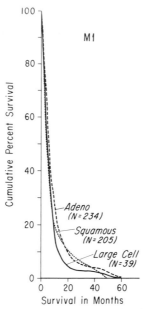

Fig. 23. Survival pattern of lung cancer patients, *distal metastasis classification M1,* distal metastasis present such as in scalene, cervical or contralateral hilar lymph nodes, contralateral lung, liver, etc., stratified by histologic type of tumor.

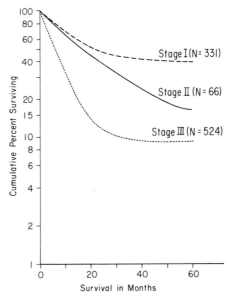

Fig. 24. Survival pattern of lung cancer patients with *squamous cell carcinoma* stratified by stage of disease (semilog plot).

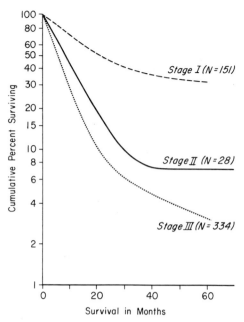

Fig. 25. Survival pattern of lung cancer patients with *adenocarcinoma,* stratified by stage of disease (semilog plot).

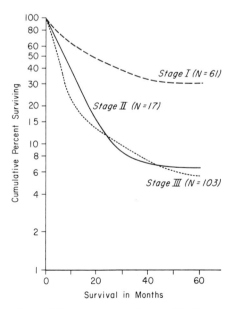

Fig. 26. Survival pattern of lung cancer patients with *large cell carcinoma* stratified by stage of disease (semilog plot).

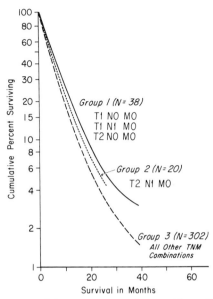

Fig. 27. Survival pattern of lung cancer patients with *undifferentiated small cell carcinoma (oat cell)* stratified by TNM groups (semilog plot).

gational therapy, the correct TNM values are assigned so that specific subsets may be targeted for therapeutic consideration.

VII. OTHER FACTORS AFFECTING SURVIVAL PATTERNS

Estimates of human survival are commonly derived from general population statistics giving consideration only to the variables of age and sex. For more accurate prediction, additional variables should be considered. These include (a) presence of developmental defects, (b) presence of serious chronic illness other than cancer, (c) race, (d) economic status, and (e) type of employment. Further refinement in the validity of estimating survival would result from consideration of (a) hereditary factors, (b) environmental factors, (c) marital status, (d) height–weight ratio, (e) social conditions. It can be shown that all of these factors correlate with longevity.

In estimating survival in lung cancer, all of the above variables remain operational. In addition, at diagnosis, there are a number of complex interacting biologic variables that are specifically tumor-related and which influence the subsequent clinical course of the disease. These include (a) the basic biological nature of a specific tumor cell type, (b) its growth and metastatic spread, and (c) host–tumor immunological relationships.

A system of classification which takes into account all variables influencing survival would be hopelessly complex and unmanageable. The number of combinations and permutations of all known or suspected variables is almost infinite. Even large series of cases would be stratified to such an extent that very few patients would be classified in any one described subset of the total population. Furthermore, it must be remembered that no two patients are completely similar nor can their characteristics be completely described. In practice, we can only group together patients who are generally alike. This is done by abstracting certain common features and disregarding or omitting other aspects that are dissimilar.

From the AJC studies, we are persuaded that indices of anatomic extent of disease, stratified morphologically, permit a simple yet valid classification that best reflects prognosis. In identifying measures of disease extent, only those that contributed most significantly to the force of mortality were selected. This was achieved by an optimization analysis of some 28 variables.

This approach led to the exclusion of a number of factors that we consider to be less significantly associated with survival. Some of these deserve comment, however, as they are judged by a few investigators to be of major significance and are incorporated into some systems of classification.

With respect to the morphologic classification, age and sex factors show a moderate intergroup variability but very little intragroup variability. This relates to the marked variation in sex ratios among the various histologic types of disease. In a statistical survey of 9865 patients, the overall male: female ratio was 7.8 : 1. The ratios by histologic types were epidermoid (squamous cell) 18.6 : 1; adenocarcinoma, 2.8 : 1; undifferentiated small cell (oat cell), 6.5 : 1; and undifferentiated large cell, 6.3 : 1. When stratifying by morphology, therefore, this factor is not highly significant and, accordingly, was excluded. The duration of symptoms, defined from date of onset to date of diagnosis, were similarly studied. When grouped by 3-month time intervals, the last being greater than 24 months, nine survival curves could be generated. The survival dynamics of all morphologic types were remarkably similar, and there were no statistically significant differences detected between the groups. It was concluded that there was no significant relationship between symptom duration and survival.

There are three significant and documentable interrelated elements in the factor of general health [8], namely, (1) physiologic parameters related to operability, (2) coexistent chronic disease unrelated to the tumor, and (3) debilitating derangements directly related to the neoplastic process.

As surgery is the only current therapy that can be considered "curative," the combination of resectability and physiologic inoperability clearly portends a diminished life expectancy in stage I and stage II disease. This does not bias end result reporting, however, as survival becomes primarily a function of therapy. This applies equally to resectable patients who refuse surgery. The occurrence of significant chronic disease appears normally distributed among the various stages of lung cancer. For the most part, this reflects the very small differences between the mean age and its standard deviation for each group. Accordingly, this element also is not a source of significant bias in end result reporting. In our studies, patients with significant systemic manifestations of disease, causally related to the primary lung malignancy, are uniformly classified as stage III and usually as M1. The 5-year cumulative survival for the various subsets describing this extent of disease ranges from 0 to 3%. It seemed unwarranted to further subdivide the entire structure of the classification scheme in order to provide for a variable which might affect such a limited range of survival. In special cases, such as phase III investigational therapeutic trials for advanced disease where the discrimination function of the comorbidity variable is judged important, it is preferrable to assign a single digit index of patient performance in accordance with the Zubrod [29] scale. The basic structure of the TNM classification is thereby preserved for general usage and appears valid under all conditions.

VIII. FLEXIBILITY OF THE TNM SYSTEM FOR SPECIALIZED USE

The basic TNM system of classification, when stratified by cell type, will meet the needs of most investigators and cancer registries for the meaningful reporting of end results. I am persuaded that the minimal requirement for publication of a manuscript should be the reporting of therapeutic results in lung cancer according to the stage of disease by histologic type of the primary tumor [18]. It is even more valid to report experience in descriptive terms of the anatomic extent of the TNM subsets, but this is practical only in relatively large series of cases. This system, nevertheless, provides for an abbreviated notation for purposes of recording and for describing targeted groups in planning treatment.

It is appreciated that, as therapeutic strategies become increasingly sophisticated, there is a corollary requirement for increasing precision in the description of select subgroups within each TNM category which may need separate consideration. This situation is encountered in current national and international collaborative clinical trials. The basic system is responsive to such needs through a decimal point system of expanded notation. A worksheet such as that shown in Table I may be amplified to identify specific subsets within each TNM category. The opportunities for further expansion, if needs develop, are limited only by the imagination. Multiple digits to the right of the decimal point may be used to describe the characteristics of each of the TNM categories. It is essential, however, that the basic rules for assigning TNM values be followed. By doing so, various

TABLE I WORK SHEET FOR STAGING LUNG CANCER[a]

No. _____ Name _____ Date _____

Directions: Encircle the T, N, and M rating following the description that is most accurate for the patient's cancer. Encircle the value for each rating and add to obtain the total value. Consult the table at the bottom of the form to determine the stage.

This form may be used for 4 staging classifications: (1) CLINICAL (2) SURGICAL (3) POST–SURGICAL (post-resection) (4) RETREATMENT (upon failure of initial treatment, patient is restaged prior to retreatment).

Check appropriate classification: Clinical ___ Surgical ___ Post-Surgical ___ Retreatment ___

	CLASSIFICATION:	
PRIMARY TUMOR – T		Value
No evidence of primary tumor	T0	0
Tumor proven by the presence of malignant cells in broncho-pulmonary secretions but not visualized roentgenographically or bronchoscopically	TX	0
Carcinoma in situ	T1S	1
A tumor that is 3.0 cm or less in greatest diameter, surrounded by lung or visceral pleura and without evidence of invasion proximal to a lobar bronchus at bronchoscopy	T1	1
A tumor more than 3.0 cm in greatest diameter, or a tumor of any size, which invades the visceral pleura or with its associated atelectasis or obstructive pneumonitis extends to the hilar region. At bronchoscopy the proximal extent of demonstrable tumor must be within a lobar bronchus or at least 2.0 cm distal to the carina. Any associated atelectasis or obstructive pneumonitis must involve less than an entire lung, and there must be no pleural effusion	T2	2
A tumor of any size with direct extension into an adjacent structure such as the chest wall, the diaphragm, or the mediastinum and its contents; or demonstrable bronchoscopically to involve a main bronchus less than 2.0 cm distal to the carina; any tumor associated with atelectasis or obstructive pneumonitis of an entire lung or pleural effusion	T3	4
REGIONAL LYMPH NODES – N		
No demonstrable metastasis to regional lymph nodes	N0	0
Metastasis to lymph nodes in peribronchial and/or the ipsilateral hilar region (including direct extension)	N1	1
Metastasis to lymph nodes in the mediastinum	N2	4
DISTANT METASTASIS – M		
No distant metastasis	M0	0
Distant metastasis such as in scalene, cervical, or contralateral hilar lymph nodes, brain, bones, lung, liver, etc.	M1	4

Cell type:

Squamous ☐   Small ☐   Adenocarcinoma ☐   Large ☐

Other (specify) _____

TOTAL VALUE	STAGE
0	Occult Carcinoma
1 or 2	I
3	II
4 or more	III

SUMMARY OF STAGING

T _____
N _____
M _____
Stage ____

If patient had a resection, indicate whether post-surgical treatment classification was based on pathological evaluation of:

primary tumor mass   ☐ yes   ☐ no   ☐ unknown
regional lymph nodes   ☐ yes   ☐ no   ☐ unknown

[a] Adopted from potocols of the National Cancer Institute, Working Party for the Study of Lung Cancer.

series can still be compared by grouping subsets to the appropriate level of specificity. This system, therefore, can be used to meet the objectives of a wide range of investigations.

With respect to the primary tumor, for example in T2 lesions, the first digit to the right of the decimal point may be the exact size of the tumor; the second digit, invasion of the visceral pleura (0 no or unknown, 1 yes); the third digit, involvement of the hilum by atelectasis or obstructive pneumonitis (0 not present, 1 involving segment, 2 involving lobe). Accordingly, a primary tumor 4 cm in greatest diameter with atelectasis involving the anterior segment of the right upper lobe might be classified T2.401.

It may be particularly appropriate to further classify T3 lesions, for investigational reasons. Because of their unique biological behavior, superior sulcus tumors form a specific targeted group for therapy. These cases can be identified by assigning the first digit to the right of the decimal point in T3 lesions to superior sulcus tumors (0 absent, 1 with painful apical syndrome, 2 with true Pancoast syndrome). This more precisely indicates the progressive extent of the primary lesion. On the basis of our current studies we take the view that T3.1 lesions are appropriately treated with preoperative irradiation and resection, while our best results in treating T3.2 lesions are by definitive irradiation. Subsequent digits may be used to identify factors relating to the extent or accompanying complications of the primary lesion. For example, the second digit may be extension into the mediastinum (0 no, 1 chest wall, 2 diaphragm, 3 pericardium, etc.). The third digit may describe involvement of the main bronchus less than 2 cm distal to the carina (0 no, 1 yes); the fourth digit, atelectasis or pneumonitis of an entire lung (0 no, 1 yes); fifth digit, pleural effusion (0 no; 1 yes, transudate negative; 2 yes, transudate positive; 3 yes, exudate negative or positive). Thus a superior sulcus tumor with extension into the chest wall might be designated T3.2100.

In our initial studies of independent variables, each of the factors that are associated with the various subgroups of T3 lesions are essentially equivalent in their contributions to the force of mortality. For example, the presence of any associated pleural effusion is a sign of an extremely poor prognosis. There are, however, slight differences in the dynamics of the survival curve according to whether the fluid was a transudate without malignant cells or a transudate with malignant cells. The survival curve for the latter case is essentially identical to that for any exudate whether or not malignant cells are identified. The T3 subgroups are not entirely mutually exclusive. Therefore, the decimal point expansion can be utilized to express the extent of disease and its accompanying complications that limit the choice of therapeutic modality.

In the same way numerical descriptors may be assigned to certain subgroups of lymph nodes within the categories of N1 and N2. In the case of N1, the first digit to the right of the decimal point may be peribronchial nodes (0 no, 1 yes); the second digit, interlobar nodes (0 no, 1 yes); the third digit hilar nodes (0 no, 1 yes). With respect to mediastinal node involvement N2, the first digit might be assigned to ipsalateral tracheo-bronchial nodes (0 no, 1 yes); the second digit, subcarinal nodes (0 no, 1 yes); the third digit, ipsalateral low paratracheal nodes (0 no, 1 yes); the fourth digit, high ipsalateral paratracheal nodes (0 no, 1 yes); the fifth digit, contralateral paratracheal (0 no, 1 yes). Thus a stage III patient with involvement of the tracheobronchial nodes and the upper paratracheal nodes might be designated N2.10010 if the needs of the investigator required such detail.

The presence or absence of metastasis to specific organs (M1) may be designated in the same way to satisfy the needs of any investigator or group of investigators. The first digit to the right of the decimal point might be assigned to the ipsalateral scalene or supraclavicular lymph nodes (0 no; 1 yes, clinical; 2 yes, histological), the second digit to the contralateral scalene or supraclavicular nodes (0 no; 1 yes, clinical; 2 yes, histological), the third digit to other cervical nodes (0 no; 1 yes, clinical; 2 yes, histo-logical), the fourth digit to contralateral hilar lymph nodes (0 no; 1 yes, clinical; 2 yes, histological), the fifth digit to brain (0 no; 1 yes, clinical; 2 yes, histological), the sixth digit to bones (0 no, 1 yes, clinical; 2 yes, histological), the seventh digit to liver (0 no; 1 yes, clinical; 2 yes, histo-logical). Thus a stage III patient with pathologically proven metastasis to the ipsalateral supraclavicular nodes and clinical evidence of metastasis to the liver but without evidence of any other metastasis might be designated M1.2000001 if the needs of the investigator or clinician required these details.

There is no unanimity of opinion regarding the advisability of resecting appropriate tumors when the mediastinal lymph nodes are involved (re-sectable T with N2, M0). The literature indicates that the 5-year survival rate is less than 10% in patients with metastatic mediastinal adenopathy following surgical resection. Our own position is that resection is a valid option whenever a tumor-free margin can be obtained and where the extent of mediastinal involvement is limited to the subcarinal nodes and/or to the nodes of the ipsalateral mediastinum adjacent to the distal half of the intrathoracic trachea (resectable T with N2.11100 M0). This applies only to squamous cell and undifferentiated large cell carcinomas where the 5-year survival is 14 and 11%, respectively. We do not resect adenocarci-noma if there is any evidence of mediastinal lymph node metastasis at mediastinoscopy. Undifferentiated small cell (oat cell) carcinoma is no longer regarded as a surgical disease regardless of its clinical extent.

Radiotherapy is generally regarded as the primary modality in the following categories: (a) T3, any N, M0, (b) any T, N2, M0, (c) any T, any N, M1 with metastasis limited to the ipsalateral and/or contralateral scalene, supraclavicular or other cervical lymph nodes. These classifications are equated with "regional" disease. Any M1 subgroup with metastasis to the contralateral lung, brain, bone, kidney, or other distant organs or lymph nodes generally is regarded as "extensive" disease, and such cases fall to the chemotherapists. Current investigational treatment plans utilize combined modalities in all stage III carcinoma and in all cases of of undifferentiated small cell carcinoma.

Both conventional treatment and investigational therapeutic strategies can be directly related to clearly identified segments of the lung cancer population. The concept of local, regional, and extensive disease also can be related to the TNM classification. All stage I and stage II disease is "local," and such cases fall to the surgeon for primary treatment. Cases of both "regional" and "extensive" disease fall into stage III. As demonstrated, with the exception of certain superior sulcus tumors, patients with these descriptive categories of disease extent display remarkably similar patterns of survival. The role of surgery, radiotherapy, and chemotherapy, as unique single modalities of treatment, will vary somewhat according to the philosophy of the attending physician.

This system of classification is specifically applicable to the clinical staging of lung cancer. It derives from the best estimate of tumor extent utilizing all clinical sources of information available to the point of exploratory thoracotomy. All patients should be initially staged on this basis, accepting the fact that such clinical evaluation, being in part judgemental in nature, is subject to error. Clearly, the accuracy of the clinical TNM classification and stage grouping is directly related to the degree of thoroughness of the preoperative evaluation of disease extent. This is one reason that we stress objective evaluation of the mediastinal contents by mediastinoscopy or mediastinotomy [19], and why we utilize the complementarity of mediastinoscopy and pulmonary angiography as routine evaluative procedures [21]. The value of objectively identifying the histologic type of disease is evident in the data presented.

Once the original clinical stage grouping is assigned, it should not be altered during the subsequent course of the disease. In patients undergoing surgery, additional objective evidence of disease extent will be obtained and may be utilized in a second classification. The term "surgical evaluative classification" is used to describe the known extent of disease following a major surgical exploration with or without biopsy. The term "postsurgical treatment classification" is used to describe the known extent of disease following examination of a therapeutically resected specimen.

There is a rising gradient of reliability and validity in the staging process as one moves from the "clinical classification" to the "postsurgical treatment classification." This relates to the increased amount of objective data available from the gross and microscopic examination of resected specimens. It is especially important to appreciate this point in comparing therapeutic results reported in the literature and especially in the design of investigational clinical trials that are to evaluate therapeutic approaches. Subsets of the lung cancer population can only be compared appropriately when the characteristics of cell type, stage of disease, and level of classification are the same for each set. Ongoing studies indicate that the proposed scheme for describing the T, N, M sets and for their grouping into stages is equally applicable to each type of classification.

IX. CONCLUSIONS

The universal goal of oncologists is to provide each cancer patient with the optimum form of treatment for his disease. With current knowledge, this goal may only be reached through orderly classification of the biological process of neoplastic disease and its response to treatment. Measures of this response may be communicated in meaningful terms and translated into therapeutic practice only if uniform evaluators are utilized. A practical and valid TNM system for the clinical classification of lung cancer has been developed to serve this purpose. This system, presented here in both a basic and a compatible expanded research format, was derived from studies of the relationship of prognosis to morphology and to the anatomic extent of disease.

These studies indicate that the four major cell types of lung cancer differ significantly from each other. In epidermoid (squamous) carcinoma, adenocarcinoma, and undifferentiated large cell carcinoma, only those clinically measurable parameters of the disease's extent which were the most powerful factors in the force of mortality were utilized to describe the extent of the primary tumor and its metastatic manifestations. With respect to the extent and complications due to the primary tumor, the data indicates that prognosis is related to tumor size and location, extent of proximal margination, and complications such as atelectasis, obstructive pneumonitis, and pleural effusion. Metastases to the regional lymph nodes, and especially to those within the mediastinum, are extremely important predictors of survival as is the presence of more distant metastases.

Involvement of the hilar nodes does not materially increase risk if the primary lesion is less than 3 cm, but it is of serious consequence if the primary is large, especially in adenocarcinoma and undifferentiated large cell carcinoma. Involvement of mediastinal nodes has dire implications.

The existence of pleural effusion, regardless of the identification of malignant cells, forewarns of a grave outcome and, if malignant cells are present, patients rarely live more than 12 months. Clinically suspicious palpable lymph nodes in the neck are a valid index of distal spread. A fatal outcome is essentially identified with evidence of direct mediastinal invasion and distal hematogenous metastasis. The survival rates for patients with squamous cell carcinoma were consistently better than for those with undifferentiated large cell and adenocarcinoma, and these differences are sufficiently great to support the opinion that in reporting groups of patients with lung cancer all cases should be stratified and analyzed by cell type. Since, however, the relationship between survival and anatomic extent was similar for the three cell types, a single set of definitions of the various categories of T, N, and M was developed [1]. The identified subsets of the population were subsequently grouped into three defined stages of disease extent. In undifferentiated small cell carcinoma no relationship could be found between the clinically demonstrated extent of disease and prognosis. Tumors of this cell type are, therefore, not staged.

In presenting this clinical classification of lung cancer, we recognize certain problems and limitations which must be kept in mind. In a given patient, the total tumor burden cannot be precisely quantitated, and the delicate balance between host defenses and the aggressiveness of the malignancy is not measurable. These, and a number of other complex interacting biological variables, which cannot be measured, will influence the subsequent clinical course of the disease. Patients can, however, be grouped together according to certain measurable common features of their disease so that each group will have a relatively unique pattern of survival. Thus, the survival experience for one population of a given cell type and stage of disease may be compared with another of a similar cell type and stage. By so doing, the results of different modalities of treatment can be compared more reliably and validly.

ACKNOWLEDGMENTS

The author wishes to express his deep appreciation to David T. Carr, M.D. for his major and invaluable contributions to this work. The contributions of members of the Task Force on Lung Cancer of the American Joint Committee are recognized with gratitude. This investigation was generously supported by grants from the American Cancer Society and the National Institutes of Health under the auspices of the American Joint Committee on Cancer Staging and End Results Reporting and by the National Cancer Institute under Contract CM-33737. Partial support was also received from the Department of Biomathematics of The University of Texas System Cancer Center, M. D. Anderson Hospital under PHS-NCI research grant CA 11430, Barry W. Brown, Ph.D., Consultant.

REFERENCES

1. American Joint Committee for Cancer Staging and End Results Reporting, Clinical Staging System For Carcinoma of the Lung, 1973.
2. Carbone, P. P., Frost, J. K., Feinstein, A. R., Higgins, G. A., and Selawry, O. S., Perspectives and prospects. *Ann. Intern. Med.* **73,** 1003–1004 (1970).
3. Carr, D. T., A report on the development of the staging system for cancer of the lung. *Nat. Cancer Conf. Proc. 6th, 1968,* pp. 877–878 (1970).
4. Cliffton, E. E., Criteria for operability and resectability, *In* "Lung Cancer" (W. L. Watson, ed.), pp. 258–262, Mosby, St. Louis, Missouri, 1968.
5. Copeland, M. M., Program of American Joint Committee on Cancer Staging and End Results Reporting. *Acta Unio Int. Contra Cancrum* **19,** 871–874 (1963).
6. Denoix, P. F., Enquete permanent dans les centres anticancereux. *Bull. Inst. Nat. Hyg.* **1,** 70–75 (1946).
7. Dold, U., Schneider, V., and Krause, F., Applicability of TNM-system on lung carcinoma: Field trial. Proposal of advanced TNM-classification including a category for diagnostic certainty degree. *Z. Krebsforsch.* **84,** 1–5 (1972).
8. Feinstein, A. R., New staging system for cancer and reappraisal of "early" treatment and "cure" by radical surgery. *N. Eng. J. Med.* **279,** 747–753 (1968).
9. Gehan, E. A., Estimating survival functions from life table. *J. Chronic Dis.* **21,** 629–644 (1969).
10. Guinn, G. A., Tomm, K. E., North, L., and Mocega, E., Clinical staging of primary lung cancer. *Chest* **64,** 51–54 (1973).
11. International Union against Cancer (UICC). Committee on TNM Classification. "Malignant Tumors of the Lung. Clinical Stage Classification and Presentation of Results." Geneva, 1966.
12. International Union against Cancer (UICC). Committee on TNM Classification. "TNM General Rules." Livre de Poche, Geneva, 1969.
13. International Union against Cancer (UICC). Committee on TNM Classification. "TNM General Rules." Geneva, 1969.
14. International Union against Cancer and American Joint Committee for Cancer Staging and End Results Reporting. "Supplement to TNM Classification of Malignant Tumors." Geneva, 1973.
15. Ishikawa, S., Staging system on TNM classification for lung cancer. *Jap. J. Clin. Oncol.* **6,** 19–30 (1973).
16. Johnston, R. N., and Smith, D. H., Symptoms and survival in lung cancer. *Lancet* **2,** 588–591 (1968).
17. Larsson, S., Pretreatment classification and staging of bronchogenic carcinoma. *Scand. J. Thorac. Cardiov. Surg., Suppl.* **10** (1973).
18. Matthews, M. J., Morphologic classification of bronchogenic cancer. *Cancer Chemother. Rep.,* **4,** 299–301 (1973).
19. Mountain, C. F., The role of mediastinoscopy in the management of lung cancer. *Cancer Conf., Proc. 6th,* pp. 829–834 (1970).
20. Mountain, C. F., Carr, D. T., and Anderson, W. A. D., A system for the clinical staging of lung cancer. *Amer. J. Roentgenol. Radium Ther. Nucl. Med.* [N.S.] **120,** 130–138 (1974).
21. Mountain, C. F., and Medellin-Lastra, H., Pulmonary angiography, azygography, and mediastinoscopy in the diagnosis and staging of bronchogenic carcinoma. *In* "Radiologic and other Biophysical Methods in Tumor Diagnosis," pp. 191–201. Yearbook Publ., Chicago, Illinois, 1975.

22. Paulson, D. L., Importance of defining location and staging of superior sulcus tumors. *Ann. Thorac. Surg.* **15,** 549–551 (1973).
23. Rakov, A. I., Kabeshev, E. N., and Lakshtanova, I. P., Evaluation of TNM clinical classification for lung cancer. *Neoplasma* **16,** 325–333 (1969).
24. Rubin, P., Unified classification of cancer: Oncotaxonomy with symbols. *Cancer* **31,** 963–982 (1973).
25. Senior, R. M., and Adamson, J. S., Survival in patients with lung cancer. *Arch. Intern. Med.* **125,** 975–980 (1970).
26. Sixth International Congress of Radiology, London, July 23–29, 1950. Abstracts of papers, radiotherapy section synopsis, method of presentation of results of treatment Abstracts 42–64, pp. 22–38 (1950).
27. Smith, T. L., Putman, J. E., and Gehan, E. A., Computer program for estimating survival functions from life table. *Comput. Programs Biomed.* **1,** 58–64 (1970).
28. World Health Organization, *World Health Org. Tech. Rep. Ser.* **25,** 22 (1950).
29. Zubrod, G., Schneiderman, M., Frei, E., Brindley, C., Gold, L. G., Shnider, B., Oviedo, R., Gorman, J., Jones, R. Jr., Johsson, U., Colsky, J., Chalmers, T., Ferguson, B., Derick, M., Holland, J., Selawar, O., Regelson, W., Lasagna, C., and Owens, A. H. Jr., Appraisal of methods for the study of chemotherapy of cancer in man: Comparative therapeutic trial of nitrogen mustard and triethylene thiophosphoramide. *J. Chronic Dis.* **11,** 7–33 (1960).

Chapter 7

Nonspecific Immunological Alterations in Patients with Lung Cancer

Lucien Israel

The immune status of patients with cancer, in general, and lung cancer, in particular, has become a field of considerable interest, and it is already too late to quote the vast number of studies published on the subject. In this chapter an attempt will be made to outline the general trends and to raise some controversial questions, the discussion of which could in turn lead to new trials and new studies.

I. PRETHERAPEUTIC IMMUNE STATUS
IN ADVANCED LUNG CANCER

Studies published by Krant *et al.* [13], Al Saraf *et al.* [1], Lopez-Cardozo [14], Ducos *et al.* [6], Wells *et al.* [20], and Brugarolas *et al.* [3, 4] have shown that in advanced lung cancer cell-mediated immunity is markedly depressed. This depression is reflected in skin tests to recall antigens (PPD,* mumps, varidase, candidin, etc.), in phytohemagglutinin (PHA) blastogenesis *in vitro,* in sensitization to dinitrochlorobenzene (DNCB), and in absolute lymphocyte counts. In contrast, serum immunoglobulin levels and antibody synthesis remain within the normal range.

In a study published in 1968 [10] we reported 52% of negative PPD skin tests in a group of 100 patients, whereas the percentage of negative tests in controls is only 17%. The proportion of positive and negative patients was the same for epidermoid carcinoma and adenocarcinoma, whereas in oat cell carcinoma the proportion of negative patients was higher.

Furthermore, PHA blastogenesis was significantly decreased in cancer patients as compared to a matched control group ($p < 0.001$). Thirty-six of the cancer patients served as donors for lymphocytes that were injected intradermally into normal recipients. In 26 cases (72%) these lymphocytes failed to induce a graft-versus-host reaction as compared to an 8% failure rate for lymphocytes from normal donors.

It may be concluded from all these studies that immune competence is definitely impaired in patients with advanced lung cancer, and in our experience this impairment has proved to be more pronounced than in other types of cancer.

II. PRETHERAPEUTIC IMMUNE STATUS
IN EARLY LUNG CANCER

Immune status in early and resectable lung cancer has not been extensively investigated. However, immune depression appears to occur even at this stage as indicated by the studies of Eilber and Morton (see Section III) and Steward (quoted by Hersh *et al.* [7]) which included cases of early lung cancer and showed that some patients converted from negative to positive immune competence after surgery.

The only quantitative study available to date was published by us in 1973 and involved only the PPD response in cases of resectable lung cancer [11]. This study showed that in a group of 323 patients with squamous

---

* PPD, purified tubercular protein derivative.

cell carcinoma, 158 had a negative response to PPD (48%) as against 17% for controls. We feel that it is important to remark that immune depression is not entirely due to widespread disease but may also be encountered in early cases with a relatively small, resectable tumor, at least in lung cancer. The logical conclusion that immediately comes to mind is that at a very early stage patients can be separated into two different groups on the basis of host–tumor relationship. This could in turn lead to different therapeutic strategies. It might be added that our study revealed no correlation between PPD response, on the one hand, and sex and age, on the other.

At this point I would like to raise a question that has been brought to light by unpublished data from our unit: in recent years our patients have been regularly tested with intradermal PPD, killed BCG, varidase, candidin, and DNCB (sensitization with 2000 μg; challenge with 0.5, 5, and 50 μg applied simultaneously). We have learned two things from this study so far: (1) Some patients who are unresponsive to PPD still respond to killed BCG, which appears to be a far more sensitive test. (2) Inability to become sensitized to DNCB is very often observed while recall antigens still elicit a good response. This suggests that the primary response, as tested by DNCB sensitization, is suppressed prior to that of the secondary response. The exact significance of this difference is still unclear at the present time.

III. PROGNOSTIC RELEVANCE OF PRETHERAPEUTIC IMMUNE STATUS

Brugarolas et al. [3] showed that using the diameter of induration to a skin test with streptokinase–streptodornase as a basis, it was possible to divide surgical patients into three prognostic groups well correlated with postsurgical survival. Our study [11], performed with PPD showed similar results (Table I), median survival being significantly higher in the PPD positive group (16+ months) than in the PPD negative group (8.6+ months).

Furthermore (Table II) 33 patients who converted from negative to positive after surgery survived longer than patients who remained negative. It is interesting to note that the prognostic value of nonspecific immune status in lung cancer patients is not confined to early cases, but applies to advanced cases as well. This has been clearly demonstrated by the studies of Krant et al. [13], Brugarolas et al. [4], and Israel [9]. Whatever the mechanism underlying the constraining effect of a good immune status on the spread of lung cancer, this mechanism remains operational even in

TABLE I

Prognostic Value of Preoperative PPD Skin Tests in 323 Adequately Resected Squamous Cells Bronchogenic Carcinomas with No Further Treatment[a, b]

Time following surgery (months)	165 PPD positive[c] patients (% surviving)	158 PPD negative[d] patients (% surviving)	Chi square	Statistical significance
3	93	84	5.38	$p < 0.02$
6	78	66	3.85	$p < 0.05$
9	66	49	5.90	$p < 0.02$
12	58	41	5.72	$p < 0.02$
18	46	30	5.42	$p < 0.02$
24	36	25	6.01	$p < 0.02$
36	27	20	7.11	$p < 0.01$
48	21	12	9.11	$p < 0.005$

[a] From Israel et al. [11].
[b] Median survival measured on actuarial curves.
[c] PPD positive: 16+ months.
[d] PPD negative: 8.6+ months.

patients with metastases—a point to be kept in mind when the relative indications of nonspecific immune stimulation are discussed.

IV. POSSIBLE CAUSES OF PRECANCEROUS IMMUNE DEFICIENCIES

Although primary immune deficiency disease [12] and iatrogenic depression in organ transplants [15] are associated with an increased incidence of cancer, Hersh et al. pointed out [7] that no case of lung cancer has ever been reported in such situations, and he raised the question as to whether temporary failure of immune surveillance is necessary for lung cancer to develop or whether prolonged contact with tobacco carcinogens, which are immunodepressants themselves, may suffice. Apart from this cause, immune depression due to nonspecific environmental factors, such as infectious viruses, may promote the development of transformed cells. It might be of interest to monitor the immune status of high risk populations, namely, adult male smokers, in order to determine whether immune de-

TABLE II

Prognostic Value of Postoperative Changes in PPD Skin Test 3 Weeks after Resection

Time following surgery (months)	69 negative remained negative (% surviving)	33 negative converted to positive (% surviving)	Chi square	Statistical significance
3	83	96	10.8	$p < 0.001$
6	63	88	18.0	$p < 0.001$
9	44	68	10.7	$p < 0.001$
12	35	60	12.5	$p < 0.001$
18	31	45	0.36	$p > 0.05$
24	23	31	0.72	$p > 0.05$
36	20	26	1.01	$p > 0.05$
48	5	26	8.66	$p < 0.005$

ficiency occurs uniformly or preferentially in subjects who ultimately develop lung cancer.

V. TUMOR-INDUCED IMMUNE DEFICIENCY

It now appears fairly well established that tumors, in general, and many lung tumors, in particular, exert a nonspecific immunodepressant effect. Hersh et al. [7] recently reviewed available data on the subject. Sherwin et al. [16], Silk [17], and others had already drawn attention to this phenomenon, and we observed, in 1968 [10], an augmentation in immune reactivity following removal of lung tumors. This finding has led us to consider this type of immune depression as a paraneoplastic syndrome. Unfortunately, the mechanism by which tumors depress immune reactivity remains entirely unknown, although it is the serum that has been shown to possess this property. Some preliminary data from our unit tend, however, to show that acute phase reactants, which are regarded by myself and others as nonspecific inhibitors of immune reactions, are found in higher levels in sera from patients with lung cancer than with many other tumors. It would be extremely important to elucidate the exact nature of this phenomenon, since this might lead to its therapeutic control. Data accumulated in large series of patients treated with *Corynebacterium parvum* strongly suggests that tumor-induced immune deficiency differs from chemotherapy-induced immune deficiency. The latter can be prevented by immune stimulants, whereas the former may occur while the patient is on immunostimulant therapy when recurrence occurs after adequate surgery.

VI. CHEMOTHERAPY AND IMMUNE STATUS

Hersh et al. [8] showed that although chemotherapy may induce a loss of immune competence, responders usually exhibit an overshoot in immune reactivity when chemotherapy is discontinued. This appears to be of great importance in the distinction between optimum and maximum schedules. Conversely, Brugarolas et al. [4] reported that patients with good immune status showed a better response to chemotherapy than patients whose immune status was deficient. These facts will undoubtedly have an important bearing on future combined modality programs, and they are also important when considering the mechanisms involved in chemotherapeutic cell killing. It appears that cooperation between immunocytes and cytostatic agents is necessary for an optimal effect and that in some circumstances chemotherapy might be immunogenic. Consequently, reliable immunological monitoring is necessary during chemotherapy in order not to overdepress the host's immune reactivity. The potential of combined immunochemotherapy will be discussed in Chapter 14; suffice it to say here that we have observed definite synergism between nonspecific immune stimulation and chemotherapy, which is reflected in higher response rates and especially in more lasting responses.

The relationship between chemotherapy and the host's immune status is not a simple one and much remains to be learned in this field.

VII. RADIOTHERAPY OF LUNG CANCER AND IMMUNE RESPONSE

Stjernsward et al. [18] reported that radiotherapy for breast cancer induces profound and long-lasting T cell depression, which might be related to thymic irradiation. The same has been reported in lung cancer by Thomas et al. [19], Check et al. [5], and Braeman and Deeley [2], although the influence of T cell depression on prognosis in these patients remains a matter of controversy. In our unit, out of 14 patients who underwent skin tests to three recall antigens and to DNCB before and after irradiation to the thymic region and 2 months thereafter, 12 showed a sharp decrease in skin reactivity, 1 patient remained positive for one test, and the last patient showed a significant increase in skin responsiveness as well as a complete response to radiotherapy. It is too early to draw any conclusions from these studies, but at this stage it appears necessary to undertake extensive cooperative trials using uniform immune monitoring to determine the exact influence of chest irradiation on immune competence as well as the influence of radiotherapy-induced immune depression on prognosis.

If the effect suggested by the above studies is confirmed, the next step would be to design trials in order to determine to what extent nonspecific immune procedures could counteract the detrimental effects of radiotherapy without weakening its beneficial effects.

VIII. HOW PATIENTS SHOULD BE TESTED

Accumulating data on immunity in cancer patients suggest the necessity for using many tests in the patient. I would like to suggest the procedure I feel to be necessary at the present time for testing and monitoring nonspecific immunity in the category of patients with which we are dealing.

A. Tests for Humoral Immunity and B Cell Function

Antibody synthesis and circulating antibody titers have been found to be within the normal range in lung cancer patients. This does not necessarily imply that humoral immunity does not play a role in this situation. B cell numbers should be measured in every case; T cell-dependent and -independent antibody synthesis should be evaluated separately; and IgG subclasses should be identified and measured.

B. Tests for T Cells

We have so far found skin tests to recall antigens and DNCB sensitization to be more useful than *in vitro* PHA induced blastogenesis, at least in predicting survival. But it remains that E rosettes should be performed, as well as lymphokins and thymic hormone assays.

C. Tests for Macrophages

Circulating monocyte numbers should be measured, and macrophage functions tested. These assays are one of the most important steps to be accomplished in the near future, but it is not that simple to test the macrophages of every patient for their phagocytic activity, their ability to become activated, and their ability to bind complement.

D. Complement and Inflammation

In our laboratory a decrease in the C3 component has been found in patients who responded clinically to nonspecific immune stimulation, while increased levels of total complement were found in patients as a whole. Different fractions of complement and components of the properdin system should be systematically investigated in a search for the lack of some components or the presence of inhibitors as well as for factors involved in inflammation. The role of these agents is often overlooked in cancer immunity. In our opinion they should be explored thoroughly because both

complement and inflammation are necessary components of several mechanisms that result in immune cell killing. As mentioned earlier, nonspecific inhibitors of immune and inflammatory reactions are found in great excess in the sera of patients with lung cancers (unpublished data). We do not know as yet whether their levels correlate with the prognosis, but this seems likely since there is a general parallelism between these levels and skin tests to recall antigens.

E. A Word about Specific Immunity

As soon as lung tumor-specific antigen from allogenic sources becomes available for the purpose of skin testing cancer patients and for measuring MIF, it should become a routine procedure. In the meanwhile the search for circulating immune complexes and for circulating tumor antigen should be given some consideration.

F. When Are These Tests to Be Repeated?

From our experience the pretherapeutic immune status of patients is of major importance in defining poor risk and good risk groups. Nevertheless, much is to be learned from repeating at least some of these tests either every 2 months, every time changes are observed in the clinical course of the disease, and/or changes are made in the therapeutic program. This could show whether there are correlations between the immune competence of the host and the benefits to be expected from different cytostatic agents or combinations. This could also show whether some changes in the clinical course can be anticipated. In a large series of patients followed after resection in our unit, disappearance of DNCB response has been found to precede metastases by 1 to 4 months.

IX. CONCLUSION

Nonspecific immune deficiency and lung cancer appear to be closely related at every stage of the disease and via different mechanisms that are not mutually exclusive and which probably induce different subtypes of immune incompetence. The data available at the present time is insufficient to enable clear definition of these relationships, but at least shows that the field of immunology can no longer be ignored by surgeons, radiotherapists, and chemotherapists who see and treat lung cancer patients. Extensive efforts are needed to introduce immunological monitoring for all patients throughout the entire history of their disease and to ensure uniformity in the exchange of information. It is fairly well established that immunity plays a major role in controlling lung cancer. In future trials, patients should be stratified into two groups with respect to immune status, and particular attention should be paid to the influence of any therapeutic procedure on this immune status. However, our efforts should not stop at this point. Having noticed these facts one would expect therapists to go a step further and try to manipulate the immune system. Some empirical efforts have already been made in these fields and they will be discussed in Chapter 14.

REFERENCES

1. Al Saraf, M., Sardesai, S., and Vaitkevicius, V. V., Clinical immunologic responsiveness in malignant disease. II. *In vitro* lymphocyte response to phytohemagglutinin and the effect of cytostatic drugs. *Oncology* **26**, 357–368 (1972).
2. Braeman, J., and Deeley, T. J., Radiotherapy and the immune response in cancer of the lung. *Brit. J. Radiol.* **46**, 446–449 (1973).
3. Brugarolas, A., and Takita, H., Immunologic status in lung cancer. *Chest* **64**, 427–430 (1973).
4. Brugarolas, A., Tin Han, Takita, H., and Minowada, J., Immunologic assays in lung cancer. Skin tests, lymphocyte blastogenesis and rosette-forming cell count. *N.Y. State J. Med.* **73**, 747–750 (1973).
5. Check, J. H., Damsker, J. I., Brady, L. W., and O'Neill, E. A., Effect of radiation therapy on mumps-delayed type hypersensitivity reaction in lymphoma and carcinoma patients. *Cancer* **32**, 580–584 (1973).
6. Ducos, J., Migueres, J., and Colombies, P., Lymphocyte response to PHA in patients with lung cancer. *Lancet* **1**, 1111–1112 (1970).
7. Hersh, E. M., Gutterman, J. V., and Mavligit, G. M., Perspectives in immunotherapy of lung cancer. *Cancer Treatment Rev.* **1**, 65–80 (1974).
8. Hersh, E. M., Whittekar, J. P., McCredie, K. B., Bodey, G. M., and Freireich,

E. J., Chemotherapy, immunocompetence, immunosuppression and prognosis in acute leukemia. *N. Engl. J. Med.* **285**, 1211–1216 (1971).

9. Israel, L., Cell-mediated immunity in lung cancer patients: Data, problems and propositions. *Cancer Chemother. Rep., Part 3* **4**, 279–281 (1973).

10. Israel, L., Bouvrain, A., Cros-Decam, J., and Mugica, J., Contribution à l'étude des phénomènes d'immunité cellulaire chez les cancéreux pulmonaires avant traitement palliatif ou chirurgical. *Poumon Coeur* **24**, 339–350 (1968).

11. Israel, L., Mugica, J., and Chahinian, P., Prognosis of early bronchogenic carcinoma survival curves of 451 patients after resection of lung cancer in relation to the results of the preoperative tuberculin skin test. *Biomedicine* **19**, 68–72 (1973).

12. Kersey, J. H., Spector, B. D., and Good, R. A., Primary immunodeficiency diseases and cancer. The immuno-deficiency cancer registry. *Int. J. Cancer* **12**, 333–347 (1973).

13. Krant, M. J., Manskopf, G., Brandrup, C. S., and Madoff, M. A., Immunologic alterations in bronchogenic cancer. *Cancer* **21**, 623–631 (1968).

14. Lopez, Cardozo, L., Immunologic behaviour before and during cytostatic treatment in bronchus carcinoma. *Oncology* **25**, 520–527 (1971).

15. Penn, I., and Starzl, T. E., A summary of the status of *de novo* cancer in transplant recipients. *Transplant. Proc.* **4**, 719–733 (1972).

16. Sherwin, R. P., Richters, A., and Richters, V., Evidence for a defective relationship between lymphocytes and documented lung cancer cells. In vivo in vitro correlation. *Proc. Int. Cancer Congr., 9th, 1966* Abst. 50072 (1967).

17. Silk, M., Effect of plasma from patients with carcinoma on *in vitro* lymphocyte transformation. *Cancer* **20**, 2088–2089 (1967).

18. Stjernsward, J., Vnaky, F., Joudal, M., Wegzell, H., and Sealy, R., Lymphopenia and change in distribution of human B and T lymphocytes in peripheral blood induced by irradiation for mammary carcinoma. *Lancet* **2**, 1352–1358 (1972).

19. Thomas, J. W., Coy, P., Lewis, H. S., and Yuen, A., Effect of therapeutic irradiation on lymphocyte transformation in lung cancer. *Cancer* **27**, 1046–1050 (1971).

20. Wells, S. A., Burdick, J. F., Christiansen, C., Ketcham, A. S., and Adkins, P. C., Demonstration of tumor-associated delayed cutaneous hypersensitivity reactions in patients with lung cancer and in patients with carcinoma of the cervix. *Nat. Cancer Inst., Monog.* **37**, 197–203 (1973).

Chapter 8

Nonspecific Causes of Death in Lung Cancer

A. Philippe Chahinian

Numerous factors, apart from the actual growth and dissemination of the tumor, contribute to the causes of mortality in patients with lung cancer. An understanding of these factors should lead to better supportive care of such patients, thus improving their chances for longer survival [12]. Without considering complications directly related to therapy, the aim of this chapter is to emphasize two nonspecific factors, namely, infection and thromboembolism. These factors may constitute a direct threat to the patient's life and may shorten survival appreciably, independently of neoplastic extension to vital organs.

I. VASCULAR ABNORMALITIES

Two types of vascular endothelial abnormalities, possibly related, may be quite nonspecifically associated with lung cancer: venous thrombosis and nonbacterial (marantic) thrombotic endocarditis.

A. Venous Thrombosis and Pulmonary Embolism

As early as 1865, Trousseau [28] was the first to report the occurrence of thrombophlebitis in association with a distant malignant lesion. This observation was remarkable in that it was made on himself, since he was afflicted with gastric carcinoma. In a series of 236 lung cancer patients, Byrd *et al.* [5] determined the incidence of clinically demonstrable thrombophlebitis to be 11%. Pulmonary embolism was noted in half of these patients, and two-thirds of the cases were fatal. However the exact incidence of these events is still a matter of debate. Any type of carcinoma may be associated with phlebitis [9]. Sproul [27], found an incidence of only 2.5% of phlebothrombosis in lung cancer patients at autopsy. This author stressed the frequency of multiple venous thrombosis in patients with carcinoma of the pancreas. Conversely, in a review of 1400 cases of phlebitis, Lieberman *et al.* [16] noted that in males the lung was the most frequently associated site for primary carcinomas and that carcinoma of the pancreas ranked second in incidence. The relative distribution of the histological types was similar to that of all surgically resected lung cancers [5].

In most of the cases reported by Byrd *et al.* [5], the occurrence of thromboembolism preceded the recognition of lung cancer, and an average of 4 months elapsed between the onset of phlebitis and establishment of the correct diagnosis. However, certain characteristic features of this type of thrombophlebitis should alert the attending physician: involvement of multiple or unusual sites including the upper trunk and arms, recurrent or migrating thrombophlebitis, and relative ineffectiveness of anticoagulant therapy [5, 9, 15]. In the presence of unexplained thromboembolic disease, bronchogenic carcinoma should be considered as the most likely cause, especially if the patient is a male cigarette smoker over 40 years of age [5]. The prognosis is poor, even when the tumor appears to be surgically excisable.

The mechanism underlying these thrombotic episodes associated with malignant disease is not clearly established. Tumor emboli or local invasion by the tumor growth appear to play a minor role. The influence of many factors has been suggested: changes in coagulation factors, decrease in fibrinolysis, fibrinoid deposits, increased platelet adhesiveness, and thrombocytosis [5, 15].

B. Nonbacterial Thrombotic Endocarditis

Nonbacterial thrombotic endocarditis (NBTE) is a pathologic entity characterized by the formation of sterile, verrucose lesions with accumulation of fibrin on the heart valves [9, 14]. NBTE occurs in a variety of chronic debilitating diseases and particularly in cancer. Most of the tumors associated with NBTE are mucin-producing adenocarcinomas [1, 9]. In a series of 75 patients with NBTE and malignant neoplastic disease, Rosen and Armstrong found the highest incidence in patients with bronchiolar carcinoma and adenocarcinoma of the lung (17 patients), the incidence being 7.7 and 7.1%, respectively [23]. Prolonged illness with marked wasting of tissues and starvation is not necessary for the development of NBTE, and about two-thirds of the patients have no underlying heart disease [23]. Thus, previously absent soft murmurs should not be dismissed as entirely insignificant in such patients [23]. The major complication of NBTE is the occurrence of arterial emboli, which usually affect the cerebral arteries [9, 14, 18]. This is the major cause of death in patients with NBTE [23]. Other complications include myocardial infarction resulting from arterial emboli, venous thrombosis with pulmonary embolism, renal failure after thrombosis of the inferior vena cava and renal veins, and liver necrosis after portal vein thrombosis [23]. Congestive heart failure is a rare cause of death. Suppurative endocarditis may develop secondarily in NBTE [23]. In all these patients, NBTE must be distinguished from metastatic cancer to the heart.

II. INFECTIOUS COMPLICATIONS

Infection and cancer are "old friends" [7]. Two types of infection can be distinguished in patients with cancer. The first type may be termed "mechanical," for example, pneumonia developing behind bronchial obstruction due to a tumor. The spectrum of microorganisms involved is not likely to be unusual, and treatment of this type of infection is related to the possibility of relieving bronchial obstruction [7]. The second type may be termed "opportunistic" and is accounted for by a weakening of host defense mechanisms. This type of infection is often caused by unusual microorganisms. In fact, these two types of infection may be combined in patients with lung cancer.

Pneumonia or a lung abscess can occur early in the course of the disease, and in about one-quarter of cases they represent the initial manifestation leading to detection of lung cancer [3]. Infection is a major cause of death in patients with lung cancer. In an autopsy study of 633 cases, Luomanen and Watson [17] found that a pulmonary infection distal to the tumor was the most common cause of death. It accounted for 271 deaths, which was 40% of the total. Klastersky et al. [12] reached similar conclusions with regard to various solid tumors and stated that bacterial infection is at present the major cause of death in cancer patients. This suggests that considerable effort should be devoted to the prevention and cure of infection in these patients.

Many factors account for this high incidence of infection. Immune de-

ficiency states, which are discussed in another chapter, are involved. Chemotherapy, radiotherapy, steroids, prolonged treatment with broad spectrum
antibiotics, and hospital environment are factors that promote infection [2,
10]. The diagnosis itself is often a difficult one. The roentgenographic picture may be confused with that of the tumor. Fever is not a constant symptom, and, furthermore, fever unrelated to infection has been reported in
47% of 17 patients with lung cancer [4].

The nature of the infection is variable but extensive epidemiologic
studies, such as those carried out in leukemia, multiple myeloma, and
Hodgkin's disease, are lacking in patients with lung cancer.

A. Bacteria

Gram-positive pathogenic bacteria, such as staphylococci, streptococci,
and pneumococci, are frequently the causative agents, but they can usually
be controlled with antibiotics [2]. *Gram-negative rods* are most frequently
responsible for severe infection and death in patients with solid tumors
[13]. The bronchial tumor itself may be the underlying site of infection
[13]. Although the exact prevalence of each species has not been systematically studied in lung cancer, it seems that *Klebsiella-Enterobacter*
group and *Pseudomonas aeruginosa* are the most commonly encountered
[11]. In their study of 36 cases of *Pseudomonas* pneumonia collected over
a 15-year period, Pennington *et al.* [22] demonstrated various underlying
neoplastic diseases, which included only one case of primary lung cancer
(oat cell). However, seven patients had tumor involvement of the upper
or lower respiratory tract. Most of the patients were leukopenic. The
mortality rate was high, reaching 81% [22], and immunoprophylaxis with
Pseudomonas vaccine seems to be effective [32]. Schimpf *et al.* [24, 25]
have emphasized the value of initial empiric therapy with carbenicillin and
gentamycin in febrile cancer patients, before culture results are available.

Bacteroides bacteremia was studied by Felner and Dowell [8] in a series
of 250 patients. Fifty-seven patients had a malignant neoplasm, and among
them three had bronchogenic carcinoma and died as a result of their infection.

B. Higher Bacteria

Nocardia asteroides is often responsible for fatal opportunistic infections. Out of the 13 cases with neoplasms and nocardiosis reported by
Young *et al.* [31], ten had hematopoietic malignancies and only three had
solid tumors. None of the patients had primary bronchogenic carcinoma.
However, these authors demonstrated the simultaneous occurrence of pul-

monary nocardiosis and tumor involvement of the lung. Diagnosis is difficult since this organism may break into fragments on sputum smears, thus
losing its characteristic structure; furthermore, it grows slowly in culture
[2].

Actinomycosis has not been shown to occur with an abnormally high
incidence in patients with neoplastic disease [2].

Tuberculosis, on the other hand, is frequently associated with cancer. Its
incidence in patients with lung cancer is reported to be between 7 and
30% [19]. This association has been discussed in Chapter 1. The disease
may be fulminant in such patients [2], with a course comparable to miliary
tuberculosis [21]. In some cases diagnosis may be difficult. Skin reactivity
to tuberculin may be suppressed because of immune deficiency related to
the underlying malignant disease [2]. Bone marrow or liver biopsy and
culture are often helpful.

C. Fungi

Candidiasis is a common fungal infection and over 90% of cancer
patients with disseminated candidiasis are on both cytotoxic drugs and
steroids [2].

Cryptococcal infection occurs most commonly in patients with leukemias
and lymphomas [2].

Invasive aspergillosis was reported in one case of lung cancer out of a
total of 93 cases encountered at the Memorial Sloan Kettering Cancer
Center [20]. Commonly associated infections were due to *Candida* species
and *Pseudomonas*. In patients with solid tumors, aspergillosis occurred
after treatment with steroids, cytotoxic therapy, or in the presence of
leukopenia. A negative serum precipitin reaction does not rule out the
diagnosis [20].

D. Viruses

Herpes simplex, herpes zoster, and cytomegalovirus are the three main
species responsible for viral infections in patients with neoplastic disease.
A fatal case of herpetic pneumonia was reported in a patient with bronchogenic oat cell carcinoma [6]. The prevalence of this disease is perhaps
not as rare as the relatively few cases in the literature would tend to indicate. Indeed, the disease usually goes undetected by both clinician and
pathologist [6]. Herpes zoster occurs in about 1.8% of patients with solid
tumors [26]. Certain factors are associated with a higher incidence of this
infection. These include tumor involvement of the central nervous system,
recent radiation therapy to nodal areas, and unresponsiveness to the
dinitrochlorobenzene (DNCB) skin test.

E. Parasites

Toxoplasmosis may give rise to abscess formation in various organs, including the brain [2].

Pneumocystis carinii is a well-known opportunistic organism and has been extensively studied in leukemias, lymphomas, and in patients with kidney transplant. Its incidence in lung cancer is unknown. No cases of underlying lung cancer were encountered in the 75 cases of *Pneumocystis carinii* pneumonia reported by Western *et al.* [30] nor in the 194 cases collected by Walzer *et al.* [29] in the United States. Among these cases, the authors found only seven patients with solid tumors: breast, 3; ovary, 1; bladder, 1; teratoma, 1; neuroblastoma, 1 [29].

III. CONCLUSION

In conclusion, the aim of this article is not to make an exhaustive review of nonspecific causes of death in patients with lung cancer but simply to draw attention to the numerous complications that threaten the patient with lung cancer and which should be detected by an alert physician. There is still a considerable lack of epidemiologic data, particularly concerning the exact type and incidence of the various infections.

Curative therapy, or even prevention, of these life-threatening nonspecific complications should improve the patients' comfort and prolong survival significantly.

REFERENCES

1. Amromin, G. D., and Wang, S. K., Degenerative verrucal endocardiosis and myocardial infarction. Report of two cases associated with mucus-producing bronchogenic carcinoma. *Ann. Intern. Med.* **50,** 1519 (1959).
2. Armstrong, D., Young, L. S., Meyer, R. D., and Blevins, A. H., Infectious complications of neoplastic disease. *Med. Clin. N. Amer.* **55,** 729 (1971).
3. Bariéty, M., Delarue, J., Paillas, J., and Rullière, R., "Les Carcinomes Bronchiques Primitifs." Masson, Paris, 1967.
4. Boggs, D. R., and Frei, E., III, Clinical studies of fever and infection in cancer. *Cancer* **13,** 1240 (1960).
5. Byrd, R. B., Divertie, M. B., and Spittell, J. A., Jr., Bronchogenic carcinoma and thromboembolic disease. *J. Amer. Med. Ass.* **202,** 1019 (1967).
6. Case Records of the Massachusetts General Hospital (Case 28-1973). *N. Engl. J. Med.* **289,** 91 (1973).
7. De Vita, V. T., and Young, R. C., Infection and cancer: Old friends. *Ann. Intern. Med.* **79,** 597 (1973).

8. Felner, J. M., Dowell, V. R., Jr., *"Bacteroides"* bacteremia. *Amer. J. Med.* **50,** 787 (1971).

9. Greenberg, E., Divertie, M. B., and Woolner, L. B., A review of unusual systemic manifestations associated with carcinoma. *Amer. J. Med.* **36,** 106 (1964).

10. Klainer, A. S., and Beisel, W. R., Opportunistic infection: A review. *Amer. J. Med. Sci.* **258,** 431 (1969).

11. Klastersky, J., Cappel, R., Debusscher, L., and Stilmant, M., Pneumonia caused by gram-negative bacilli in hospitalized patients presenting malignant disease. *Eur. J. Cancer* **7,** 329 (1971).

12. Klastersky, J., Daneau, D., and Verhest, A., Causes of death in patients with cancer. *Eur. J. Cancer* **8,** 149 (1972).

13. Klastersky, J., Weerts, D., Hensgens, C., and Debusscher, L., Fever of unexplained origin in patients with cancer. *Eur. J. Cancer* **9,** 649 (1973).

14. Knowles, J. H., and Smith, L. H., Extrapulmonary manifestations of bronchogenic carcinoma. *N. Engl. J. Med.* **262,** 505 (1960).

15. Levin, J., and Conley, C. L., Thrombocytosis associated with malignant disease. *Arch. Intern. Med.* **114,** 497 (1964).

16. Lieberman, J. S., Borrero, J., Urdaneta, E., and Wright, I. S., Thrombophlebitis and cancer. *J. Amer. Med. Ass.* **177,** 542 (1961).

17. Luomanen, R. K. J., and Watson, W. L., Autopsy findings. *In* "Lung Cancer. A Study of Five Thousand Memorial Hospital Cases" (W. L. Watson, ed.), pp. 504–510. Mosby, St. Louis, Missouri, 1968.

18. McDonald, R. A., and Robbins, S. L., The significance of nonbacterial thrombotic endocarditis. Autopsy and clinical study of 78 cases. *Ann. Intern. Med.* **46,** 255 (1957).

19. McQuarrie, D., Nicoloff, D. M., Van Nostrand, D., Rao, K., and Humphrey, E. W., Tuberculosis and carcinoma of the lung. *Dis. Chest* **54,** 427 (1968).

20. Meyer, R. D., Young, L. S., Armstrong, D., and Yu, B., Aspergillosis complicating neoplastic disease. *Amer. J. Med.* **54,** 6 (1973).

21. Neff, T., Ashbaugh, D., and Petty, T., Miliary tuberculosis and carcinoma of the lung. Successful treatment with chemotherapy and resection. *Amer. Rev. Resp. Dis.* **105,** 111 (1972).

22. Pennington, J., Reynolds, H. Y., and Carbone, P. P., *Pseudomonas* pneumonia: A retrospective study of 36 cases. *Amer. J. Med.* **55,** 155 (1973).

23. Rosen, P., and Armstrong, D., Nonbacterial thrombotic endocarditis in patients with malignant neoplastic diseases. *Amer. J. Med.* **54,** 23 (1973).

24. Schimpff, S. C., Greene, W. H., Young, V. M., and Wiernik, P. H., *Pseudomonas* septicemia: Incidence, epidemiology, prevention and therapy in patients with advanced cancer. *Eur. J. Cancer* **9,** 449 (1973).

25. Schimpff, S. C., Satterlee, W., Young, V. M., and Serpick, A., Empiric therapy with carbenicillin and gentamicin for febrile patients with cancer and granulocytopenia. *N. Engl. J. Med.* **284,** 1061 (1971).

26. Schimpff, S. C., Serpick, A., Stoler, B., Rumack, B., Mellin, H., Joseph, J. M., and Block, J., Varicella-zoster infection in patients with cancer. *Ann. Intern. Med.* **76,** 241 (1972).

27. Sproul, E. E., Carcinoma and venous thrombosis: The frequency of association of carcinoma in the body and tail of the pancreas with multiple venous thrombosis. *Amer. J. Cancer* **34,** 566 (1938).

28. Trousseau, A., "Clinique Médicale de l'Hôtel-Dieu de Paris," 5th ed., Vol. 3, p. 94. Baillière et fils, Paris, 1877.
29. Walzer, P. D., Perl, D. P., Krogstad, D. J., Rawson, P. G., and Schultz, M. G., *Pneumocystis carinii* pneumonia in the United States. Epidemiologic, diagnostic, and clinical features. *Ann. Intern. Med.* **80,** 83 (1974).
30. Western, K. A., Perera, D. R., and Schultz, M. G., Pentamidine isethionate in the treatment of *Pneumocystis carinii* pneumonia. *Ann. Intern. Med.* **73,** 695 (1970).
31. Young, L. S., Armstrong, D., Blevins, A., and Lieberman, P., *Nodardia asteroides* infection complicating neoplastic disease. *Amer. J. Med.* **50,** 356 (1971).
32. Young, L. S., Meyer, R. D., and Armstrong, D., *Pseudomonas aeruginosa* vaccine in cancer patients. *Ann. Intern. Med.* **79,** 518 (1973).

Chapter 9

The Logical Basis of Radiation Treatment Policies in the Multidisciplinary Approach to Lung Cancer

Philip Rubin, Carlos A. Perez, and Bowen Keller

The major strategy for the treatment of lung cancer is a multidisciplinary approach. Rather than emphasize the inability of each method to cure, or analyze the insignificant differences in survival rates with changes in each modality, the time has come to recognize that each form of treatment is limited but not ineffective. Therefore, the reorganization of treatment for lung cancer should be based upon a combined modalities approach with each method utilized and timed for optimal effectiveness. A form of total treatment by the various disciplines for each stage of this disease should replace the hierarchical approach of first the surgeon, then the radiotherapist, and lastly the chemotherapist. The initial management decision is the most important and should be be made cooperatively.

Lung cancer is not one disease. It is conditioned by the large number of histopathologic possibilities that exist both in tumor type and in tumor grade. This pathologic diagnosis indicates tumor behavior, invasiveness, and aggressiveness for the oncologist. The next step is to determine the extent of overt disease with sampling of potential metastatic sites for microspread. An assessment of the host's pulmonary function and general state of health is critical. The essential first step in interdisciplinary decision making is the classification of the cancer into specific target groups. Each target group needs to be individualized as to treatment. To individualize treatment is to begin the optimization of treatment in a combined modalities approach.

I. DEFINING THE TARGET GROUP

A. TNM Categories: Anatomic Extent

One of the most important achievements in lung cancer has been the categorization of patients by all disciplines into an acceptable classification. The TNM classification developed by Mountain and Carr and issued by the AJCCS [3, 13, 40] deserves widespread acceptance and utilization (see Table I). The primary tumor is characterized by its size and its confinement to the bronchi or lung of origin. Refinements, such as location, geographic position, associated atelectasis, and pneumonitis, are of lesser importance in the definition of T1 and T2. The essential criterion for advancement is extension beyond the confines of the lung of origin, i.e., pleural invasion or effusions, invasion of adjacent mediastinal structures, chest wall invasion. Bone destruction and nerve involvement alter the prognosis significantly, rendering the cancer a T4. T3 has many subcategories for investigational purposes. The utilization of decimal points to

TABLE I

The Definitions of T, N, and M Categories for Carcinoma of the Lung[a, b]

T Primary Tumors

T0   No evidence of primary tumor

TX   Tumor proven by the presence of malignant cells in bronchopulmonary se-
     cretions but not visualized roentgenographically or bronchoscopically

T1   A tumor that is 3.0 cm or less in greatest diameter, surrounded by lung or
     visceral pleura and without evidence of invasion proximal to a lobar
     bronchus at bronchoscopy

T2   A tumor more than 3.0 cm in greatest diameter, or a tumor of any size
     which, with its associated atelectasis or obstructive pneumonitis, extends
     to the hilar region. At bronchoscopy the proximal extent of demonstrable
     tumor must be at least 2.0 cm distal to the carina. Any associated atelec-
     tasis or obstructive pneumonitis must involve less than an entire lung, and
     there must be no pleural effusion

T3   A tumor of any size with direct extension into an adjacent structure such
     as the chest wall, the diaphragm, or the mediastinum and its contents; or
     demonstrable bronchoscopically to be less than 2.0 cm distal to the carina;
     any tumor associated with atelectasis or obstructive pneumonitis of an
     entire lung or pleural effusion

N Regional Lymph Nodes

N0   No demonstrable metastasis to regional lymph nodes

N1   Metastasis to lymph nodes in the ipsilateral hilar region (including direct
     extension)

N2   Metastasis to lymph nodes in the mediastinum

M Distant Metastasis

M0   No distant metastasis

M1   Distant metastasis, such as in scalene, cervical, or contralateral hilar lymph
     nodes, brain, bones, lung, liver, etc.

---

[a] Each case must be assigned the highest category of T, N, and M which describes
the full extent of disease in that case.
[b] From Ref. [3].

further categorize and individualize subcategories has been advanced by
those oncologists engaged in developing cooperative protocols [40].

The modification of T categories offered by Rubin [52] is designed to
split the advanced group into those in which local control by irradiation is
a possibility from those in which the disease is extremely advanced and
palliation is the only goal. This is translated into therapeutic approaches on
the investigational level. The division into T3 and T4 categories rests upon
the advanced intrathoracic, intrapulmonary disease characterized by invasion of pleura and the extension into adjacent structures, fixing but not
deeply invading vital viscera, nerves, and organs. The invasion and destruc-

TABLE II

Modifications of T Categories as Proposed by Radiation Therapy Groups at Lung Cancer Working Party

T3	(Extrapulmonary limited and intrathoracic): This group includes primary lesions which invade through the visceral pleura and are adherent to the parietal pleura. Localized bronchogenic cancers within 2 cm of the carina are essentially extrapulmonary. There is no evidence of visceral, vascular neurologic, osseous, or cardiac (including pericardial) invasion
T3.1	Primary lesion meeting above criteria and limited to one lobe including associated atelectasis and infiltration
T3.2	Primary lesion meeting above criteria and limited to two lobes
T3.3	Primary lesion meeting above criteria and limited to one main bronchus without atelectasis
T3.4	Primary lesion meeting above criteria with associated pleural effusion with negative cytology, indicating extensive mediastinal adenopathy and venous compression. This type of lesion is modified by virtue of nodal involvement and is not necessarily an advanced lesion
	It is important to recognize that thoracic exploration may be required to identify T3 lesions. Such categories as T3.1, T3.2, and T3.3 represent T1, T2, and T3 lesions clinically and radiographically assessed, which are beyond resection due to location or evidence of extrapulmonary invasion uncovered at the time of surgery
T4	(Extrapulmonary and/or extrathoracic): This group includes very extensive primary lesions invading into the nerves, major vessels, and cardiac and osseous sites. They are beyond the parietal pleura and are in the chest wall, viscera, and deep mediastinal structures
T4.1	Associated with total collapse of involved lung with and primary lesion
T4.2	Positive pleural effusion cytology with any primary lesion
T4.3	Superior vena caval obstruction with any primary lesion

tion of bone, nerves, pericardium and heart, and esophagus advance the lesion to T4 (see Table II).

The nodal categories are determined by hilar or mediastinal involvement. N1 is hilar involvement; N2 is mediastinal involvement but is most often characterized as superior mediastinal and subcarinal involvement. The scalene node is often located in the upper mediastinum but is considered with supraclavicular nodes. The contralateral nodes, diaphragmatic nodes, and supraclavicular nodes are considered beyond the scope of surgery but not beyond that of radiation by oncologists. Thus, a further categorization was made into N3 and N4, distinguishing regionally advanced nodes from those more distant nodes, such as those which are mid- and high cervical, coeliac, and axillary in location (see Table III).

Metastases are a poorly subcategorized group that in most classifications is neglected. Clustering or segregating specific metastatic sites is important for the development of treatment policies as will be demonstrated in this

TABLE III

Nodal Categories as Proposed by Radiation Therapy Groups at Lung Cancer Working Party

N0	No demonstrable spread to lymph nodes
N1	Ipsilateral hilar nodes
N2.1	Subcarinal (ipsilateral) and lower mediastinal (ipsilateral) involvement
N2.2	High mediastinal involvement
N2.3	Contralateral, hilar, and mediastinal nodes
N2.4	Posterior mediastinal nodes and diaphragmatic and pericardial involvement
N3	Supraclavicular nodes and scalene nodes

report. The frequency of a site or viscera becoming the first relapse of disease demands the appropriate sharpness of definition. The ability to eradicate occult or solitary metastases by present modalities is the requisite for this detailing. Finally, there is the need to cluster the TNM categories, since each component is critical to outcome. The stage grouping is the basis for the determination of treatment policy and outcome (see Table IV).

B. Histopathologic Categories

The lack of uniformity in lung cancer histopathologic nomenclature has been recently reviewed by Sobin (Table V). However, the most widely utilized classification of lung cancer according to histopathologic types is the WHO listing [60] (see Table VI). This large list of tumors can be reduced to four major types: epidermoid cancer, adenocarcinomas, large cell anaplastic cancer, and small cell anaplastic cancer with the remainder clustered into a miscellaneous group. As noted in Table VI, the other tumor types are benign and are statistically insignificant in survival outcome

TABLE IV

Metastatic Categories as Proposed by Radiation Therapy Groups at Lung Cancer Working Party

M (Distant metastasis)	
M1	Solitary, isolated metastasis confined to one organ or to one anatomic site
M2	Multiple metastatic foci confined to one organ system or one anatomic site (ie, lungs, skeleton, liver, etc.) resulting in minimal or no functional impairment
M3	Multiple organs involved anatomically resulting in minimal to moderate or no functional impairment
M4	Multiple organs involved anatomically resulting in moderate to severe functional impairment

TABLE V

Categories Enumerated in Classifications Used for Studies on Carcinoma of the Lung

Series[a]	Epidermoid squamous	Small cell	Bronchogenic adenocarcinoma	Adenocarcinoma	Alveolar	Large cell	Undifferentiated anaplastic	Others	Number of therapy studies	Number of other studies	% total studies
1	+			+			+		10	5	24
2	+	+	+		+	+			6	6	21
3	+	+	+		+		+		4	4	14
4	+	+		+			+		4	3	12
5	+	+		+		+			2	3	9
6	+		+		+		+		2	1	5
7	+	+	+		+				1	—	2
8	+	+		+					1	—	2
9	+			+			+	Simplex	—	1	2
10	+							+	1	—	2
11	+	+		+				polygonal	1	—	2
12	+	+	+			+		Cylindri-cal, solid	1	—	2
13	+	+	+			+	+	Clear cell	1	—	2
									34	23	100

[a] Specific references to this study are listed in Sobin's article [60].

reports. A typical plotting of histopathologic tumor type versus survival [3] is seen in Fig. 1; the order of survival, i.e., aggressiveness, is epidermoid cancer, adenocarcinoma, large cell anaplastic, and small cell anaplastic. This has been confirmed by numerous authors independent of treatment modality [57, 61, 67]. The relationships of tumor cellular type to the incidence of blood vessel invasion and lymph node metastases of cancer of the lung in resected specimens [61] follows the survival pattern noted previously according to Spjut *et al.* Epidermoid cancer and adenocarcinomas had similar degrees of involvement, but anaplastic tumors had a much greater degree of vascular invasion. Selawry's and Hansen's [57] thorough analysis of the world literature has shown that mediastinal node involvement at mediastinoscopy correlates better with survival according to histopathologic type than do scalene nodes. The incidence of metastases to liver, bone, and brain is clearly higher with small cell anaplastic tumors followed by large cell anaplastic and adenocarcinomas, and epidermoid cancer (Table VII).

TABLE VI

WHO Classification of Lung Cancer According to Histopathologic Types

I. Epidermoid carcinomas
II. Small cell anaplastic carcinomas
    1. Fusiform cell type
    2. Polygonal cell type
    3. Lymphocyte-like ("oat cell") type
    4. Others
III. Adenocarcinomas
    1. Bronchogenic
       a. Acinar
       b. Papillary
    2. Bronchioloalveolar
IV. Large cell carcinomas
    1. Solid tumors with mucinlike content
    2. Solid tumors without mucinlike content
    3. Giant cell carcinomas
    4. "Clear" cell carcinomas
V. Combined epidermoid and adenocarcinomas
VI. Carcinoid tumors
VII. Bronchial gland tumors
    1. Cylindromas
    2. Mucoepidermoid tumors
    3. Others
VIII. Papillary tumors of the surface epithelium
    1. Epidermoid
    2. Epidermoid with goblet cells
    3. Others
IX. "Mixed" tumors and carcinosarcomas
    1. "Mixed" tumors
    2. Carcinosarcomas of embryonal type ("blastomas")
    3. Other carcinosarcomas
X. Sarcomas
XI. Unclassified
XII. Mesotheliomas
    1. Localized
    2. Diffuse
XIII. Melanomas

II. TREATMENT POLICIES BASED UPON ANATOMIC–HISTOPATHOLOGIC CLASSIFICATION

A. Anatomically Defined Target Groups: TNM Groups for Treatment

General agreement as to TNM categories allows for the assignment of target groups for treatment. If the TNM classification is to be meaningful and useful, this fundamental criterion must be met. Table VIII presents the

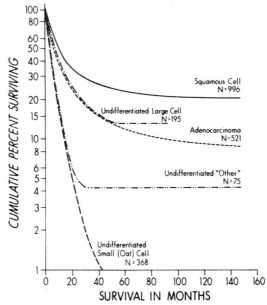

Fig. 1. Bronchogenic carcinoma survival by histologic type. N is number of cases. From Mountain *et al.* [40]. Courtesy of Charles C. Thomas, Publisher.

recommended treatment by stage grouping. For the resectable and operable group of lung cancers (T1 and T2), lobectomy or pneumonectomy, depending upon location and size of the lesion, is the standard procedure for achieving tumor ablation. When hilar nodes are negative, no further treatment is advised, but if these first station nodes are positive, mediastinal

TABLE VII
Incidence of Metastatic Involvement

	Post-surgical survival 5 years (%)	Incidence of metastatic involvement (%)				
		Mediastinal nodes	Scalene nodes	Hepatic	Osseous	Brain
Epidermoid	30	27	22.8	30	24	22
Large cell anaplastic	50	42.3	46.5	38	30	24
Adenocarcinoma	25	46.6	48.3	45	39.9	34
Small cell anaplastic	5	10.8	32	60	35	40

TABLE VIII

Recommended Treatment by Stage Grouping

Stage No.	TNM	Surgery	Target of radiation therapy	Chemotherapy
0	T0 N0 M0	Lobectomy when found	None	None
I	T1 N0 M0	Lobectomy if possible; pneumonectomy if necessary	None	None
I	T1 N1 M0	As above plus hilar node resection	Mediastinal nodes recommended (4500–5000 rad)	None
I	T2 N0 M0	As above	Mediastinal nodes optional	None
II	T2 N1 M0	Lobectomy/pneumonectomy plus hilar node resection	Mediastinal nodes recommended	None
III	T3,2, N0 M0	None but biopsy; resection of diaphragm and chest wall not advised	Definitive radiation therapy; 5000–6000 rad to T, plus mediastinal nodes (4000–5000 rad)	None
III	T1,2 N2 M0	Surgery optional	Definitive radiation therapy 5000–6000 rad to T, mediastinal and supraclavicular nodes (4500–5000 rad)	None
III	T3 N2 M1	None	As above	None
IV	T$_{any}$ N$_{any}$ M1	None	Palliative radiation therapy to T— 4000 rad/split course, 2000/week–2–3 rest–2000/week	None
IV	T$_{any}$ N$_{any}$ M1	None	Palliative to T, palliative to isolated metastases simultaneously	Cytoxan
	M to brain		Palliative 3000 rad/2 weeks (whole bone)	CCNU
	M to bone		Palliative 3000 rad/2 weeks (small field)	Cytoxan
	M to liver		Palliative 3000 rad/2 weeks	Cytoxan
Special problems			Rapid daily dose 400 × 3 = 1200 rad; then 150–5000 rad	None
Superior vena cava obstruction		None		
Pleural effusion			Radiocolloid ^{32}P—rarely	Intrapleural alkylating agent

irradiation is a logical supplemental treatment. Stages I and II are managed in a similar fashion except for adjuvant treatment.

For the advanced T3 lesion invading the pleura and/or pleural space, or nodal advancement into mediastinal stations (N2), radical surgery is not warranted and irradiation is the principal modality for tumor reduction. For a very extensive involved primary (T4) or remote nodes (N3), radiation therapy is palliative, as reflected in lower doses, concentrated fractionation and split course schedules. Although there is no specific chemotherapeutic agent that is most effective, Cytoxan is frequently recommended for most tumor types [56]. Protocols are available for study of 2 or 3 day schedules, but no combination has emerged as superior for a specific tumor type, either in combination with irradiation or alone.

Special problems requiring different dose schedules and management include superior vena caval obstruction and pleural effusion. A rapid high daily dose schedule of 400 rads per day for 3 days combined with diuresis utilizing Lasix or Diuril is adequate to control this emerging clinical problem. Intrapleural alkylating agents are preferred over radiocolloids for pleural effusions.

B. Histopathologic Basis of Treatment

1. SQUAMOUS CELL CARCINOMA

Despite the great technical advances in radiotherapy and the improved knowledge of the biology of lung cancer in the past 30 years, little improvement in the prognosis of the disease has been achieved.

a. Operable and Resectable Lesions. It is known that surgical procedures (lobectomy and pneumonectomy) yield 2-year survival rates in the range of 50% in patients with tumors localized to the primary site without nodal metastasis and 25% in patients with hilar node metastasis. Smart [40, 59] reported a 22% 5-year survival rate in a carefully selected group of 40 patients with early bronchogenic carcinoma who were treated to doses of 5000–5500 rads in 7 to 8 weeks for squamous cell carcinoma and 4900–5500 rads for anaplastic tumors. These results were comparable to those of reported surgical series. Morrison *et al.* [39] carried out a prospective randomized study of 58 patients who had bronchial carcinoma confined to the thorax without gross evidence of distant metastasis, and who were treated either by surgery or supervoltage irradiation (8 MeV X-rays). Of 20 patients with squamous cell tumors treated by surgery, 30% survived 4 years, whereas only 1 of 17 patients treated by radiation therapy (6%) survived as long. Patients with anaplastic lesions showed no significant difference in survival after either method of treatment. The dose given to patients treated by irradiation was only 4500 rads over 4 weeks, a dose that is considered inadequate for sterilization of squamous cell carcinoma.

b. *Unresectable Tumors.* Guttman [25] reported on a group of 103 patients with tumors found to be unresectable at operation; they were subsequently treated to the entire involved lung and adjacent mediastinum with 4 MeV X-rays to 5000 rads tumor dose over 5 weeks. Fifty-seven and two-tenths percent of the patients survived 1 year, 17.4% 3 years, and 8.7% more than 5 years. The average survival time of these patients was raised to 27 months, compared to 6 months in the untreated patients reported in the literature.

Roswit et al. [49] reported a slight improvement in survival at 1-year (22.2%) in a group of 308 patients treated with orthovoltage X-rays to doses in the range of 4000–5000 rads, compared with a group of 246 controls who were given an inert placebo (a 16% 1-year rate in survival).

2. OAT CELL CARCINOMA.

Miller et al. [38] reported on a group of 144 patients who had oat cell carcinoma of the lung and who were randomly treated by surgery (71 patients) or radical radiation therapy (73 patients). In 34 of the 71 patients treated by surgery, a pneumonectomy was performed. Radical radiation therapy was given to 62 of the 73 patients in that group. Three of the 73 irradiated patients survived 5 years (4%), as opposed to only 1 patient in the surgical group. This patient was inoperable and received palliative radiation therapy. He survived 60 months, at which time brain and rib metastases developed [22]. Metastasis was the most common cause of failure, being noted in 81% of the 71 surgical patients and 91% of the 73 irradiated patients.

No reliable information is available on the potential benefit of radiation therapy alone or in combination with chemotherapy to the prolongation of survival in patients with widespread tumor dissemination at the time of treatment.

3. OTHER HISTOLOGICAL TYPES

Even though some feel that adenocarcinoma and large cell anaplastic carcinoma are not particularly sensitive to radiation, others have reported no significant difference in radiation response or survival in these.

III. THE MEASUREMENT OF RESPONSE
TO IRRADIATION

A. Survival as a Measure

The measure of response to treatment has often been survival. The assumption that effective treatment means better survival is simplistic and an inadequate answer to the question of the ability of irradiation to control lung cancer. Several authors, among them Guttman [25], Rubenfeld [51], and Rubin et al. [53] have correlated higher tumor doses with better survival rates. Admittedly, a certain degree of selection exists in a number of these patients, the more favorable cases receiving the higher doses.

Roswit et al. [50] failed to observe a difference in survival in patients receiving doses over 5000 or 6000 rads as compared with others receiving lower doses. A poor survival was observed in patients receiving less than 4000 rads.

Of interest is the report by Deeley [18], describing better survival rates in a group of 51 patients receiving 3000 rads in 20 sessions over 4 weeks as compared to a group of 51 patients receiving 4000 rads with the same fractionation. The survival rate was 6% at 2 years in the 3000-rad group as opposed to no survival in the 4000-rad group. It was felt that this was probably due to a greater incidence of fibrosis in the patients treated with higher doses. There was no significant difference in the incidence of distant metastases or residual carcinoma in the chest in these two groups. The difference between a 6% versus a 0% survival suggests that neither dose level is adequate.

B. Tumor Sterilization as a Measure

If sterilization of the primary tumor and nodes is utilized as the criterion for response, irradiation can be shown to be more effective. Examination of surgical specimens has provided evidence of primary tumor sterilization of 30–54% at 5000–6000 rads level and nodal sterilization of 77% [9]. Despite the improvement in staging, no true gain in survival has been demonstrated with high dose preoperative irradiation. Some recent studies suggest it may have, in fact, reduced survival time. In a well-documented postmortem study, in which death was unrelated to therapy, Rissanen et al. [47] demonstrated tumor ablation in epidermoid cancer in 55%, adenocarcinoma in 50%, large cell anaplastic in 70%, and small cell cancer in 75% of patients.

C. Radiographic Measurements

The prediction of radiation response based upon histopathologic analysis is just beginning to be documented. The lack of data exists due to the inaccurate radiographic evaluation of tumor response and the small number of postmortem correlations. Radiographic analysis is difficult due to associated pneumonitis and atelectasis, which make the true margins of an infiltrative carcinoma often impossible to identify. The endobronchial aspect of the carcinoma is often not apparent on films, although tomograms may be helpful. A dramatic clearance of the pulmonary shadow may be due to the clearance of secondary pulmonary changes, i.e., atelectasis and pneumonitis. Nevertheless, some investigators have scored tumor resolution or response versus dose. The tumor regression has ranged from 54% at 4000 rads to 87% at 6500 rads. At the 5000-rad range frequently employed, the regressions have been reported to be 50% by Rubin [53], 30% by Hall [26], and 86% by Fernholtz and Muller [21]. The dose–response curve of Pereslegin [45] is most interesting in that dose levels from 3800–9500 rads were explored, yielding an optimum regression of 92% at 6500 rads. The "highest dose" survival rate is as poor as the "lowest dose" survival rate, producing a bell-shaped curve (Fig. 2). Although this "optimal" dose is beyond the level usually prescribed in the American literature, if tissue inhomogeneity was corrected, the dose of 5000 rads commonly chosen would be increased to 6000 rads due to increased pulmonary trans-

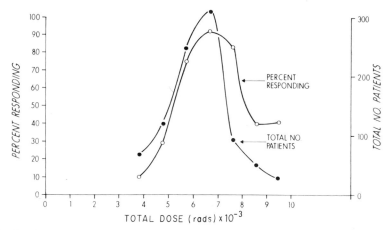

Fig. 2. The radiation responsiveness of lung cancer patients to irradiation. (On the left are the percent of responders, and on the right, the total number of patients. The open circles are the percent responding, and the solid circles, the total number of patients.) (Adapted from Pereslegin [45], with permission.)

mission of supervoltage irradiation. Also, grid techniques were utilized [45] revealing a lack of homogeneity in dose, and they account for the delivery of these higher doses.

Radiation response has been correlated with histology as seen in Carr and Child's [14] report: epidermoid 36%, adenocarcinoma 32%, and large cell anaplastic 25% in contrast to small cell anaplastic 82%. The exquisite radiation sensitivity of oat cell cancer is well recognized and has discouraged the use of survival as a measure of radiation response in lung cancer. This concept was challenged by Rubin [53] who showed that survival was related to response in different tumor types, although it was not a totally reliable prognosticator (Fig. 3). If less than 50% of the pulmonary shadow disappeared, then the chance of one-year survival was less than even, whereas greater than 50% pulmonary shadow clearance improved the survival odds to better than 50%.

The radiographic evaluation after irradiation is further complicated by the later development of radiation pneumonitis, fibrosis, and scarring. This further stresses the need for correlative radiographic and pathologic studies in order to assess and establish the criteria for tumor response and tumor control.

D. New Parameters

A correlated approach of radiography and an immunologic or chemical test for residual cancer would be an important development. Although carcinoembryonic antigen (CEA) is not specific for lung cancer, a test such as this could serve to measure response to treatment by lowering of the titer.

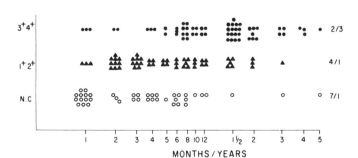

Fig. 3. Tumor regression. This graph represents the radiation responsiveness of patients treated for lung cancer. The scoring is 1+ to 4+ depending upon each 25% shadow disappearance on the film. (The numbers on the right relate to the ratio of nonsurvivors to survivors.)

Additional studies to ascertain local T and N control by histopathology would also be essential. Careful integration of all methods of analysis will be a significant aid to the prediction of treatment effectiveness. Such a CEA study is in progress in lung cancer patients in Radiation Therapy Oncology Group (RTOG) protocols [16].

IV. BEST TECHNIQUE OF RADIATION THERAPY IN LUNG CANCER

A. The Search for the Optimal Total Dose

If one utilizes the criterion of tumor sterilization, then the optimum dose level lies beyond 6000 rads if the aim is to achieve a sterilization rate of 95%. Bromley and Szur [11] demonstrated that localized lung cancer can be destroyed in about 40% of the cases with orthovoltage radiation at moderate dose levels (4700 rads average). Bloedorn et al. [9] reported that in a group of 26 patients receiving 6000 rads preoperatively in 6 weeks to the chest, careful study of multiple sections of operative specimens showed no recognizable tumor cells in the primary site in 54% of the patients or in the mediastinal lymph nodes in 92%. Survival rates were dose related, with a greater percentage of survivors beyond 1 year if doses above 5000 rads were given, according to Rubin et al. [53] (Fig. 4).

Rissanen et al. [47] analyzed 67 patients with histologically verified inoperable lung cancer. In 18 patients receiving tumor doses between 4800–6250 rads over 5 to 10 weeks, no carcinoma was demonstrated in the treated area. In contrast, 26 patients showing clearly viable carcinoma in the treated area had received doses in the range of 2000–3000 rads. In another study, 24 preoperatively irradiated patients with cancer of the lung were treated to tumor doses of 5500–6000 rads in $5\frac{1}{2}$ to 6 weeks and were

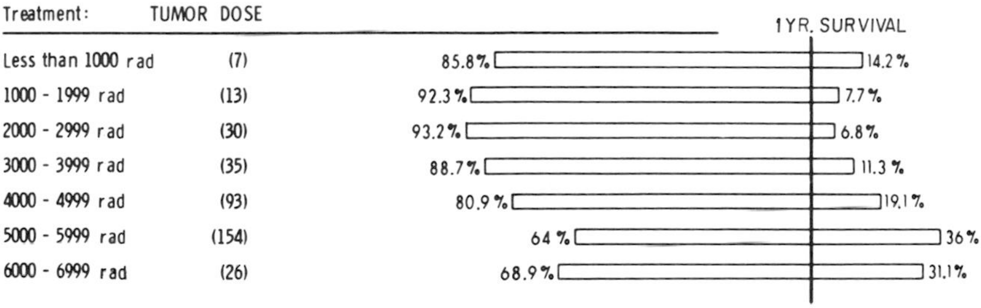

Treatment:	TUMOR DOSE		1YR. SURVIVAL
Less than 1000 rad	(7)	85.8%	14.2%
1000 - 1999 rad	(13)	92.3%	7.7%
2000 - 2999 rad	(30)	93.2%	6.8%
3000 - 3999 rad	(35)	88.7%	11.3%
4000 - 4999 rad	(93)	80.9%	19.1%
5000 - 5999 rad	(154)	64%	36%
6000 - 6999 rad	(26)	68.9%	31.1%

Fig. 4. Survival rates seen in relation to dose. A greater percentage of survivors beyond 1 year is seen in the group receiving doses above 5000 rads. Numbers in parentheses are number of cases.

operated on 4 to 8 weeks later [47]. Seven patients showed no evidence of any residual primary and of 15 patients with preoperative radiographic evidence of hilar or mediastinal adenopathy, only three showed residual tumor on microscopic sections.

B. The Optimal Fractionation Schedule

Most of the patients with bronchogenic carcinoma have been irradiated with continuous courses of therapy. A few authors have explored the potential of split course radiation therapy. This type of radiation would allow for increased reduction of tumor mass, improved vascularization, better repair of normal tissues, and reoxygenation of initially hypoxic tumor cells [54]. Interrupted or split schedules offer advantages in assessing the combination of chemotherapy with radiation therapy.

Levitt et al. [34] reported no difference in symptomatic relief or survival between two groups of patients randomly treated, one (15 patients) with a split course consisting of three doses of 600 rads tumor dose delivered in three consecutive days and repeated 28 days later, and the other (14 patients) receiving daily fractionated radiation to a dose of 6000 rads given over 6 to 8 weeks. Dutreix [19] reported satisfactory palliative results with a regime consisting of two doses of 1650 rads given in 48 hours followed by 3 weeks rest and then nine fractions of 300 rads given three times weekly. Deeley [18] conducted a comparative trial of twice weekly irradiation, giving a total of 2400 rads in 28 days (8 fractions of 300 rads) for anaplastic tumors, 3200 rads in 28 days (8 fractions at 400 rads) for squamous cell carcinoma, 3000 rads in 28 days for anaplastic tumors and 4000 rads in 28 days for squamous cell carcinoma in five fractions per week. No difference in survival, morbidity, or metastatic spread was found in preliminary analysis at 2 years.

On the other hand, Abramson and Cavanaugh [1,2] reported a significantly better survival rate (43% at 1 year) in a group of patients treated with 2000 rads tumor dose in five fractions over 1 week followed by 3 weeks rest and 2000 rads given in a similar fashion, compared with a 14% 1 year survival in a control group receiving 6000 rads in 6 weeks, five fractions per week (Fig. 5). Holsti and Vuorinen [31] employed split course therapy, delivering 5000–6000 rads in 5 to 6 weeks in a continuous course, six fractions per week and split course irradiation giving 5–10% more dosage with an additional 2 to 3 weeks overall time interposed between the fractions. The survival rates were slightly higher at 6 months than at 1 and 2 years for the patients treated with split course therapy (70, 35, and 10%, respectively), in contrast with the patients treated by continuous irradiation (54, 33, and 4%, respectively).

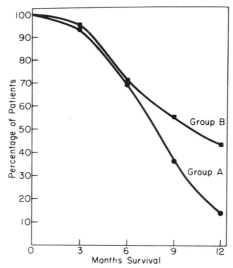

Fig. 5. Survival rates seen in relation to fractionation schedule. The control group A received 6000 rads in 6 weeks, five fractions per week. Group B received 2000 rads in five fractions the first week, rested for 3 weeks, and then received 2000 rads in a similar fashion. (From Abramson and Cavanaugh [1], reproduced with permission.)

Rissanen *et al.* [48] described a higher incidence of tumor sterilization in a group of 38 patients on whom autopsies were performed following megavoltage split course irradiation. Fourteen out of the 38 patients (37%) treated with this regime had complete microscopic destruction of the tumor, whereas only four of 29 patients treated by continuous irradiation (14%) showed no tumor in the treated area. The incidence of distant metastasis in the split course group was 76% in contrast to the 93% in the continuous group.

C. The Optimal Treatment Plan

Radiation therapy remains the mainstay for palliation of patients with limited disease, about 75% of the patients show significant tumor regression with doses over 4000 rads. In some series, the treated patients survived about 25% longer than the treated controls [49].

Rubin *et al.* [53], in an analysis of the controversial status of the management of lung cancer, pointed out that there is an obsession about the length of survival when the results in the treatment of bronchogenic carcinoma are analyzed rather than an assessment of local control of thoracic disease or the quality of survival.

As was stated previously, there are conflicting reports in the literature as to whether irradiation prolongs the survival of patients with lung cancer whether they are treated for cure or palliation. Randomized studies, such as the one reported by Roswit *et al.* [49] (radiation alone) and Krant *et al.* [32] (radiation and nitrogen mustard compared with radiation or mustard alone) [33] have shown no improvement in survival. When skillfully administered, radiation therapy may be quite effective in palliating distressing symptoms in these patients, but whether this prolongs their useful life or not remains to be determined.

1. PORTALS OF IRRADIATION

There are no definite criteria regarding the volume to be irradiated in carcinoma of the lung because of the poor survival results. However, an analysis of the patterns of spread of the tumors indicates that in a curative plan, the regional lymph nodes should be irradiated. So, depending on whether the lesions are in the upper, middle, or lower lobes, different volumes of the hilar and mediastinum should be treated (Fig. 6). The portal arrangements apply to both adenocarcinoma and squamous cell carcinoma where they are well or poorly differentiated. Furthermore, if the lesions are located in the upper lobes, regardless of the histology, and as in oat cell carcinoma, probably regardless of its anatomical location, the inclusion of the supraclavicular nodes in the irradiated field is a reasonable step (Fig. 7). The validity of this practice is difficult to analyze in the light of our present knowledge. Oat cell cancer may include generous fields for primary and regional nodes, as well as elective fields for suspected metastasis (see Fig. 16).

When using supervoltage energies to treat patients palliatively, usually opposing AP and PA ports are adequate to deliver 4000–5000 rads midplane to the tumor. In order to decrease the dose to the spinal cord to below 4000 rads in 4 weeks, 20 fractions, and an unequal loading, favoring the anterior port (2:1 or 3:1) may be used. However, when using medium range megavoltage (1 to 4 MeV), the treatment planning should be carefully executed to prevent delivering doses of over 5000 rads to the entire heart, since this increases the incidence of pericarditis and heart damage [62].

When higher doses are indicated, as in curative cases, more complicated portal arrangements are required, using either oblique ports to avoid the spinal cord or, when anatomically feasible, rotational therapy. In these instances, it is crucial to avoid delivering more than 2000 rads to large volumes of normal lung, since this will cause undesirable physiological pulmonary complications.

SQUAMOUS CELL CANCER AND UNDIFFERENTIATED

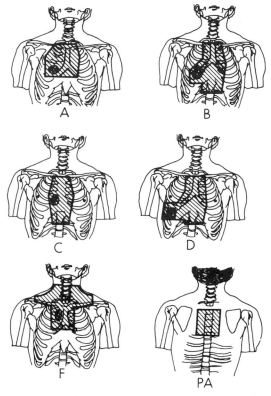

AP-PA (Except F- Supraclavicular Port)

(MIRROR IMAGE FOR TUMORS IN LEFT LUNG)

Fig. 6. Portal arrangements. Spread pattern of tumor and site of lesion for squamous cell carcinoma and adenocarcinoma, both well and poorly differentiated varieties. A, B, C, D, and F are portal arrangements. PA, posteroanterior.

2. TOLERANCE OF NORMAL STRUCTURES TO MAXIMUM DOSES

The thorax is occupied by a significant number of viscera wtih rather limited tolerance to ionizing radiation. The following is a suggested maximum limit of doses to be administered to these organs:

Ipsilateral normal lung: no more than 4000 rads, unless involved by tumor

Contralateral normal lung: no irradiation, unless absolutely unavoidable. In this case, 2000 rads T.D. (tumor dose) maximum. Radiation

APICAL   TUMORS

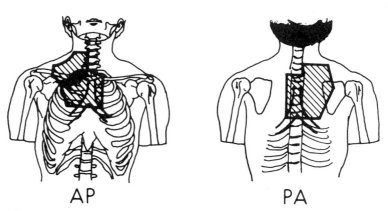

AP   PA

Fig. 7. Portal arrangements. When lesions are located in the upper lobes, inclusion of the supraclavicular nodes in the irradiated field is reasonable, regardless of histologic type and/or anatomical location.

pneumonitis and subsequent fibrosis of the lung will occur in all patients receiving 4500 rads to the lung, usually within 3 to 6 months after initiation of treatment

Entire heart: 4500 rads T. D., 5 weeks maximum. Less than 50% of the heart may receive 5500 rads maximum in 6 weeks

Spinal cord: 4500 rads T. D., 5 weeks maximum; 2500 rads T. D. with split radiation regime.

Esophagus: 5500 T. D. 5 weeks maximum.

Reversible alopecia, skin pigmentation, and esophagitis are expected side effects of radiotherapy. Radiation induced pericarditis and myocarditis or transverse myelitis rarely occur at dosages lower than 5500 rads.

Radiotherapy shoud be continued in the presence of moderate induced hematologic toxicity, but discontinued when WBC falls to 2000/mm^3 and/ or platelets fall to 60,000/mm^3, until hematologic recovery above these levels takes place.

Of course, the above doses must be modified whenever chemotherapeutic agents are administered because of the additive or synergistic effect they may have with irradiation.

3. DOSIMETRY TREATMENT PLAN GUIDELINES

The following information was compiled in an attempt to provide examples of minimum acceptable treatment planning for the Radiation Therapy Oncology Group (RTOG) Lung Cancer Protocols. These suggestions are made to indicate how mediastinal nodes, as well as the primary target volume, might be treated without exceeding dose tolerance to the spinal cord, heart, and contralateral lung. There are acceptable alternate plans, and the plans offered here should not be considered definitive in every case.

Isodose distributions at the midplane of the tumor shall be submitted. (For the purpose of calculating this distribution, it can be assumed that the central axis is the midplane of the tumor) (Fig. 8).

In addition to this distribution, calculation of the dose to two specific points is recommended.

    a. The spinal cord dose 1 cm below the superior margin of field should be calculated.

    b. When the supraclavicular nodes are treated, the dose at a 3 cm depth from the anterior field at the site of these nodes should be calculated

Calculations at these points should be corrected for

    a. Beam unflatness at distances from the central axis

    b. Changes in source surface distance (SSD) due to surface curvature of the patient. If tissue compensation is not used, spinal cord tolerance at the superior margin of the field may be the limiting factor. Therefore, it is recommended that tissue compensation be utilized where large increases in SSD occur

4. TREATMENT PLANNING

The treatment plans listed below are all for ^{60}Co teletherapy. Only cobalt distributions are presented because the general principles can be demonstrated with the use of one energy. Cobalt represents a fairly common denominator in radiation therapy, and if the distribution is acceptable with cobalt, the same beam arrangements at higher photon energies generally will produce better results.

From the point of view of the sample treatment plans, 5000 rads to the target volume was chosen. The relative percentage isodose values are also included as these treatment plans can be used for other lung protocols.

Following the treatment plans, an example of the dosage calculation for one of the two aforementioned points is included. There are acceptable alternate methods of calculation, and the method used here should not be considered the only one.

a. Parallel-Opposed Fields (Fig. 9). This plan without a spinal cord block is *unacceptable*. In order to reach the doses prescribed for the mediastinal nodes, the spinal cord will receive a dose in excess of 4500 rads. This criticism appears to be valid for photon energies up to 25 MV.

b. Parallel-Opposed Fields with Spinal Cord Block (Fig. 10). Parallel-

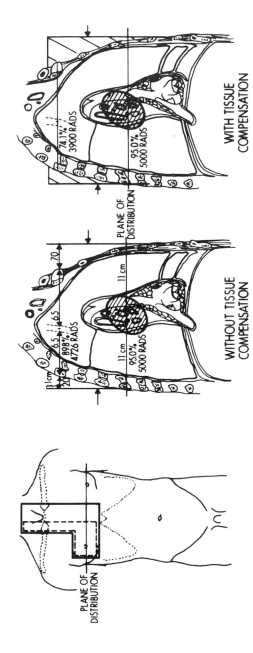

Fig. 8. Cobalt-60 teletherapy, dosage calculations in a posterior field, with and without tissue compensations. The former is preferred. Due to variations in normal lung volume, no attempt is made to calculate for tissue inhomogeneity.

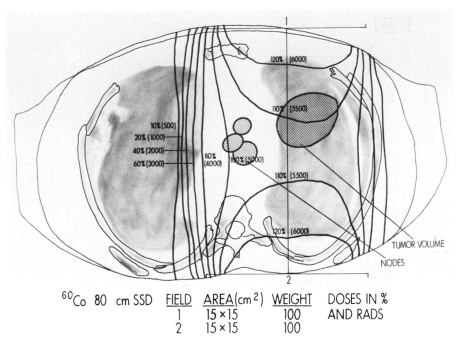

^{60}Co 80 cm SSD

FIELD	AREA(cm^2)	WEIGHT	DOSES IN %
1	15×15	100	AND RADS
2	15×15	100	

Fig. 9. Cobalt-60 teletherapy, parallel-opposed field without a spinal cord block is found *unacceptable*.

opposed fields with a spinal cord block or reduced posterior field or a beam wedge, are considered to be acceptable. The dose to the mediastinal nodes is not entirely homogeneous, but is considered to be adequate. The dose to the heart and contralateral lung is acceptable. Care must be taken when using this technique to adequately shield the spinal cord, when using the block or wedged field.

   c. Anterior field with a Posterior Oblique Wedged Field (Fig. 11). An anterior field with a posterior oblique wedge field (biased 1 : 1.2) is an acceptable arrangement for treating the primary target volume and nodes without overdosing the heart or contralateral lung. A slightly higher dose is delivered to the contralateral lung with improved dose homogeneity in the mediastinal nodes. There may be difficulty in determining the proper placement of the oblique field, especially with beam shaping.

   d. Parallel-Opposed Fields with Posterior Oblique Boost (Fig. 12). Parallel-opposed fields with a posterior oblique boost is an acceptable arrangement. The posterior oblique field is essentially a booster field and will be used just to include the target volume without beam shaping. Similar arrangements are shown for 4 MeV and 22 MeV X-rays and illustrate the

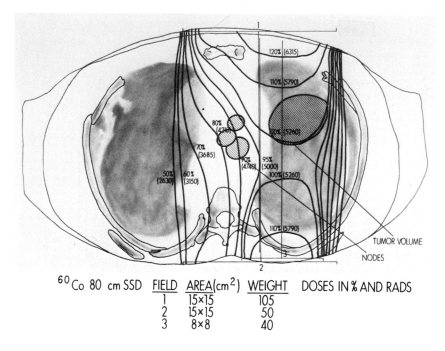

^{60}Co 80 cm SSD

FIELD	AREA(cm²)	WEIGHT	DOSES IN % AND RADS
1	15×15	105	
2	15×15	50	
3	8×8	40	

Fig. 10. Cobalt-60 teletherapy, parallel-opposed field with a spinal cord block.

improvement in dose homogeneity in target tumor volume. (Figs. 13 and 14).

e. Sample Dosage Calculation.   The dosage calculation refers to the parallel-opposed field arrangement with a spinal cord block or reduced posterior field (Fig. 10). Dosage calculations are done with and without tissue compensating filters (Figs. 8 and 15). (See Appendix for dose calculations [39].)

D. Complications of Irradiation

It is well known that fractionated doses of radiation over 2500 rads may produce permanent damage to the alveolar endothelium and interstitial fibrosis of the lung parenchyma [8]. It must be remembered that a large proportion of these patients are chronic smokers with chronic obstructive lung disease [10, 23]. Germon and Brady [23] studied a group of 30 patients with bronchogenic carcinoma receiving doses in the range of 6000 rads in 5 to 6 weeks. Prior to treatment, the pulmonary function tests showed some abnormality in all of the patients, most of them having some

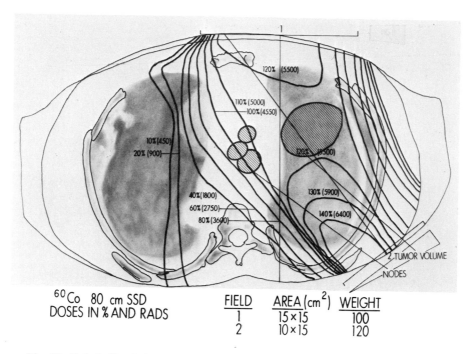

^{60}Co 80 cm SSD
DOSES IN % AND RADS

FIELD	AREA (cm^2)	WEIGHT
1	15 × 15	100
2	10 × 15	120

Fig. 11. Cobalt-60 teletherapy, anterior field with a posterior oblique wedged field.

degree of obstructive lung disease, increased residual volumes greater than 40% of the total lung capacity, abnormal distribution of alveolar ventilation, and reduced diffusing capacity of CO_2. Severe respiratory disability attributable to radiation pneumonitis and fibrosis did not develop in any of the patients. Decreased vital capacity and diffusing capacity were observed after irradiation as well as significant alterations in pulmonary arterial perfusion. These were demonstrated prior to therapy in areas larger than those suspected radiographically, but the greater impairment was noted after irradiation, probably due to capillary damage.

Teates and Cooper [64] reported on 16 patients followed up to 40 months after thoracic irradiation. Twenty-five percent showed definite evidence of ventilatory function reduction and 50% radiographic findings consistent with radiation effects in the lung.

Since these sequelae must be accepted after radical irradiation of the lung, it is imperative to establish definitely that the benefits of irradiation will outweigh the undesirable effects on an already impaired pulmonary function.

The effects of irradiation of the thoracic viscera can be considered as acute–transient, of minor clinical significance, and unavoidable, although

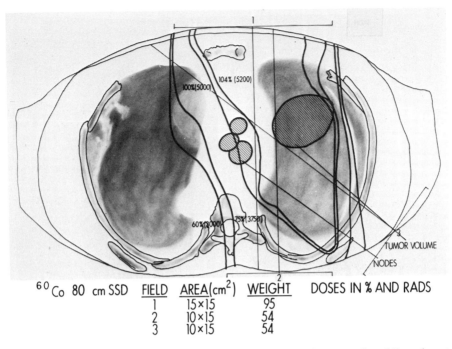

Fig. 12. Cobalt-60 teletherapy, parallel-opposed field with a posterior oblique boost field.

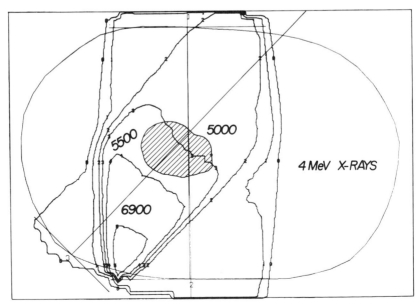

Fig. 13. Same arrangement as ⁶⁰Co teletherapy in Fig. 12 (parallel-opposed field with a posterior oblique boost) shown instead for 4 MeV X-rays.

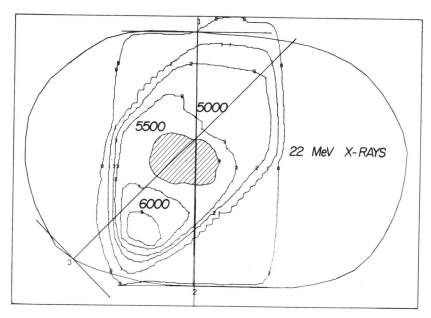

Fig. 14. Same arrangement as ^{60}Co teletherapy in Fig. 12, shown instead for 22 MeV X-rays.

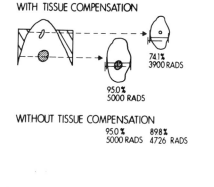

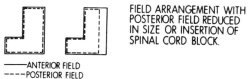

Fig. 15. Dosage calculations with and without tissue compensations.

the symptomatology can be diminished by appropriate supportive measures. Later major complications, that should be avoided by all means with accurate treatment planning and impeccable treatment techniques, are permanent and if sufficient lung volume is irradiated are of major clinical significance.

Sore throat, difficulty swallowing, and even some erythematous changes of the skin are not uncommon. This can be managed with appropriate diets, analgesics, and topical lubrication of the skin. Nausea and, at times, vomiting are not rare, but they can be prevented or decreased with phenotiazine compounds. Mild radiation pneumonitis may be manifested by dry cough, pleuritic chest pain, and clear expectoration. Fever may be noted, and if persistent, can be highly suggestive of superimposed viral or bacterial infection. In this case, bed rest, antibiotics (if positive cultures are found), and steroids may be indicated.

More clinically significant acute side effects include a more severe degree of pneumonitis, which is essentially treated as outlined above, or a serous pericarditis. The same therapeutic measures may be effective in this case. The spinal cord may give rise to some symptoms secondary to radiation characterized by a paresthesias of the trunk and extremeties and a sensation of electric shock with hyperflexion of the vertebral column (Lhermitte's syndrome). Usually, this is a transient phenomenon, not related to the subsequent development of more severe radiation myelopathy [36].

Doses above 2500 rads will produce clinical and radiographic evidence of pneumonitis, and 100% of the patients receiving higher doses will develop fibrosis of the irradiated pulmonary tissues with impairment of pulmonary function [7]. This sensitivity is increased when irradiation is associated with chemotherapeutic agents, such as actinomycin D. The subject has been thoroughly reviewed both experimentally and in clinical situations by Phillips and Margolis [46].

The occurrence of serous or fibrotic pericarditis has been reported following the administration of doses over 4500–5000 rads to varying volumes of the heart. Associated changes of the myocardium and endocardium have been described [62].

High doses of irradiation are known to produce mucosal atrophy and degeneration of the muscular layers of the esophagus. This has been reported with doses over 5000–6000 rads in 5–6 weeks.

Radiation myelopathy has been described in patients receiving greater than 4000 rads at the rate of 1000 rads per week or smaller fractions in shorter periods of time. It is felt that the degenerative demyelinization of the spinal cord is secondary to radiation injury of the small capillaries of this organ. The symptomatology is related to the segment of degenerative cord and is irreversible [36]. Necrosis of the chest wall (bone or soft tissues) has been rarely described with high doses of irradiation (over 6000 rads).

V. NEW STRATEGIES

A. Combined Modalities

The results of combination treatment have been relatively ineffective as measured by survival.

1. PREOPERATIVE IRRADIATION

Several randomized studies have been reported, evaluating the potential usefulness of preoperative irradiation in the treatment of cancer of the lung. None of the reports, except for those dealing with the rare apical lung cancer (Pancoast tumor) [44], have shown significant benefits in terms of survival or tumor control.

Paulson et al. [44] and Hilaris et al. [30] have observed 3- to 5-year survival rates in the range of 30% in selected groups of patients with apical tumors treated with moderate doses of preoperative irradiation (3500–4000 rads tumor dose in 3 to 4 weeks) followed by en bloc resection of the tumor.

2. POSTOPERATIVE IRRADIATION

This can be expected only to inhibit the growth of microscopic tumor deposits or residuum in the hilar and mediastinal nodes. However, it would not affect the already disseminated foci outside of these volumes, which may not be clinically apparent at the time of the operation.

Several studies with relatively small groups of patients have failed to show any significant improvement in survival in patients operated upon for bronchogenic carcinoma and irradiated postoperatively. Bangma [5] reported on a group of 73 patients randomly allocated after pneumonectomy to two groups, one receiving postoperative irradiation (36 patients) and the other group (37 patients) serving as control. A dose of 4300–4500 rads was given in approximately 5 weeks. The two groups did not significantly differ in their mortality rate or frequency of tumor metastases. A higher mortality within the first postoperative year was noted among the irradiated patients (six out of eight) than among the controls (one out of six). In neither the lobectomy nor the pneumonectomy group did postoperative irradiation influence the outcome of the patients. It was interesting, however, that of eight patients treated by lobectomy receiving postoperative irradiation, only two developed intrathoracic metastases, whereas six had extrathoracic tumor dissemination. In the nonirradiated control group, five patients developed intrathoracic metastases, and only one had extrathoracic tumor dissemination.

3. IRRADIATION AND CHEMOTHERAPY

Numerous prospective and nonrandomized studies have been carried out over the past 20 years to explore the potential benefits of chemotherapeutic agents in the treatment of bronchogenic carcinoma. Multiple studies with single agents, including nitrogen mustard, vinblastine, cyclophosphamide, actinomycin D, 5-fluorouracil, and hydroxyurea, have failed to show any significant improvement in survival of tumor control [12, 14, 15, 17, 24, 33, 56, 58, 63, 65, 66]. Bergsagel et al. [7] reported a slight prolongation of survival in a group of patients who received repeated doses of cyclophosphamide combined with irradiation, as compared with a control group of patients who were treated with irradiation alone.

Cell kinetic studies by thymidine labeling index in 12 patients with oat cell carcinoma showed that the labeling index was 16.7%, in comparison with a 2.5% for epidermoid carcinoma [41]. This indicates a high proliferation rate in oat cell carcinoma, which would make it more sensitive to phase or cycle specific chemotherapy agents or radiation therapy [55].

Multiple drug therapy has been shown to produce a maximum cell kill with the appropriate drugs, optimal schedule, and adequate duration of maintenance treatment. A combination of cyclophosphamide, CCNU, (cyclohexylchloroethyl nitrosourea), and methotrexate showed statistically significant superiority over other combinations of cyclophosphamide and methotrexate in patients with small cell carcinoma, when the groups were treated to equal toxicity [27].

Maurer et al. [37] and Eagen et al. [20] reported improved survival with the use of several combinations of chemotherapeutic schedules in the treatment of small cell carcinoma of the lung, combined with 3300 rads tumor dose in ten treatments over 12 days.

4. EFFECTIVE AND EFFICIENT RADIATION TREATMENT

The new strategy is to measure response by tumor reduction and tumor sterilization. That is, each modality needs to be utilized optimally to reduce the tumor burden and thereby to set the stage for the next therapeutic modality. Radiation treatment should be given to that dose that is effective in tumor ablation and low in complications. This means careful dosimetry and histopathologic studies correlated with doses in three-dimensional studies. Such investigations are currently in progress.

B. Treatment of Occult Metastases

The effectiveness of irradiation in eradicating occult metastases is well established for both squamous cell carcinoma and adenocarcinoma. Levels of 4500 rads have controlled nodal sites with high risk of metastases. Utilizing Herring's model [29] for tumor size and cell number, lower dose could be utilized if tumor emboli in the premetastatic stage were present. Tumor cell collections of 103 or 104 would require doses of 2000–3000 rads to sterilize. At issue is what sites require prophylactic treatment. This can be garnered from autopsy and pathologic analysis.

Nohl [42] has published a comprehensive review of lymph node spread of bronchogenic carcinoma, which is quite frequent to the hilar and mediastinal nodes (over 50% of the cases). The nodal involvement is approximately 40% in patients with squamous cell carcinoma as opposed to 80–90% in patients with oat cell or undifferentiated lesions, which have a high incidence of nodal involvement, similar to that of the other anaplastic lesions [35,43]. In a group of 680 autopsies of patients with bronchogenic carcinoma, Line and Deeley [44] reported a high incidence of metastatic lesions to the lymph nodes, liver, adrenals, bone, and brain. The incidence of metastasis was almost twice as frequent in patients with oat cell, anaplastic, and adenocarcinomas in comparison with the patients with squamous cell carcinoma.

Over 50% of patients with small cell carcinoma had evidence of locally distant metastasis at autopsy. This was significantly higher than in the epidermoid carcinoma patients [68]. Hansen *et al.* [28] demonstrated the value of routine biopsies of the posterior iliac crest, bone marrow, and liver in patients with bronchogenic carcinoma. Forty-six percent of the patients with small cell carcinoma had positive bone biopsies in contrast to 18% of the patients with adenocarcinoma and 2.6% of the patients with epidermoid carcinoma.

These authors reported eight positive bone marrow needle biopsies of the posterior iliac crest in eight out of 20 patients with limited (intrathoracic) small cell carcinoma (40%).

Maurer *et al.* [37] and Eagan *et. al* [20] found 14 positive bone marrow aspirations in 35 patients with oat cell carcinoma (41%). Hansen [27] reported that the development of brain metastasis in ten out of 22 patients with limited oat cell carcinoma of the lung treated by a combination of chemotherapeutic agents, in addition to 5000 rads to the primary lesion and mediastinal hilar nodes (45.5%). Neurological manifestations became the major symptomatic feature in eight of these patients.

Bell [6] found metastases in 17 of 88 patients with known bronchogenic carcinoma (19.3%) on whom abdominal laparotomies were performed; most of these were to the liver (12 cases) or the lymph nodes in the upper abdomen (3 cases).

Since, as indicated by Onuigbo [43], there may be a centrifugal distribution of metastasis in lung cancer, the more distant the organ from the primary pulmonary growth, the lower the probability of developing metastasis. If there is an orderly pattern of dissemination from more proximal to distant organs, it would be of theoretical value to prevent the development of metastatic deposits in these areas of high risk. Also, since the majority of the chemotherapeutic agents do not cross the blood–brain barrier, the central nervous system may be considered a sanctuary for tumor cells that would not be affected by circulating chemicals, so that prophylactic irradiation of the brain may be considered in special groups of patients, such as those with oat cell carcinoma. This approach has been found to be effective in childhood acute lymphoblastic leukemia. [4].

Thus, the new strategy would be to treat potential metastatic sites before overt metastases appear with tolerable doses, such as 2000–3000 rads given in a fractionated schedule of 150 rads daily. It would entail treatment of large segments of the anatomy (Fig. 16). The treatment schedule would last approximately 3–4 weeks with interruptions of 2 weeks to allow for bone marrow recovery and utilization of chemotherapy. It is essential that the radiation and medical oncologists integrate their techniques of irradiation, chemotherapy, and immunotherapy to reduce toxicity while reducing the tumor burdens. The new strategy is to learn to utilize the therapeutic efficacy of our colleagues as effectively as our own.

VI. APPENDIX: EXAMPLE OF CALCULATION
OF SPINAL CORD DOSE

A. Primary Considerations

1. The spinal cord, in this calculation, is at the midline of the patient at the superior margin of the lung fields (Fig. 8). This may not always be the case.

2. The treatment plan used is Plan B (see transverse dosimetry plan B; Fig. 10).

3. The posterior field is blocked, shielding the spinal cord, as described in the text. However, some contribution from scatter reaches the spinal cord from this field.

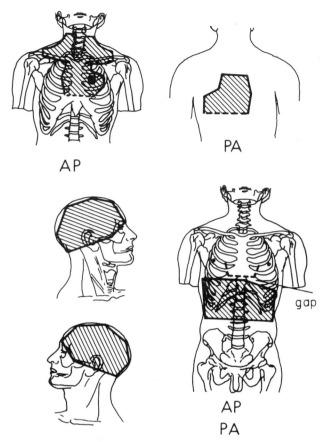

AP

PA

gap

AP
PA

Fig. 16. Oat cell cancer is known to include generous fields for primary and regional nodes, as well as elective fields for suspected occult metastasis in brain, liver, kidney and adrenals.

B. With Tissue Compensation

1. ANTERIOR FIELD

(a) Depth (6.5 cm of tissue plus 7.0 cm of compensation) = 13.5 cm

(b) The anterior field DD% (depth dose percent), 1 cm dose inside the superior margin of the posterior field (see Fig. 8) and corrected for beam unflatness off-axis = 38.0% at a 13.5 cm depth. [This depth dose is obtained from an isodose curve for ^{60}Co, 80 cm SSD, 15 × 15 cm² field at a depth of 13.5 cm, 1 cm from the geometrical edge of the field at the surface. All depth doses in the following calculation have been determined this way.]

2. Posterior Field

(a)   Depth (6.5 cm of tissue plus 2.0 cm of compensation) = 8.5 cm

(b)   The posterior field DD%, one cm inside the superior margin of the posterior field (see Fig. 8) and corrected for beam unflatness off-axis = 54.0% at a 8.5 cm depth.

3. Posterior Blocked Field

(a)   Depth = 8.5 cm
(b)   DD% corrected for unflatness = 18.0%

4. Bias Correction

Anterior: 38.0% × 1.05 bias = 39.9%
Posterior: 54.0% × 0.5 bias = 27.0%
Posterior
   blocked: 18.0% × 0.4 bias =   7.2%
Total Corrected Depth Dose = 74.1%

5. Dose Calculation

(a)   Prescribed tumor dose = 500 rads to 95.0% line
(b)   Given dose = 5000/95.0% rads × 100 = 5263 rads
(c)   Spinal cord dose = 5263 rads × 0.741 = 3900 rads

C. Without Tissue Compensation

1. Anterior Field

(a)   The Increase in SSD = 7.0 cm
(b)   Depth = 6.5 cm
(c)   DD% correction for an increase in SSD
    38.0% + [38.0% × (7 cm × 4.5%)] = 50.0%

Reference: "The Effective Attenuation Coefficient Method," International Commission on Radiological Units and Measurements (ICRU) Report 10d, Handbook 87, p. 23. U.S. Nat. Bur. Stds., Washington, D.C., 1963.

For alternate methods see:

"Effective SSD Method" (see handbook above).

H. E. Johns and J. R. Cunningham, "The Physics of Radiology," 3rd ed., pp. 332–334. Thomas, Springfield, Illinois, 1971.

J. Cundiff *et al.*, A method for the calculation of dose in the radiation treatment of Hodgkin's disease. *Amer. J. Roentgenol., Radium Ther. Nucl. Med.* [N.S.] **117**, 30–44 (1973).

J. Holt *et al.*, Extension of the concept of TAR to high energy X-rays. *Radiology* **96**, 437–446 (1970).

2. POSTERIOR FIELD

(a) Increase in SSD = 2.0 cm
(b) Depth 6.5 cm
(c) DD% correction for an increase in SSD
     $54.0\% + [54.0\% \times (2\text{cm} \times 4.5\%)] = 58.9\%$

3. POSTERIOR BLOCKED FIELD

(a) Increase in SSD = 2.0 cm
(b) Depth = 6.5 cm
(c) DD% = 18.0%
(d) $18.0\% + [18.0 \times (2\text{cm} \times 4.5\%)] = 19.6\%$

4. BIAS CORRECTION

Anterior: $50.0\% \times 1.05$ bias = 52.5%
Posterior: $58.9\% \times 0.5$ bias = 29.5%
Posterior
  blocked: $19.6\% \times 0.4$ bias = ___7.8%___
Total Corrected Depth Dose = 89.8%

5. DOSE CALCULATION

(a) Prescribed tumor dose = 5000 rads to 95.0% line
(b) Given dose = $5000/95.0\%$ rads $\times 100 = 5263$ rads
(c) Spinal cord dose = 5263 rads $\times .898 = 4726$ rads

REFERENCES

1. Abramson, N., and Cavanaugh, P. J., Short-course radiation therapy in carcinoma of the lung. *Radiology* **96**, 627–630 (1970).
2. Abramson, N., and Cavanaugh, P. J., Short-course radiation therapy in carcinoma of the lung, a second look. *Radiology* **108**, 685–687 (1973).

3. Anderson, W. A., chairman, "Clinical Staging System for the Carcinoma of the Lung." American Joint Committee for Cancer Staging and End Results Reporting, 1973.
4. Auer, R. J. A., Simone, J. B., Hustu, H. O., and Verzosa, M. S., A comparative study of central nervous system irradiation and intensive chemotherapy early in remission of childhood acute lymphocytic leukemia. *Cancer* **29**, 381–391 (1972).
5. Bangma, P. J., Post-operative radiotherapy. *In* "Modern Radiotherapy—Carcinoma of the Bronchus" (T. J. Deeley, ed.), pp. 163–170. Appleton, New York, 1971.
6. Bell, J. W., Abdominal exploration in one-hundred lung carcinoma suspects prior to thoracotomy. *Ann. Surg.* **167**, 199–203 (1968).
7. Bennett, D. E., Million, R. R., and Ackerman, L. V., Bilateral radiation pneumonitis, a complication of the radiotherapy of bronchogenic carcinoma. *Cancer* **23**, 1001–1018 (1969).
8. Bergsagel, D. E. *et al.*, Lung cancer: Clinical trial of radiotherapy alone versus radiotherapy plus cyclophosphamide. *Cancer* **30**, 621–627 (1972).
9. Bloedorn, F. G., Cowley, R. A., Cuccia, C. A., Mercado, R., Jr., Wizenberg, M. J., and Linberg, E. J., Preoperative irradiation in bronchogenic carcinoma. *Amer. J. Roentgenol. Radium Ther. Nucl. Med.* [N.S.] 92, 77–87 (1964).
10. Brady, L. W., Germon, P. A., and Cander, L., The effects of radiation therapy on pulmonary function in carcinoma of the lung. *Radiology* **85**, 130–134 (1965).
11. Bromley, L. L., and Szur, L., Combined radiotherapy and resection for carcinoma of the bronchus: Experiences with 66 patients, *Lancet* **2**, 937–941 (1955).
12. Carbone, P. P., Frost, J. K., Feinstein, A. B., Higgins, G. A., and Selawry, O. S., Lung cancer: Perspectives and prospects. *Ann. Intern. Med.* **73**, 1003–1024 (1970).
13. Carr, D. T., Keynote Address on Diagnosis, Staging and Criteria of Response to Therapy for Lung Cancer. *Cancer Chemother. Rep.* **4**, 17 (1973).
14. Carr, D. T., Childs, D. S., Jr., and Lee, R. E., Radiotherapy plus 5-FU compared to radiotherapy alone for inoperable and unresectable bronchogenic carcinoma. *Cancer* **29**, 375–380 (1972).
15. Carter, S. K., Some thoughts on surgical adjuvant studies in lung cancer. Prepared for Chemotherapy Committee, Lung Cancer Working Party, 1972. *Cancer Chemotherapy Reports* Part 3, Vol. 4, pp. 109–111, March 1972.
16. Concannon, J., A study of CEA antigen in lung cancer patients treated with irradiation. *RTOG Protocol* (1973).
17. Coy, P., A randomized study of irradiation and vinblastine in lung cancer. *Cancer* **26**, 803–807 (1970).
18. Deeley, T. J., A clinical trial to compare two different tumour dose levels in the treatment of advanced carcinoma of the bronchus. *Clin. Radiol.* **17**, 299–301 (1966).
19. Dutreix, J., Schlienger, M., and le Peigneux, M., Irradiation en deux séries et irradiation pré-opérative en deux jours. *J. Radiol., Electrol., Med. Nucl.* **48**, 167–172 (1967).
20. Eagan, R. T., Maurer, L. H., Forcier, R. J., and Tulloh, M., Combination chemotherapy and radiation therapy in small cell carcinoma of the lung. *Cancer* **32**, 371–379 (1973).
21. Fernholz, H. J., and Muller, G., Ergebnisse and komplikationen der telekobalttherapie beim bronchialkarzinom. *Strahlentherapie* **137**, 381–392 (1969).

22. Fox, W., and Scadding, J. G., Medical Research Council comparative trial of surgery and radiotherapy for primary treatment of small-celled or oat-celled carcinoma of the bronchus, ten-year follow-up. *Lancet* **2**, 63–65 (1973).

23. Germon, P. A., and Brady, L. W., Physiologic changes before and after radiation treatment for carcinoma of the lung. *J. Amer. Med. Ass.* **206**, 809–814 (1968).

24. Green, R. A., Hunthley, E., Close, H., and Pateno, M. E., Alkylating agents in bronchogenic carcinoma. *Amer. J. Med.* **46**, 516–524 (1969).

25. Guttman, R., Radical supervoltage therapy in inoperable carcinoma of the lung. *In* "Modern Radiotherapy—Carcinoma of the Bronchus" (T. J. Deeley, ed.), pp. 181–195. Appleton, New York, 1971.

26. Hall, T. C. *et al.*, A clinical pharmacologic study of chemotherapy and x-ray therapy in lung cancer. *Amer. J. Med.* **43**, 186–193 (1967).

27. Hansen, H. H., Keynote address on chemotherapy for lung cancer. *Cancer Chemother. Rep.* **4**, 25–28 (1973).

28. Hansen, H. H., Muggia, F. M., Andrews, R., and Selawry, O. S., Intensive combined chemotherapy and radiotherapy in patients with nonresectable bronchogenic carcinoma. *Cancer* **30**, 315–324 (1972).

29. Herring, D., "The Degree of Precision Required in the Radiation Dose Delivered in Cancer Radiotherapy," Rep. No. EMI-216. Enviro-Med Inc., California, 1970.

30. Hilaris, B. S., Luomanen, R. K., and Beattie, E. J., Jr., Integrated irradiation and surgery in the treatment of apical lung cancer. *Cancer* **27**, 1369–1373 (1971).

31. Holsti, L., and Vuorinen, P., Radiation reaction in the lung after continuous and split-course megavoltage radiotherapy of bronchial carcinoma. *Brit. J. Radiol.* **40**, 280–284 (1967).

32. Krant, M. J. *et al.*, Comparative trial of chemotherapy and radiotherapy in patients with non-resectable cancer of the lung. *Amer. J. Med.* **35**, 363–373 (1963).

33. LePar, E., Brady, F. L., and Beckloff, G. L., Clinical evaluation of the adjunctive use of hydroxyurea (NSC-32065) in radiation therapy of carcinoma of the lung. *Radiol. Clin. Biol.* **36**, 32–40 (1967).

34. Levitt, S. H., Bogardus, C. R., and Ladd, G., Split-dose intensive radiation therapy in the treatment of advanced lung cancer. *Radiology* **88**, 1159–1161 (1967).

35. Line, D. H., and Deeley, T. J., The necropsy findings in carcinoma of the bronchus. *Brit. J. Dis. Chest* **65**, 238–242 (1971).

36. Locksmith, J., and Powers, W. E., Permanent radiation myelopathy. *Amer. J. Roentgenol., Radium Ther. Nucl. Med.* [N.S.] **102**, 916–926 (1968).

37. Maurer, L. H., Tulloh, M., Eagan, R. T., Forcier, R. J., and House, R., Combination of chemotherapy and radiation therapy for small cell carcinoma of the lung. *Cancer Chemother. Rep.* **4**, 171–176 (1973).

38. Miller, A. B., Fox, W., and Tall, R., Five-year follow-up of the Medical Research Council comparative trial of surgery and radiotherapy for the primary treatment of small-celled or oat-celled carcinoma of the bronchus. *Lancet* **2**, 501–505 (1969).

39. Morrison, R., Deeley, T. J., and Cleland, W. P., The treatment of carcinoma of the bronchus. A clinical trial to compare surgery and supervoltage radiotherapy. *Lancet* **1**, 683–684 (1963).

40. Mountain, C. F., Carr, D. T., and Anderson, W. A. D., A system for the clinical staging of lung cancer. *Amer. J. Roentgenol., Radium Ther. Nucl. Med.* **120,** 130–138 (1974).
41. Muggia, F. M., Correlation of histologic types with cell kinetic studies in lung cancer. *Cancer Chemother. Rep.* **4,** 69–71 (1973).
42. Nohl, H. C., An investigation into the lymphatic and vascular spread of carcinoma of the bronchus. *Thorax* **11,** 172–185 (1956).
43. Onuigbo, W. I. B., Centrifugal metastasis in lung cancer. *Brit. J. Dis. Chest* **55,** 86–90 (1961).
44. Paulson, D. L., Shaw, R. R., Kee, J. L., Mallams, J. T., and Collier, R. E., Combined preoperative irradiation and resection for bronchogenic carcinoma. *J. Thorac. Cardiov. Surg.* **44,** 281–294 and 305–308 (1962).
45. Pereslegin, I. A., "Radiotherapy of Lung Cancer." Meditsina, Moscow, 1963.
46. Phillips, T. L., and Margolis, L., Radiation pathology and the clinical response of lung and esophagus. *Front. Radiat. Ther. Oncol.* **6,** 254–273 (1972).
47. Preoperative irradiation of cancer of the lung: Preliminary report of a therapeutic trial. *Cancer* **23,** 419–429 (1969).
48. Rissanen, P. M., Tikka, U., and Holsti, L. R., Autopsy findings in lung cancer treated with megavoltage radiotherapy. *Acta Radiol., Ther., Phys., Biol.* **7,** 433–422 (1968).
49. Roswit, B., Patno, M. E., Rapp, R., Veinburgs, A., Feder, B., Stuhlbarg, J., and Reid, C. B., The survival of patients with inoperable lung cancer: A large-scale randomized study of radiation therapy versus placebo. *Radiology* **90,** 688–697 (1968).
50. Roswit, B., Higgins, G. A., Shields, W., and Keehn, R. J., Preoperative radiation therapy for carcinoma of the lung: Report of a national VA controlled study. *Front. Radiat. Ther. Oncol.* **5,** 163–176 (1970).
51. Rubenfeld, S., and Kaplan, G., Treatment of bronchogenic cancer with conventional x-rays according to specific time-dose pattern. *Radiology* **73,** 671–678 (1959).
52. Rubin, P., Radiotherapy for lung cancer. *Cancer Chemother. Rep.* **4,** 311–315 (1973).
53. Rubin, P., Ciccio, S., and Setisarn, B., The controversial status of radiation therapy in lung cancer. *Nat. Cancer Conf., Proc., 6th, 1968.* pp. 855–866.
54. Sambrook, D. K., Split-course radiation therapy in malignant tumors. *Amer. J. Roentgenol., Radium Ther. Nucl. Med.* [N.S.] **91,** 37–45 (1964).
55. Schabel, R. J., Jr., The use of tumor growth kinetics in planning "curative" chemotherapy of advanced solid tumors. *Cancer Res.* **29,** 2384–2389 (1969).
56. Selawry, O. S., Monochemotherapy of bronchogenic carcinoma with special reference to cell type. *Cancer Chemother. Rep.* **4,** 177–188 (1973).
57. Selawry, O. S., and Hansen, H. H., Lung cancer. *In* "Cancer Medicine" (J. Holland and E. Frei, eds.). Lea & Febiger, Philadelphia, Pennsylvania, 1973.
58. Slack, N. H., Bronchogenic carcinoma: Nitrogen mustard as a surgical adjuvant and factors influencing survival. *Cancer* **25,** 987–1002 (1970).
59. Smart, J., Can lung cancer be cured by irradiation alone? *J. Amer. Med. Ass.* **159,** 1034–1035 (1966).
60. Sobin, L. H., Multiplicity of lung tumor classifications. *Recent Results Cancer Res.* **39,** 29–35 (1967).
61. Spjut, H. J., Roper, C. L., and Butcher, H. R., Jr., Pulmonary cancer and its prognosis. *Cancer* **14,** 1251–1258 (1961).

62. Stewart, J. R., Cohn, K. E., Fajardo, L. F., Hancock, E. W., and Kaplan, H. S., Radiation-induced heart disease, a study of twenty-five patients. *Radiology* **89,** 302–310 (1967).
63. Study of cytotoxic chemotherapy as an adjuvant to surgery in carcinoma of the bronchus. Medical Research Council Working Party. *Brit. Med. J.* **2,** 421–428 (1971).
64. Teates, D., and Cooper, G., Jr., Some consequences of pulmonary irradiation: A second long-term report. *Amer. J. Roentgenol., Radium Ther. Nucl. Med.* [N.S.] **96,** 612–619 (1966).
65. Tucker, R. D., Sealy, R., Van Wyk, C., Le Roux, P. L. M., and Soskolne, C. L., A clinical trial of cyclophosphamide (NSC-26271) and radiation therapy of oat cell carcinoma of the lung. *Cancer Chemother. Rep.* **4,** 159–160 (1973).
66. von Essen, C. F., Kligerman, M. M., and Calabresi, P., Radiation and 5-Fluorouracil: A controlled clinical study. *Radiology* **81,** 1018–1027 (1963).
67. Weiss, W., Boucot, K. R., and Cooper, D. A., The Philadephia Pulmonary Neoplasm Research Project: Survival factors in bronchogenic carcinoma. *J. Amer. Med. Ass.* **216,** 2123 (1971).
68. Yesner, R., Observer variability and reliability in lung cancer diagnosis. *Cancer Chemother. Rep.* **4,** 55–58 (1973).

Chapter 10

Problems of Best Supportive Therapy in Lung Cancer

Lucien Israel

The problem of determining the best supportive therapy should occupy a prominent place in all chapters of medical oncology. However the problem is of particular importance in lung cancer for two reasons.

1. The situation of the lungs is such that it makes them a particularly susceptible target for nonspecific causes of death, namely, infection and pulmonary embolism. It is quite obvious that any therapeutic program that neglects these aspects is necessarily inadequate even if it is perfect from a purely oncological standpoint.

2. Lung cancer is one of the rare cancers for which there is no significant difference in survival between responders and nonresponders to chemotherapy and radiotherapy. In Chapter 3, it was shown that tumor regression means going back in time with regard to the tumor's natural course, and this should necessarily be reflected in a corresponding increase in survival. The discrepancy between objective response and survival clearly indicates that patients die of causes other than their cancer, or to be more precise death does not result simply from an increase in the population of malignant cells.

199

It thus appears that application of procedures designed to prevent death from nonspecific causes in lung cancer should make considerable progress possible in terms of survival, even if no corresponding advances are made in specific therapy. Below, we shall briefly discuss some of the therapeutic methods that should be submitted to controlled trial in the very near future.

I. CORRECTING ADRENAL INSUFFICIENCY

It is well known that prednisone shortens survival in lung cancer patients, when compared to a placebo [6]. But it is also well known that prednisone is an immunodepressant which, when administered alone to lung cancer patients, can only promote opportunistic infections.

The same is not true of hydrocortisone, for example, which corrects adrenal insufficiency in doses that are not immunosuppressive. Of course we do not advocate comparing supportive therapy to a placebo while the cancer progresses, but rather the best specific therapy versus this therapy combined with the best possible nonspecific therapy. It is from this angle that the investigation of steroids in lung cancer should be reconsidered, in view of the high incidence of adrenal insufficiency during the course of the lung cancer even when metastasis to the adrenal glands does not occur. We have clinical data suggesting that the addition of 0.5 mg/kg/day of hydrocortisone administered orally reduces weight loss, orthostatic hypotension, and general weakness in our patients on chemotherapy so that they can tolerate more aggressive treatment for a longer period of time.

II. WEIGHT LOSS, IMMUNE DEFENSE MECHANISMS, BONE MARROW FUNCTION, AND ANDROGENS

Bone marrow insufficiency is a common occurrence in cancer patients. One of the consequences of this condition is a decrease in the number of available immunocytes. It is also known that androgens may exert a beneficial effect on bone marrow function [1, 2, 4, 5] as well as on weight. This makes androgens a good candidate for inclusion in a program of best supportive therapy. In male cancer patients, high doses of androgens can be expected to produce only beneficial effects. It is our practice to administer 250 mg of a long-acting form of testosterone every 2 weeks to our patients on chemotherapy. This treatment is well tolerated and appears to exert a beneficial effect on bone marrow resistance to chemotherapy as well as on weight. However we have not performed any controlled trials, and we are unable to say exactly what the precise role of androgens in therapy might be. The aim of controlled trials would be to answer this question.

III. SPECIFIC PROPHYLAXIS FOR OPPORTUNISTIC MICROBIAL INFECTIONS

We have no experience with this type of prophylaxis, but the high incidence of pulmonary infections in cancer patients treated by radiotherapy or chemotherapy suggests that it is of considerable importance. Since the almost complete eradication of rheumatic fever during 1950's through administration of low daily doses of sulfanamides, we know that chemoprophylaxis of infection is possible with low doses. Here again, controlled trials would be necessary to determine whether any advantage is to be derived from combining specific anticancer treatment with routine antibiotic therapy directed against the most commonly encountered organisms.

IV. SPECIFIC PROPHYLAXIS FOR OPPORTUNISTIC FUNGAL INFECTIONS

Such prophylaxis is all the more necessary in this context of immunodepression when antimicrobial agents are prescribed. The same principle as that mentioned for antimicrobial chemotherapy could be applied to test the efficacy of antifungal prophylaxis, namely, daily administration of low doses.

V. NONSPECIFIC PROPHYLAXIS FOR OPPORTUNISTIC INFECTIONS

In a previous chapter, we mentioned that regular administration of *Corynebacterium parvum* resulted in a considerable decrease in the incidence of bacterial and viral infections in our patients. This finding is hardly surprising, since the immune stimulation thus achieved is not selective for anticancer immune mechanisms. Wider use of immune stimulation methods in patients on chemotherapy would result in more effective control of opportunistic infections.

There is also another method that may be used which involves repeated administration of high doses of γ-globulins. This therapy has proved to be effective in preventing infection. Although nontreated cancer patients tend to exhibit predominant depression of cell-mediated immunity, cytotoxic chemotherapy affects also humoral immunity. This is a good indication for administration of γ-globulins, which we investigated some years ago, and warrants reconsideration and trial on a wider scale [3].

VI. PROPHYLAXIS FOR PULMONARY EMBOLISM

In Chapter 13 Dr. Elias shows why pulmonary embolism is so common in patients with lung cancer. In view of the high incidence and the gravity of this accident at all stages of the disease, it seems unbelievable that no routine procedure has yet been advocated to try to prevent pulmonary embolisms. It is still not known with certainty whether heparin or fibrinolytic agents would be preferable to aspirin. But the properties of the latter and its ease of administration make it one of the best candidates for controlled clinical trials designed to establish the most effective therapeutic procedures for preventing pulmonary embolisms in patients being treated for lung cancer.

VII. CONCLUSION

We feel it is important to place strong emphasis on the idea that the slow progress achieved in treating lung cancer, as compared to other forms of cancer, is due partly to the existence of nonspecific causes of death, namely, opportunistic infections and pulmonary embolism. A very important task lies ahead, namely, the determination of the best possible procedures for preventing these complications in all cancer patients, irrespective of disease stage. The aim of such procedures would not only be to counter the immune depression and hypercoagulability induced by the tumor itself but also to combat therapeutic immunodepression and post-radiotherapeutic thrombosis in order to enable existing forms of treatment to exert their full effect with a minimum of adverse effects. The number of drugs proposed for clinical trials in various types of infections and in pulmonary embolisms is so great that successive trials designed to investigate and compare the results achieved with different associations are not feasible. In view of this situation, discerning judgment has to be used in designating trials that are feasible and potentially successful. In our experience, hydrocortisone, androgens, aspirin, and γ-globulins have proved to be relatively simple, effective, and coherent supportive therapy drugs that have the same right to clinical trial as the new, potentially active, chemotherapeutic agents.

REFERENCES

1. Brodsky, I., Dennis, L. H., De Castro, N. A., Brady, L., and Kahn, S. B., Effect of testosterone enanthate and alkylating agents on multiple myeloma. *J. Amer. Med. Ass.* **193**, 874 (1965).
2. Brodsky, I., Reimann, H. A., and Dennis, L. H., Treatment of cyclic neutropenia with testosterone. *Amer. J. Med.* **38**, 802 (1965).
3. Israel, L., Effet protecteur et curatif des gamma-globulines humaines vis-à-vis des infections virales, microbiennes et mycosiques, apparaissant sous chimiothérapie anticancéreuse. *Med. Interne* **5**, 297 (1970).
4. Israel, L., La fluoxymestérone quotidienne au cours des chimiothérapies anticancéreuses prolongées. *Rev. Med.* **33**, 2041 (1971).
5. Shadidi, N. T., Morphologic and biochemical characteristics of erythrocytes in testosterone induced remission in patients with acquired and constitutional aplastic anemias. *J. Lab. Clin. Med.* **62**, 294 (1963).
6. Wolf, J., Spear, P., Yesner, R. *et al.,* Nitrogen mustard and the steroid hormones in the treatment of inoperable bronchogenic carcinoma. *Amer. J. Med.* **29**, 1008. (1960).

Chapter 11

On Chemotherapy of Lung Cancer

Oleg S. Selawry

I. INTRODUCTION

The 5-year survival of patients with bronchogenic carcinoma remains at 8–10%, and 50% of the patients have recognized, extrapulmonary metastases at the time of diagnosis [33]. Hence, chemotherapy is potentially indicated in 50% of the patients at the time of diagnosis and in close to 90% of all patients at some later time in the course of their disease. What, then is the current status of chemotherapy in the treatment of lung cancer, including successes, limitations, and prospects?

The attempt is made to answer some of these questions based on an updated review of results and concepts of chemotherapy for lung cancer, intended for the practicing physician and for the clinical investigator in their striving for more effective treatment. It is assumed that the reader is familiar with basic aspects of cancer chemotherapy. Details on drug dosage, schedule, and toxicity are therefore omitted, except for instances where drugs were used in an unusual way.

The subject is conveniently divided into sections on general aspects, monochemotherapy, oligo- and polychemotherapy, regional treatment, and combination of chemotherapy with surgery and radiotherapy, respectively. Combination of chemotherapy with immunotherapy is described in Chapter 10.

II. GENERAL ASPECTS

The most widely accepted indication for chemotherapy includes the palliation of the inoperable symptomatic patient with complaints beyond control of radiotherapy. This indication includes two categories of patients: (1) those with symptoms related to metastatic spread beyond one hemithorax, including ipsilateral scalene and lower cervical lymph nodes and (2) those with symptomatic, local recurrence after maximal dosage of radiotherapy.

It is widely held, however, that patients with earlier disease have a better chance to respond than patients with far advanced cancer. Preliminary data seem to validate this concept for bronchogenic small cell carcinoma, but not for epidermoid carcinoma of the lung [3]. Hence, chemotherapy might also be indicated for treatment of the asymptomatic patient with small cell carcinoma and possibly other types of lung cancer, depending on the expected benefit to the patient as weighed against the untoward side effects of the treatment.

Everyone familiar with lung cancer knows how difficult it is to define "benefit to the patient," "objective response," and "progressive disease" because of the crudeness of currently applied methods [106]. This warrants a short discussion of criteria for evaluation of response.

Survival as the sole measure of "patient benefit" appeared foolproof and definitive [50, 129]. It was shown, however, that median survival of successive cohorts of 60 or more patients treated by the same physicians with placebo varied by more than 50%, even when patients were staged and divided into those with regional disease, limited to one hemithorax with or without ipsilateral scalene or lower cervical lymph node involvement, and those with distant metastases [108]. This observation is in sharp contrast to the excellent, world-wide comparability of surgical end results [108] and might be related to limitations in the methods of staging and to differences in the composition of the patient cohorts as to microscopic type of lung cancer, performance status, and other prognostic factors. In treated patients, the situation might be further complicated if prolonged survival of patients with objective tumor response were counterbalanced by shortened survival of nonresponders exposed to potentially toxic drugs. Moreover, it might be ethically difficult to continue obviously ineffective treatment in the presence of progressive disease and in sight of other non-cross-resistant, potentially effective drugs.

Some of these problems can be minimized by stratification of patients by known prognostic factors and by inclusion of concomitant, prospectively randomized controls [50] treated to an earlier end point such as "progressive disease" [109]. This approach requires approximately 20 patients in each treatment arm for detection of a 100% difference in median time to progression. This number would increase to around 50 patients for detection of a 50% difference and to about 230 patients if a 20% difference was looked for [43, 106].

Objective tumor shrinkage as sole criterion of response appears adequate for the initial therapeutic trial of new drugs. Most authors accept a regression of at least 50% of well-outlined intrathoracic tumor lesions as reproducible and reliable evidence of objective response and use the product of the longest and the widest perpendicular diameters for tumor measurement [105, 106]. A marked (estimated 75%) change of poorly outlined pulmonary lesions is likewise accepted as objective response. Regression of 25% can be measured reproducibly in well-outlined palpable lesions. These criteria were used for the current review, if at least one evaluable or measurable lesion regressed and if there was no progression (increase by 50% of a well-outlined lesion or by 100% for an evaluable not measurable lesion) or occurrence of new lesions elsewhere. All eligible patients were included, irrespective of longevity. Therefore, the data of this review are sometimes at variance with those authors who excluded patients who died within 2 or 3 weeks from onset of treatment. Even then, there might be wide fluctuations of response rates reported by individual investigators. This is exemplified in a summary of the overall rate of objective response as compared to response rates reported in individual publications on monochemotherapy with the five most widely used drugs against lung cancer (Table I). The drugs are listed in sequence of popularity as judged by the number of patients reported. The overall rate of objective responses ranges from 12 to 31% and has no direct relation to popularity. More importantly, the response rates reported in individual publications range from 0 to 60+% for each of the two most widely used drugs. Indeed, response rates vary considerably, depending on microscopic type of tumor (Tables II–V), stage of disease [3], performance status of the patient [130],

TABLE I

Objective Response of Lung Cancer to the Five Most Popular Drugs[a]

Drug	Number of patients treated	Percent responding		References
		All patients	Range[b]	
Cyclophosphamide	1513	20	0–63	[7, 37, 111]
Mechlorethamine	1442	31	0–68	[7, 8, 32, 37, 73, 92, 120]
Hexamethylmelamine	485	18	10–30	[122, 128]
Methotrexate	416	22	3–43	
Bleomycin	331	12	0–20	[14, 88–90, 119]

[a] From [105].
[b] Range of response rates in individual publications.

prior treatment, age, and possibly immunologic status of the patient [121; also Chapter 7]. Optimal use of drugs as to dosage and schedule will likewise influence results. Thus, data on objective tumor regression have to be seen against the background of the above-mentioned factors, and the rule of thumb, by which at least 14 patients need to be treated in order to exclude an objective response rate of 20% with a rejection error of 5% [43], depends on proper patient selection and on treatment to definite, reversible toxicity.

Improved methods for measurement of objective response are within reach. Israel and Chahinian noted that volume doubling times of measurable pulmonary lesions are reasonably constant in a given tumor. Decreased volume doubling time, short of partial or complete regression, might thus become an early and more sensitive indicator of response or failure within 1 to 3 weeks from the onset of treatment.

Endobronchial estimation of tumor size in addition to serial chest films

TABLE II

Objective Response of Epidermoid Carcinoma of the Lung to Single Drugs[a]

Drug	% Responding	Patients treated	References
Methotrexate	25	140	
Dibromodulcitol	23	39	[86]
Emetine, dehydroemetine	22	9	[61]
Mechlorethamine	21	183	[37]
Cyclophosphamide	20	232	[7]
Adriamycin	19	70	[14, 28, 87]
CCNU	17	58	[36, 45]
Vinblastine	16	20	
1-Methyl-1-nitrosourea	15	14	
Bleomycin	13	265	[12, 119]
Procarbazine	13	55	[18]
Hexamethylmelamine	12	68	
Busulfane	7	61	
BCNU	6	34	[96]
Methyl-CCNU	6	36	
Aminochrysene	0	11	[66]
Carbazilquinone	0	17	[72, 100]
Colchicine	0	11	
Mercaptopurine	0	16	
Mitomycin C	0	22	
Acetyl picolinoylhydrazine	0	4	[127]
Streptonigrin	0	10	

[a] Data from Selawry [105].

TABLE III

Objective Response of Small Cell Carcinoma of the Lung to Single Drugs[a]

Drug	% Responding	Patients treated	Reference
1-Methyl-1-nitrosourea	65	26[b]	[70, 92]
Methotrexate	39	79	
Mechlorethamine	39	80	
Cyclophosphamide	31[c]	296	[37]
Hexamethylmelamine	26[c]	54	[122]
Adriamycin	25[c]	48	
Procarbazine	25	44[b]	[18]
BCNU	21[c]	19	
Methyl-CCNU	21	19	
Dibromodulcitol	20	15[b]	
Epipodophyllotoxin, ethylidine glucoside	20	10	
CCNU	19[c]	31	[36, 93]
Busulfane	18	17	
Emetine, dehydroemetine	11	19	[61]
Carbazilquinone	11	9	
Mercaptopurine	11[c]	9	
Vinblastine	33[d]	9	
Vincristine	33	6	
Mitomycin	9	11	
Bleomycin	0	27	
Aminochrysene	0	8	
Sarcolysine	0	6	[92]

[a] From Selawry [105].
[b] Includes large cell anaplastic carcinomas.
[c] Includes complete regressions.
[d] Three patients surviving for 1+ years. No measurements given.

improved the reliability of measurements [17, 18, 88–90; A. Pirogov and A. Trakhtenberg, personal communication] and helped to determine the status of tumor growth in areas with pneumonitis or fibrosis following radiotherapy [91]. Fiberoptic bronchoscopy makes this approach more acceptable to the patient. Cytology, which can be obtained routinely or in connection with bronchoscopy, was reported to give further clues for response to certain drugs [27, 71]. Marker substances such as ectopically produced hormones and tumor-related antigens might also prove useful for estimation of tumor response [95].

Finally, the design of chemotherapeutic studies in lung cancer can make results more comparable, by the use of a "standard" treatment in addition to the "experimental" treatment. Y. Kenis', suggestion to use cyclophospha-

TABLE IV

Objective Response of Adenocarcinoma of the Lung to Single Drugs[a]

Drug	% Responding	Patients treated	References
Methotrexate	32	25	
Mechlorethamine	28	86	[92]
Mitomycin C	27	11	
Cyclophosphamide	21	48	[7, 37]
Procarbazine	19	16	
Adriamycin	15	53	
Hexamethylmelamine	15	39	
Bleomycin	13	30	
CCNU	13	55	[36, 45, 94]
Methyl-CCNU	13	39	[13, 36, 97, 121]
Colchicine	14	7	
Emetine, dehydroemetine	14	7	[61]
Epipodophyllotoxin,			
ethylidine glucoside	25	4	[39]
1-Methyl-1-nitrosourea	22	9	[70, 92]
Vinblastine	17	6	
Dibromodulcitol	8	12	
Busulfane	4	28	
BCNU	0	22	
Carbazilquinone	0	11	[72]
Mercaptopurine	0	9	
Sarcolysine	0	3	[92]

[a] From Selawry [105].

mide (CTX), 1100 mg/m^2 every 3 weeks i.v. as "standard," found general acceptance at the International Workshop for Treatment of Lung Cancer at Airlie House, 1972 [130] and should be supported where clearly superior treatment is lacking.

Tumor shrinkage per se is not necessarily related to patient benefit, especially when responses are short or when there are pronounced side effects from treatment. Therefore, duration of response is given, where possible, and survival of responders is compared with that of nonresponders for selected studies.

Furthermore, comparative controlled clinical trials are emphasized, except for monochemotherapy, because of the difficulty of relying on historical controls (*vida infra*). Publications that have been included in previous reviews are usually quoted [10, 11, 45, 105–108]. The data of subsequent sections of this chapter should be seen against the background of these methodologic considerations.

TABLE V
Objective Response of Large Cell Carcinoma of the Lung to Single Drugs[a]

Drug	% Responding	Patients treated	References
Procarbazine	35	17	
Mechlorethamine	26	148	[37]
Adriamycin	25	28	
Cyclophosphamide	23	22	
Hexamethylmelamine	18	39	
CCNU	17	41	[36, 45, 94]
Methyl-CCNU	17	23	[13, 97, 121]
Methotrexate	12	104	
Busulfane	17	6	
Mitomycin C	50	2	
Streptonigrin	14	7	
Vinblastine	100	2	
BCNU	9	22	
Mercaptopurine	3	29	
Colchicine	0	12	
Bleomycin	0	2	[119]
1-Methyl-1-nitrosourea	0	1	[92]

[a] From Selawry [105].

III. MONOCHEMOTHERAPY

The response to individual single drugs varies considerably, depending on the microscopic type of lung cancer. Thus, important responses to one particular cell type, especially a less common one, can be obscured in reports on large series of patients, when data are not given by cell type (see Table X). Hence, the efficacy of chemotherapeutic agents will be discussed by cell type whenever possible, while overall responses by drugs are published elsewhere [105].

Objective tumor regression was most widely reported as prime criterion for response and will therefore be stressed in the subsequent discussion.

A. Epidermoid Carcinoma

Five drugs induced responses in 20% of the patients or better (Table II). Methotrexate (MTX) leads the list with 25% of 140 patients responding. The available data do not permit a correlation of response to dose schedule of methotrexate. It appears, however, that treatment with widely spaced doses (every 2–3 weeks) are inferior to other dose schedules, because of considerable variability of individual tolerance to the drug and because of the usually rapid recurrence of tumor after unmaintained responses. This is readily understandable for a drug that inhibits growth, predominantly during S phase and hits, therefore, only a minority of cells during each individual treatment [46, 47].

Attempts to improve the therapeutic index by use of high doses of methotrexate (1000–12,000 mg/m²/dose i.v.) followed by leucovorin ("citrovorum factor")—in order to "rescue" rapidly proliferating normal tissues, such as oral and intestinal mucosa, from methotrexate toxicity—are controversial [35, 74]. The morbidity is high. Renal failure of undetermined origin was recently reported in five patients so treated (A. Skarin, personal communication). This interesting approach might best be limited to further cautiously monitored investigative study rather than to treatment of individual patients.

Dibromodulcitol is probably cross-resistant to bifunctional, alkylating agents, such as mechlorethamine (nitrogen mustard, HN_2) and cyclophosphamide (Cytoxan, Endoxan); has a narrow therapeutic margin; and can cause delayed hematologic toxicity. The drug might be advantageous, however, for treatment of cerebral metastases because it crosses the blood–brain barrier.

Emetine and dehydroemetine warrant further study and might be of special interest for combination chemotherapy, where this nonmyelosuppressive agent could be used at full dose.

Mechlorethamine and cyclophosphamide, as the most widely used agents, are definitely effective. The virtually identical response rates of 21 and 20%, respectively, are in possible disagreement with data of the Veteran's Administration Lung Group [50] (Table X), where mechlorethamine induced a statistically significant doubling of median survival from 3 months for placebo-treated patients to 6 months for drug-treated patients, but showed only marginal survival benefit for small cell carcinoma; in contrast, cyclophosphamide failed to prolong survival in patients with epidermoid carcinoma but significantly increased median survival of patients with small cell carcinoma from a median of 1.4 months to a median of 4.0 months.

Adriamycin, CCNU (cyclohexylchloroethyl nitrosourea), and vinblastine are close seconds and might be of interest because of lack of cross-resistance to the five more effective agents.

Bleomycin was extensively studied because of reported efficacy in well-differentiated epidermoid carcinoma of the head and neck. The overall response rate of 13% of 265 patients is disappointing. It should be noted, however, that one author reports an encouraging survival gain (*vida infra*). The low incidence of hematologic toxicity of this drug made it a favorite for combination chemotherapy [13], thus far without proved success.

Drugs with response rates of less than 10% might be ineffective, especially when responses are short lasting, because such response rates were occasionally reported for placebo-treated patients (Eastern Coopera-

tive Oncology Group, unpublished data of a comparative study of methotrexate versus placebo), possibly related to transient clearance of atelec-
tatic areas that might be difficult to distinguish from adjacent tumor lesions.
The reverse might also be true; the negative data for some of these agents
might be "false negatives," where the number of patients is small or where
the study is limited to patients with prior chemotherapy and far advanced
disease (vida supra).

B. Small Cell Carcinoma

Small cell carcinoma is the most sensitive to chemotherapy. Eleven
drugs induced objective response in at least 20% of the patients, four of
these drugs showed response rates of more than 30%, and at least six
drugs induced occasional complete tumor regression (Table III).

Soviet studies with 1-methyl-1-nitrosourea lead the list of effective agents
and would be well worth pursuing because the data include patients with
both large and small cell anaplastic carcinoma [70, 92, 105, 106]. Interest
in a comparison of 1-methyl-1-nitrosourea with the other clinically used
nitrosoureas [bischloroethylnitrosourea (BCNU), cyclochloroethythylni-
trosourea (CCNU), and methyl-CCNU] might be further enhanced because of their apparently different ranking in the four major types of lung
cancer (Tables II–V) and in animal tumors, because of their lack of cross-
resistance with classic bifunctional, alkylating agents, and because of an
apparent more than additive effect when combined with cyclophosphamide
in the treatment of patients with small cell carcinoma (vida infra) and in
certain animal tumors [79].

Methotrexate, as a cell cycle-sensitive agent, and mechlorethamine are
the next two most effective drugs, with cyclophosphamide as a close third.

Hexamethylmelamine would be of interest, if it lacks cross-resistance
with alkylating agents. Clinical studies are underway because preclinical
data are controversial.

Adriamycin, procarbazine (PROC), and "VP16" (4'-demethyl-epipodo-
phyllotoxin ethylidene glucoside, VP16-213) are worth consideration because of apparent lack of cross-resistance with preceding agents.

Carbazilquinone, mercaptopurine (or thioguanine?), and the Vinca
alkaloids—vincristine and vinblastine—warrant further study because of
impressive results in small numbers of patients. The paucity of data on
Vinca alkaloids is particularly surprising because of their widespread use
in polychemotherapy. Bleomycin might be the only adequately studied
"ineffective" drug thus far studied in small cell carcinoma, if one discounts
tumor regression of < 50% [14], which does not qualify for inclusion in
Table III (vida supra).

C. Adenocarcinoma

Four drugs produced response in more than 20% of the patients, including the "usual," methotrexate, mechlorethamine, and cyclophosphamide and the "unusual," mitomycin C, albeit in a small number of patients (Table IV).

Again, the list is extended by six additional drugs, four of them without apparent cross-resistance against the four most active agents. Five additional drugs warrant further exploration, because of observed tumor regression in a small number of patients treated.

D. Large Cell Carcinoma

The composition of patient samples with large cell carcinoma is somewhat variable because of the varying proportions of patients with poorly differentiated epidermoid and adenocarcinomas in this group [77].

Procarbazine might be the most effective agent, followed by mechlorethamine, adriamycin, and cyclophosphamide, all with response rates of more than 20% (Table V).

Methotrexate is only marginally effective, in contrast to other cell types. Mitomycin C, streptonigrin, and vinblastine warrant further exploration because of activity in the small numbers of patients thus far treated and because of expected lack of cross-resistance with the drugs of established efficacy.

E. Drugs with Insufficient Data on Effect by Cell Type

Depending on minimum criteria for "initial therapeutic trials" [106] only 9 to 12 of 56 antineoplastic agents listed in this chapter were at least marginally studied in all four major types of bronchogenic carcinoma. These agents include adriamycin, cyclophosphamide, hexamethylmelamine, mechlorethamine, methotrexate, the three nitrosoureas (BCNU, CCNU, and methyl-CCNU), and procarbazine. 1-Methyl-1-nitrosourea, mitomycin C, and vinblastine could be added if even one single response in the smallest number of patients were regarded as adequate.

Twenty-three additional drugs received attention but remained "inadequately" tested by cell type (Table VI). The best known among these drugs are cytarabine, the tumor-inhibiting antibiotics, except for adriamycin and, possibly mitomycin (*vida supra*), fluorouracil, hydroxyurea, the thiopurines, and vincristine (VCR).

Closure of these gaps, at least for drugs of novel structure and/or novel action, would broaden the basis of monochemotherapy and would, therefore, be highly desirable.

TABLE VI
**Objective Response of Lung Cancer to Single Drugs
with Insufficient Data on Response by Cell Type[a]**

Drug	Percent responding		Patients treated	Reference
	All patients	Range		
Acetyl picolinoylhydrazine	0	—	10	[127]
Aminochrysene	0	—	19	[66]
Busulfane	9	7–21	169	
Chlorambucil	5	—	21	
Colchicine	3	0–4	30	
Cytarabine	0	—	19	
Dactinomycin	0	—	16	
Daunorubicin	7	—	14	
Dichloromethotrexate	9	—	22	[5]
Emetine, dehydroemetine	17	—	35	
Flourouracil	7	0–36	157	
Hydroxyurea	16	0–26	88	[30]
Ifosfamide	80	—	20[b]	[103]
Imidazole carboxamide, dimethyl triazeno	11	10–25	132	[69]
Melphalan, sarcolysine	7	3–11	67	
Mercaptopurine	3	0–4	105	
1-Methyl-1-nitrosourea	31	22–63	93	
Mithramycin	0	—	23	
Mitomycin C	23	8–27	203	[44, 67]
(cis-) Platinum diamminodichloride	11	—	9	[68, 98]
Podophyllotoxins	8	0–16	66	[85]
Porfiromycin	7	—	42	
Streptonigrin	11	0–29	53	
Thiopeta	15	7–32	141	
Vinblastine	7	0–20	239	
Vinchristine	14	5–33	43	[56]

[a] From Selawry [105].
[b] Limited to small cell carcinoma. Some patients might have also received radiotherapy.

F. Drugs Not Tested for Objective Response in Lung Cancer

An additional group of 21 drugs remain untested against lung cancer (Table VII). Of these, L-asparaginase was compared with cyclophosphamide for survival only, with equivocal results: suggestive superiority, equality and inferiority, respectively, against epidermoid carcinoma in three subsequent trials by the same investigators (Table X).

L-Asparaginase, as most of the other drugs in this group, shows novel chemical structure and/or action. Four of these drugs are also nonmyelo-

TABLE VII

Some Drugs Untested for Objective Response in Lung Cancer[a]

Drug	Reason for interest	
	Nonmyelosuppressive	Novel structure
L-Asparaginase	+	+
Acronyazine	+	+
Aminothiadiazole		+
Anguidine		+
Azacytidine		+
Baker's antifole		+
Camptothecin		+
Cycloleucine		+
Diglycoaldehyde		+
Gallium nitrate		+
Guanazole		+
ICRF 159 (Diketopiperazine)		+
Neocarzinostatin		+
Phosphoramide		+
Piperazinedione		+
Prospidine		+
Pyrazomycin		+
Streptozotocin	+	+
Tetrandrine		+
Thalicarpine	+	+
Trityl cysteine		+

[a] Information on source, availability, and tolerance of drugs can be obtained through Dr. M. Slavik, Chief, Investigational Drug Branch, CTE, DCT, National Cancer Institute, Building 37, Room 6E20, Bethesda, Maryland 20014.

suppressive and would lend themselves readily for combination with myelo-suppressive agents. Several drugs might show lack of cross-resistance to agents of known therapeutic value and might enrich our armamentarium of clinically useful tumor inhibitory agents.

G. Relation of Objective Response to Survival

Objective response to monochemotherapy lasts for a median of 3 months [108] and is usually associated with prolonged survival. The most surprising data in this respect are reported for bleomycin in epidermoid carcinoma (Table VIII), where 44 patients received 15–30 mg twice weekly i.v. or i.m. to a total of about 300 mg. Response was documented by chest film, bronchoscopy, and pulmonary function studies for each patient [88–90]. The objective response rate was 30%. Twelve of the 13 responders were alive at a median of 14+ months as compared with a median survival of only 3 months for the nonresponders. Only 7 of 31 nonresponders

TABLE VIII

Effect by Cell Type of Objective Response on Survival of Patients with Lung Cancer

Drug	Cell type	Median survival (months)		No. of patients		$p \leqslant 05$	Reference
		Responders	Nonre-sponders	Responders	Nonre-sponders		
Bleomycin	Epidermoid	14+	3	12/31[a]	7/31	+	[88–90]
	Adenocarcinoma	28+	2	2/2	0/5	b	
Mechlorethamine							[92]
Cyclophosphamide	Epidermoid	12	6	11	109	+	
Ethylenimines	Small cell	6.7	2.9	23	57	+	
Sarcolysine	Adenocarcinoma	4.5	not given	1	37	−	
1-Methyl-1-nitrosoureas	Large cell	7.5	4	2	6	−	
Antibiotics							
Antimetabolites							
as single events							
CTX + MTX[c]	Epidermoid	4.5	1.7	2	17	b	[52, 109]
	Small cell	7.3	3.1	8	15	+	
	Adenocarcinoma	8.6	4.0	1	16	b	
CTX + MTX + CCNU[c]	Epidermoid	5.7	3.1	2	15	b	
	Small cell	8.8	3	18	13	+	
	Adenocarcinoma	8.1	6.1	6	14	−	
CTX + MTX + VCR + PROC	Epidermoid	6.5	3.3	12	19	−	4
simultaneously	Small cell	7.8	2.5	29	11		

[a] Patients surviving/patients treated.
[b] No statement on significance.
[c] Mechlorethamine used instead of CTX for epidermoid and large cell carcinoma.

were alive at the time of publication. These results are supported by a much smaller series of patients; 7 of 12 patients with epidermoid carcinoma and 1 of 2 patients with anaplastic carcinoma had regressions of pulmonary lesions of 25% to less than 50%, regressions that are otherwise discounted for the tables of this chapter. The "responders" lived for a median of 12 months, the nonresponders for median of 3.5 months [119]. The high response rates in these studies might be related to the relatively early stage of disease of the patients and, in the case of the second study, to the more lenient criteria for response.

Most other studies also show—at times statistically significant—prolongation of survival of responders over nonresponders (Tables VIII and IX) and, in support of Israel, survival gain for patients with arrest of tumor growth short of objective regression. Data on combination chemotherapy are included in Table VIII to obviate the need for repetition.

Two studies are notable exceptions and show no survival gain of responders over nonresponders (adenocarcinoma treated with CTX + MTX + CCNU, Table VIII, and adriamycin, Table IX). This is not readily explained, since there was no apparent undue toxicity that could have counterbalanced the potential benefits of objective response, and the treatments were no more immunosuppressive than in other studies.

The difficulties of using survival as the only criterion for response were already discussed. This is illustrated in five controlled clinical trials (Table X). The first two trials showed statistically significant superiority of cyclophosphamide over placebo for small cell carcinoma and of mechlorethamine for epidermoid carcinoma. Thus, it appeared that different bifunctional alkylating agents can have different tumor spectra. This concept was later widely advanced for other classes of drugs, such as the *Vinca* alkaloids (vinblastine and vincristine), the nitrosoureas, (BCNU, CCNU, and methyl-CCNU), and the anthracyclines (adriamycin and rubidomycin).

The remaining three trials in Table X represent successive studies by the same investigators comparing a "low" dose of asparaginase with cyclophosphamide as standard drug. It will be noted how variable the data are from study to study, in part, probably because of the relatively small number of patients.

IV. OLIGO- AND POLYCHEMOTHERAPY

However encouraging and important the data on the almost 9000 patients included under monochemotherapy, it is only a minority of the patient population that responds. The survival gain of responders is

TABLE IX

Effect (Including All Cell Types) of Objective Response on Survival in Patients with Lung Cancer

Drug	Survival (months)		No. of patients		$p \leq 05$	Reference
	Responders	Nonresponders	Responders	Nonresponders		
Adriamycin	7.3	6.3	11[a]	12[a]	—	[22]
CCNU or methyl-CCNU	12.6	6.3 Static 2.3 Progressive	6	39 Static 79 Progressive		[36]
Hexamethylmelamine	33 CR[e] 8.4 PR[e]	6 Static 2.6 Progressive	1 12	16 41	b	[108]
Hexamethylmelamine	10.9	3.3	10	10	c	[122]
Mechlorethamine	7	3.5	8	13	—	[62]
Mechlorethamine[d]	7.2	3.3	24	121	—	[37]
Methotrexate	6.7	4.0	9	50	b	[108]
Thiotepa	17.3	7.9	5	43	c	[2]

[a] Patients without prior chemotherapy.
[b] Difference between responders and nonresponders significant.
[c] No statement on significance.
[d] Mechlorethamine or cyclophosphamide alone, or in combination, i.e., HN_2 + CCNU or CTX + CCNU.
[e] CR, complete tumor regression; PR, partial tumor regression.

TABLE X

Response of Lung Cancer to Single Drugs as Measured by Survival[a]

Drug	Survival, median (months)				Patient number				Reference
	Epidermoid carcinoma	Small	Adeno-carcinoma	Large cell carcinoma	Epidermoid carcinoma	Small cell carcinoma	Adeno-carcinoma	Large cell carcinoma	
Cyclophosphamide	2.7	4.0[b]	2.5	2.5	81	57	69	139	[50]
Placebo	2.6	1.4[b]	2.6	1.7	124	87	101	204	
Mechlorethamine	6	2.5	1.9	2.8	66	70	38	91	
Placebo	3	1.8	2.8	2.0	229	127	136	300	
Cyclophosphamide[c]	4.8	3.3	2.4	2.5	22	14	14	11	[64]
L-Asparaginase[d]	6.3	4.1	3.5	1.5	7	4	6	7	
Cyclophosphamide[c]	2.6	1.5	3.1	2.8	16	10	21	17	
L-Asparaginase[d]	2.7	2.7	2.0	1.1	30	12	18	10	
Cyclophosphamide[c]	3.6	2.8	2.8	3.5	58	34	26	34	
L-Asparaginase[d]	1.3	0.9	1.1	1.5	14	8	11	6	

[a] Controlled Clinical Trials by the Veteran's Administration Lung Group.
[b] Difference statistically significant.
[c] Cyclophosphamide dose 1100 mg/m² every 3 weeks. i.v.
[d] L-Asparaginase dose 150 IU/kg/week for 6 weeks, i.v.

usually measured in months instead of years. And long-term survival is too anecdotal to distinguish it from the small number of patients with an unusually bland natural course of disease.

Moderate improvements are within reach by better use of established agents [optimal dose, optimal schedule for cell cycle phase-specific drugs and possibly for nitrosourea [16, 60], optimal duration of treatment] and by vigorous exploration of hitherto untested and new drugs. A major breakthrough, however, is highly unlikely with the use of single drugs in patients with advanced cancer. Thus, the experience with monochemo-therapy becomes the indispensable stepping stone for oligo- and polychemo-therapy and for combination of chemotherapy with other modalities of treatment, notably surgery, radiotherapy, and immunologic manipulation.

The use of two or more drugs, simultaneously or in short succession, received the greatest impetus from antimicrobial chemotherapy. The basic pharmacologic principles were empirically applied to cancer in man and yielded survival comparable with that of healthy persons for a spectrum of tumors, notably Wilms' tumor and acute leukemia of children and Hodgkins' disease and malignant trophoblastic tumors in adults. Lesser, although impressive, results were obtained in common types of solid tumors, such as breast cancer [22].

The term oligochemotherapy might be used for combination of two or three drugs, polychemotherapy for administration of four or more agents. There is no precedent for strict definitions. Both terms are used in contra-distinction to combination chemotherapy as the combination of chemo-therapy with other modalities of treatment, such as surgery, and/or radio-therapy.

The minimal requirements for successful oligo- and polychemotherapy are met for all four major types of lung cancer, foremost for small cell carcinoma; they include the following.

a. The criterion of the established antitumor activity of each component drug is applied to the 56 drugs listed in the preceding section. Exceptions are conceivable: sequential use of methotrexate and leucovorin, its anti-dote, was already mentioned [34, 35, 74] and is based on conclusive ani-mal experiments [47]. Another example includes a pilot study where 25 patients with lung cancer were randomized to either a five-drug combina-tion alone or the identical five drugs plus anticoagulant doses of heparin for 1–2 weeks. Eight of the 12 patients on heparin experienced objective response; none of the 13 patients on five-drug combination alone re-sponded [38]. A larger prospective controlled study is currently underway.

b. Different mode of action and lack of cross-resistance are usually preferable for combination chemotherapy. The biochemical [102] and experimental [46] backgrounds are discussed elsewhere.

c. Divergent toxicity is desirable for administration of full or close to full doses of each component drug, lest polychemotherapy fails for lack of adequate dosage of effective agents. This consideration explains the wide use of drugs that partially spare the bone marrow, notably bleomycin, cyclophosphamide, and vincristine. For the same reason would it be desirable to explore the antitumor activity of nonmyelosuppressive drugs (Table VII).

Another aspect of divergent toxicity includes the time sequence after drug administration during which toxicity occurs and the expected effect on cell kinetics of dose limiting normal tissue and of tumor tissue. This consideration leads to the combination of cell cycle stage nonspecific drugs with delayed toxicity, notably the nitrosoureas, with cell cycle phase-specific agents with fast occurrence of toxicity, such as methotrexate [52, 109].

The author has 46 current clinical trials with two or more drugs on record, including well over 2000 patients. It might be expected, therefore, that most major conceptual alternatives are covered. This is not the case. Moreover, only 18 trials are controlled, some with duplication of effort.

Because of difficulties in the evaluation of smaller, uncontrolled studies, the following discussion will be limited to the four controlled clinical trials included in Table XI, amplified with separately listed uncontrolled data for one of the studies [3].

The first study shows statistically significant increase of objective response of small cell carcinoma to cyclophosphamide plus CCNU as compared to cyclophosphamide alone [37]. The effect is more than additive and does not extend to identically treated patients with adenocarcinoma. Combination of cyclophosphamide with a nitrosourea, in this and other studies, was based on superior results against Lewis lung tumor in mice, when compared to maximal response to the component drugs [79]. Combination of mechlorethamine with CCNU is of no advantage for patients with epidermoid and large cell carcinomas, when compared to mechlorethamine alone. The latter drug had been chosen for combination because of apparent superiority over cyclophosphamide as shown in Table X [50].

The second study implies more than additive superiority of another two-drug combination, procarbazine plus fluorouracil, over procarbazine alone for patients with epidermoid carcinoma and, possibly, adenocarcinoma, but no apparent advantage for patients with small cell carcinoma [15]. The data fall short of statistical significance.

Significant superiority of a three-drug combination of CCNU plus cyclophosphamide plus methotrexate over the latter two drugs alone was seen in the increase of time to progressive disease (time to change of treatment regimen) from 3 to 6 months accompanied by an increase of median

TABLE XI
Oligo- and Polychemotherapy of Lung Cancer

Drugs	Response by cell type[a]				No. of patients by cell type[a]				Reference
	Epid.	Small	Adeno.	Large	Epid.	Small	Adeno.	Large	
CTX	—	28[b]	15	—	—	88	26	—	[37]
CTX + CCNU	—	45	5	—	—	83	21	—	
Mechlorethamine	10	—	—	16	41	—	—	19	
Mechlorethamine + CCNU	3	—	—	6	39	—	—	17	
Procarbazine	12	50	0	45	8	2	5	11	[15]
Procarbazine + fluorouracil	55	44	83	40	11	9	6	10	
CTX + MTX	—	31	6	—	—	23	17	—	[52, 109]
CTX + MTX + CCNU	—	57	30	—	—	31	20	—	
Mechlorethamine + MTX	11	—	—	8	19	—	—	13	
Mechlorethamine + MTX + CCNU	12	—	—	11	17	—	—	9	
PROC + CTX + MTX + VCR									
Sequentially every 2 weeks	14	27	0	0	22	11	2	3[c]	[3, 4]
Simultaneously	39	69[b]	0	0	18	16	3	1[c]	
Simultaneously, random + nonrandom	28	62	71	50	46	53	7	19[c]	

[a] Epid., epidermoid carcinoma; Small, small cell carcinoma; Adeno., adenocarcinoma; Large, large cell carcinoma.

[b] Statistically significant superiority.

[c] Includes large cell anaplastic and "other" bronchogenic carcinomas.

survival from 5.7 to 8.3 months for small cell carcinoma and a significant prolongation of median survival from 4.5 to 8 months for patients with adenocarcinoma. In each case, there was also an impressive increase in response rate and a marked prolongation of survival in responders as compared to nonresponders (Table VIII). Results could be further improved by more frequent administration of CCNU [16, 60] and by scheduling of methotrexate in accordance with cell kinetic considerations (M. Straus, personal communication). Again, all advantage was lost, when mechlorethamine was used instead of cyclophosphamide for treatment of epidermoid and large cell carcinomas in otherwise identical drug regimens —either these two types of lung cancer are less responsive or cyclophosphamide renders itself particularly well to combination with CCNU. The latter possibility does not bear out, however, for treatment of adenocarcinoma, as noted in Table VIII, CTX + MTX + CCNU entries.

There are no published data for comparison of a four-drug combination with a smaller number of drugs. Combination of three myelosuppressive drugs requires already substantial decreases in dosage (and efficacy?), when compared to monochemotherapy. Thus, increase of the number of drugs per combination above an "optimum" might yield diminishing returns, except for inclusion of marrow-sparing drugs and for thorough planning (*vida supra*). Instead, a controlled trial of four-drugs is presented, where procarbazine, cyclophosphamide, methotrexate, and vincristine were used simultaneously or in sequential, 2-week courses [3, 4]. Simultaneous drug administration was significantly superior to sequential treatment for objective response in small cell carcinoma and was suggestively superior for epidermoid carcinoma. Uncontrolled data in adeno- and large cell carcinoma are also worth following. The responders lived longer than the nonresponders (Table VIII). Other drug combinations look promising, notably for treatment of small cell carcinoma [78].

In summary, definite progress has been made, proving superiority of oligochemotherapy with up to 3 drugs over monochemotherapy for all but large cell carcinoma. Substantial improvements seem to be within reach, especially for small cell carcinoma and, possibly, for adenocarcinoma.

V. REGIONAL DRUG ADMINISTRATION

Three approaches to regional or topical chemotherapy are considered: injection of drugs into the pleural or pericardial cavity for control of carcinomatous effusion, intraarterial infusion, and endobronchial, topical drug administration. In each case, it is hoped to achieve higher drug concentrations in the tumor and less toxicity to the host.

Intrapleural and intrapericardial chemotherapy are indicated when other measures of treatment [drainage, systemic chemotherapy, injection of a sclerosing agent such as quinacrine of insufflation of talcum into the pleural cavity (not into the pericardium), radiotherapy, where indicated, or radioactive isotopes) fail.

Mechlorethamine, 0.2–0.4 mg/kg, or thiotepa, 0.4–0.8 mg/kg, are the most commonly used drugs for control of pleural carcinomatosis after removal of all fluid. Both agents are local irritants in addition to their tumoricidal effect. Mechlorethamine has the added advantage of rapid inactivation and, perhaps, less hematologic toxicity, when given intrapleurally. Nevertheless, systemic toxicity is common. Therefore, the dosage of repeated treatments is adjusted to hematologic toxicity and is usually administered within no less than 1 week after the first treatment.

Data on intrapericardial instillation of drugs are anecdotal because pericardial involvement is usually asymptomatic; in our own hospital, pericardial tumor involvement was noted at autopsy in 20% of 126 patients with epidermoid carcinoma, in 18% of 102 patients with small cell carcinoma, and in 25% of 110 patients with adenocarcinoma and 80 patients with large cell carcinoma, respectively [77]. Yet, symptoms and/or signs compatible with pericardial effusion were noted in less than one-third of the patients, and the diagnosis was confirmed by the presence of tumor cells in the cytocentrifugate of the effusion in only 7% of the patients. Local chemotherapy was rarely indicated. We hesitated to use mechlorethamine, thiotepa, or quinacrine because of their local irritant effect, in spite of the precedent in the literature with reports of good tolerance and therapeutic benefit [116]. We saw occasionally good responses with methotrexate, 10–20 mg/m² body surface area in repeat doses, adjusted to systemic toxicity. Another nonirritant drug of potential benefit is fluorouracil, in doses of 500 mg. Cyclophosphamide has also been used, but is clearly not indicated because it has to be activated in the liver.

Intrathecal administration of methotrexate, 12 mg/m² once or twice weekly, for treatment of the occasional carcinomatous meningeopathy is mentioned en passant.

Intraarterial drug administration was usually attempted through the bronchial artery [51]; preference for the bronchial artery is based on evidence that all or most of the blood supply to primary bronchogenic carcinomas is supplied through this channel, in contrast to metastatic lesions in the lung, which might receive part or all of their arterial blood from the pulmonary artery [76].

The methodology for arterial catherization is difficult. Currently available data give little evidence for superiority of this approach over systemic chemotherapy (Table XII).

TABLE XII

Intraarterial Chemotherapy for Lung Cancer

Drug	Dose (mg)	Artery	Patients		Reference
			No.	%	
Fluorouracil	1000/24 hour	Bronchial	55	13	[40]
	250/course	Bronchial	5	"40"?	[84][a]
	60–90/kg/course	i.v.	157	7	Table VI
Mechlorethamine	0.4–0.6/kg	Bronchial	21	33[b]	[26]
	10–20	Bronchial	5	20	[123]
	0.3–0.4/kg/initial course	i.v.	1442	31	Table I
Methotrexate	50–125, 2–3 daily	Pulmonary	5	40	[51]
then leucovorin	Miscellaneous	i.v.	416	22	Table I
Mitomycin	10/course	Bronchial	22	37	[84][a]
	50/course	i.v.	203	23	Table VI

[a] Treatment preoperative.

[b] One patient died 3¾ years later without tumor at autopsy.

It stands to reason that radiotherapy is superior to chemotherapy for control of regional disease [108] and that drugs for intraarterial administration should have a half-life time of a few seconds or fractions thereof, rather than minutes or hours, to achieve high concentrations in the tumor and low concentrations in the rapidly equilibrating, systemic circulation which carries the drugs to the dose-limiting normal host tissues. The picture is further complicated by the extensive anastomoses between the bronchial and the pulmonary vessels of the lung, permitting arterial blood supply from either system, especially in the periphery of the lung and under unphysiologic conditions of differential arterial pressure (cough, extrinsic pressure).

Topical treatment by means of aerosol chemotherapy might be more promising than intraarterial treatment, especially for bronchiolar carcinoma with extensive bronchial spread or for carcinoma *in situ*, in situations where surgery or radiotherapy might be contraindicated, because high topical concentrations can be achieved and little or no systemic toxicity might be seen, especially when poorly soluble drugs are used.

Studies with aerosols of tantalum dust for bronchography showed excellent distribution of this agent, with proper particle size [41]. The use of an aerosol (particle size less than 8 μm) of two double-stranded RNA preparations from a mycophage in mice showed prolonged survival in a carcinogen-induced fibrosarcoma and statistically significantly fewer pulmonary metastases of subcutaneously implanted Lewis lung tumor when compared to untreated controls [53]. It would be interesting to expand these studies to permit extension into the clinic.

VI. COMBINATION CHEMOTHERAPY

This section will be limited to the combination of chemotherapy with surgery and with radiotherapy, respectively, with a focus on randomized clinical trials. No controlled clinical studies are on record for the combination of chemotherapy with hyperthermia, fever, or ultrasound; and combination of immunotherapy with other modalities of treatment is described elsewhere in this book.

The rationale of combination chemotherapy is based on solid experimental evidence in carcinogen-induced and in transplantable rodent tumors. These experiments indicate that chemotherapy (as well as radiotherapy) induce proportional cell kill: a certain *proportion* of sensitive cells are killed per drug dose [114]. Hence, micrometastases are more likely to be "cured" than large tumor masses.

Clinical experience tends to support this concept. This is well illustrated in patients with malignant lymphoma who relapse after induction of complete regression; relapse occurs frequently at those sites that had the most bulky tumor masses prior to initiation of therapy.

Hence, combination of chemotherapy with surgery and/or radiotherapy might be indicated in three situations: as adjuvant to local eradication of cancer, when micrometastases are suspected; as primary treatment of metastatic cancer, when radiotherapy (or reductive surgery) offer adjuvant control of bulky tumor masses; for local, adjuvant treatment of metastatic sites, such as the meninges and possibly the brain, which are poorly accessible to certain drugs.

A. Adjuvant Chemotherapy

At present, there is no hard evidence for the superiority of surgical adjuvant chemotherapy over surgery alone: the only study with positive outcome includes the postsurgical treatment of small cell carcinoma with prolonged courses of cyclophosphamide (Table XIII). At least twice as many treated patients survived 2, 3, 4 and 5 years, respectively, than the untreated controls. The numbers of patients are too small to reach statistical significance. These positive data would have remained unrecognized if results had not been evaluated by cell type.

Eight controlled clinical trials including 5019 patients showed no ad-

TABLE XIII

Controlled Trial of Surgical Adjuvant Chemotherapy with Probably Positive Outcome in Patients with Small Cell Carcinoma[a]

Treatment	2	3	4	5	No. of patients
Cyclophosphamide[b]	28	22	16	9	32
Placebo	22	8	4	4	26

[a] From Heyes and Catherall [53] and Selawry *et al.* [109].
[b] Eight mg/kg/day five times i.v. every 5 weeks for 18 months.

vantage for chemotherapy (Table XIV); a first series of studies were designed to attack circulating tumor cells, which might have been dislodged in the course of surgery. Chemotherapy was, therefore, given for only short periods of time, including mechlorethamine [54, 115] and vinblastine [31].

The failure of these studies was explained with insufficient cell kill during the short treatment periods. Subsequent studies featured chemotherapy for $1\frac{1}{2}$ to 4 years, shorter in case of recurrent disease, and were directed toward micrometastases. One of these studies showed a distinct disadvantage of cyclophosphamide over placebo, with earlier and more common relapse in the treated patients [19, 20]. This important observation might imply suppression of immunologic or other host factors by weekly courses of cyclophosphamide for 8 weeks, alternating with equal time periods without treatment. Disadvantage extended to all cell types.

We conclude that surgical adjuvant chemotherapy should be limited to prospective clinical trials, with the possible exception of small cell carcinoma. Widely spaced doses or treatment courses (3–6 week intervals) might be less immunosuppressive than daily or weekly medication. Combinations of drugs might be used, when they are superior to single agents, in patients with advanced disease. Failure of one trial with combination chemotherapy as adjuvant [63] might also have been due to limited efficacy of the drug combination when used alone in advanced disease. More extensive discussions of the subject are presented in three excellent reviews [24, 65, 82].

Combination of chemotherapy and radiotherapy was investigated in 23 prospective, randomized trials, including more than 2000 patients. Important background information is available in recent reviews [10, 93].

The results are more encouraging with reports of significant superiority of combination therapy over radiotherapy alone in three trials (Table XV). These three studies included full doses of radiotherapy, combined with full courses of chemotherapy, given to moderate toxicity.

TABLE XIV

Controlled Clinical Trials of Surgical Adjuvant Chemotherapy with Negative Outcome

Treatment	Drug dose (mg)	Schedule	No. of patients	Reference
Cyclophosphamide	8/kg/day 5 times	Every 5 weeks for 18 months	504[a]	[54]
Placebo	Same		621	
Cyclophosphamide	12/kg/week 8 times	Every 4 months for 2 years	70	[19, 20]
Placebo	Same		69	
Cyclophosphamide	200/day p.o. 10 times, then 150/day	For 2 years	259	[80]
Busulfane	4/day p.o. 10 times, then 31/day	For 2 years	254	
Placebo	Same		249	
Cyclophosphamide[b]	8/kg/day 5 times	Every 5 weeks for 18 months	96	[110]
Cyclophosphamide + methotrexate	10/kg/day 5 times, alternating with CYCL every 5 weeks	Every 5 weeks for 18 months	103	
Placebo	Same		110	
Cyclophosphamide	12/kg			
Methotrexate	0.5/kg weekly 3 times		55	[63]
Fluorouracil	12/kg every 4 weeks to a total of 13/year			
Vinblastine	0.1/kg			
Placebo	Same		27	
Mechlorethamine	0.4/kg subdivided doses before and at surgery		620	[54]
Placebo	0.3/kg day after surgery		623	
Mechlorethamine	0.4/kg subdivided doses before and at surgery, later reduced to a total dose of 0.3/kg		588	[114]
Placebo	Same		604	
Vinblastine	0.1/kg/week i.v., to individual tolerance[c]	For 3 months	86	[31]
Placebo	Same		81	

[a] Excluding patients with small cell cancer.
[b] Preliminary data.
[c] Possible advantage for small cell cancers.

TABLE XV

Controlled Trials with Positive Outcomes of Combination of Chemotherapy and Radiotherapy in Lung Cancer

Treatment	Survival (months)	$p \leqslant 0.05$	No. of Patients	Reference
RT 400–500 R/4–5 wks	7.2 median	+	42	[9]
RT + CTX 1 gm/m² every 3 weeks, 4 times			38	
RT + CTX 1 gm/m² every 3 weeks, 8 times	10.2 median		35	
RT 6000 R/6 weeks	31% 1 year	+[b]	48[b]	[17]
RT + CTX 200 mg/day 5 times per week	35% 1 year		46	
RT 5000 R/5 weeks	4.9 mean	+	15	[59]
RT followed by chlorambucil[a] 2–8 mg/day	7.6 mean		15	

[a] Dose adjusted to WBC 2000 to 4000/mm³.
[b] Superior objective response, when evaluated by chest film plus bronchoscopy.

All three studies are of methodologic interest. The first study indicates a modest, 42% gain in median survival for patients on radiotherapy and cyclophosphamide over radiotherapy alone. The survival gain for the subgroup of patients with small cell carcinoma exceeds 100% (from 5 to 10+ months), as might be expected because of the known sensitivity of this tumor to either component of this treatment. Spacing the drug doses at 3 week intervals was less immunosuppressive than daily or weekly medication. Interestingly, the use of eight drug doses was not better than limitation to four doses of cyclophosphamide. This attests to the importance of the optimal duration of chemotherapy, in addition to optimal dose and optimal schedule.

The second study advanced our knowledge of the methodology of tumor measurements: superiority of adjuvant chemotherapy would have been missed if only routine chest films had been used for determination of tumor regression. Endobronchial observation alone indicated a higher response rate for combined treatment. Combination of chest films and endobronchial observation led to discordant findings in several patients (endobronchial regression without regression of chest films or vice versa). Elimination of the discordant patients from evaluation showed a statistically significant difference of tumor regression from 29% for radiotherapy alone to 78% for combined treatment [17, 18]. Unfortunately, this difference was not reflected in 1-year survival (Table XV).

The third study might support the contention of increased efficacy of drugs in early diseases [59]; "standard" radiotherapy was compared with radiotherapy plus chlorambucil. The drug was given to toxicity (white blood cell count of 2000 to 4000/mm³) over prolonged time periods. The choice of chlorambucil for adjuvant treatment was clearly suboptimal, with a reported objective response rate of only 5% (Table VI). Nevertheless, there was a 50% increase in median survival of patients on adjuvant chemotherapy, which was regarded to be statistically significant.

The trials with "negative" outcome showed either no advantage for combination chemotherapy or statistically insignificant advantage or disadvantage.

Review of some of these "negative" data is rewarding. The discussion follows the sequence of trials as they are listed in Table XVI.

TABLE XVI

Controlled Clinical Trials with Negative Outcomes of Combination of Chemotherapy and Radiotherapy in Lung Cancer

Drug	Comment	Reference
Cyclophosphamide	20–40 mg/kg/day	[104]
	50 mg/kg/day 1 + 35, increased median survival of small cell carcinoma[a]	[125]
	80 mg/kg/day 5 times, every 5 weeks	[50]
	400 mg total dose i.v., then 100 mg/day increase survival	[55]
	400 mg total dose/day p.o., no control of radiotherapy only	[48, 49]
Dactinomycin	—	[108] (Hosley)
Fluorodeoxyuridine	Improved survival for low dose fluorouracil[a]	[108]
Fluorouracil (FU) 10 or 12 mg/kg/day five times	FU + 2000 R superior to 2000 R alone but not to 4000 R alone for objective tumor response. No change of median survival. Treatment of 2 or more metastatic lesions in the same patient	[108]
	No difference for first 2 years— 2/21 adjuvant—patients survive 5 years	[58]
	Suggestive advantage for adenocarcinoma only	[108] (Carr) [108] (Hosley)
Mechlorethamine	Simultaneously or before radiotherapy	[108] (Krant)
	Only 3 doses of chemotherapy	[108] (Durrant)
	Single dose before radiotherapy for superior vena caval obstruction	[108] (Levitt)

TABLE XVI (continued)

Drug	Comment	Reference
Methotrexate (MTX)	—	[108] (Hosley)
	MTX immediately before each radiotherapy treatment. Median survival increased from 8 to 12 months; 1 year survival from 12.5 to 42% epidermoid carcinoma only[a]	[124]
Methotrexate + cyclophosphamide	Suggestive disadvantage of response and survival in adenocarcinoma No advantage for small cell cancer	[52, 109]
Methotrexate + mechlorethamine	Disadvantage for epidermoid (significant) and large cell carcinoma	
Methotrexate + cyclophosphamide + vincristine	More complete remissions, longer survival[a]	[77]
Procarbazine	—	[101]
	Statistically insignificant disadvantage	[75]
Vinblastine	—	[29]

[a] Small number of patients.

The positive data on cyclophosphamide as adjuvant [9] are in contra-distinction to a very similar study [104]. Five to seven spaced doses of cyclophosphamide, 20–40 mg/kg (or 700–1600 mg/m^2) were given to a total dose of 10–14 gm. Neither median nor long-term survival favored cyclophosphamide. The reason for this discrepancy remains unresolved. One other study, with a different dose schedule of cyclophosphamide, also shows no benefit of adjuvant treatment [50].

Two other studies suggest superiority of adjuvant cyclophosphamide over radiotherapy alone but fall short of statistical significance [55, 125].

The role of dactinomycin and of fluoropyrimidines as adjuvants is diffi-cult to assess because data on response by cell type are unavailable and because both agents are either ineffective or only marginally effective against lung cancer (Table VI). Neither agent shows superiority over treatment with full doses of radiotherapy alone. Suggestive advantage for adjuvant fluorouracil in bronchogenic adenocarcinoma needs confirmation [107].

Strongly suggestive disadvantage for adjuvant oligochemotherapy with prolonged courses of methotrexate and either cyclophosphamide or me-chlorethamine [52, 109] in all but small cell carcinoma is disappointing.

In summary, then, chemotherapy as adjuvant to radiotherapy remains experimental and controversial but worth further exploration. The use of full doses of both treatment modalities appears currently desirable. Chemotherapy might best be given in spaced doses. Leads on the promise of cyclophosphamide for epidermoid and small cell carcinoma and for fluorouracil in adenocarcinoma are worth following and might provide good stepping stones for improvement of therapy. Sequential use of both modalities might provide kinetic advantages [126]. More detailed discussions are presented in recent reviews [10, 57, 58].

B. Chemotherapy and Adjuvant Reductive Treatment of the Primary Tumor Site

No published data are available on surgery or radiotherapy as adjuvants to chemotherapy for treatment of lung cancer.

Adjuvant, reductive surgery might be considered, where surgical cure rates are low because of early metastatic spread, such as in small cell carcinoma. Radiotherapy might be preferred as treatment of choice for local control because of the sensitivity of small cell carcinoma to ionizing rays, as evidenced by apparent equality of radiotherapy to surgery as prime treatment for small cell carcinoma [81]. Yet, combination of both modalities for treatment of "resectable" small cell carcinoma in an uncontrolled study of 29 patients yielded an astounding 4-year survival of 24% [6], as compared to 3–5% for surgery alone [108] and 7% for radiotherapy alone [81], despite the relatively low presurgical radiation dose of 1750 rad midplane dose (MPD) in daily increments of 250 rad in 8 day's overall time.

Adjuvant radiotherapy is included in several comparative clinical trials for treatment of small cell carcinoma. Results should soon be available.

C. Chemotherapy and Adjuvant Radiotherapy for Cerebral Metastases

Little is known about the uptake of systemically administered antineoplastic agents by tumor cells of cerebral metastases. Progression of cerebral metastases in the presence of objective response of primary tumor and of extracerebral metastases is particularly common in patients with prolonged systemic response of small cell carcinoma. Such lesions are usually well controlled with corticosteroids for symptomatic relief and with radiotherapy. The value of elective radiotherapy to the brain in asymptomatic patients with metastatic small cell carcinoma is currently evaluated in controlled clinical trials. Results are expected soon.

VII. SUMMARY AND OUTLOOK

Chemotherapy is of established value for palliative treatment of patients with lung cancer. The choice of treatment and the response depends to a great extent on the cell type of bronchogenic carcinoma. Symptomatic improvement and tumor regression can be expected in approximately 20% or more of the patients and will last for a median of 2–3 months. Moreover, objective response is usually associated with prolongation of survival. Oligo- and polychemotherapy are superior to monochemotherapy for treatment of small cell carcinoma and of adenocarcinoma.

Combination of chemotherapy with surgery is controversial and should be reserved for controlled clinical trials. Benefit is likely for small cell carcinoma. Harm is possible with continuous administration of immuno-suppressive drugs for prolonged time periods.

Chemotherapy as adjuvant to radiotherapy appears to have proved value in some studies, but is of doubtful status in others. It appears to be worth trying, especially in small cell carcinoma, because of good efficacy of both radiotherapy and chemotherapy when used alone.

Pending future trials, it appears advisable to give chemotherapy to definite, well-reversible toxicity and for the duration of response. The latter is usually defined as the time to progression of disease. Time to maximum tumor response might prove to be a better alternative.

Eradication of nonresectable cancer is within reach for small cell carcinoma and, possibly, for adenocarcinoma. Efforts in this direction might be supported by some of the following steps: initial therapeutic studies of unevaluated drugs by cell type; development of mutually non-cross-resistant drug combinations for intensive, sequential use; and improved quantitation of response with endobronchial observation, marker substances, and, possibly, cytology in addition to standard techniques. Moreover, it might become possible to explore nonsurgical treatment of second primary carcinomas *in situ* and of bronchiolar carcinoma by topical endobronchial treatment, where surgery and radiotherapy may be contraindicated.

Finally, progress in experimental studies of anticarcinogenesis might advance sufficiently to permit prospective clinical trials in high risk groups of patients, such as uranium miners [1] and heavy smokers, especially where increasing data on the time intervals from marked atypia to carcinoma *in situ* and to invasive carcinoma become available [99].

ACKNOWLEDGMENTS

The excellent secretarial help of Ms. Tamara Voss is gratefully acknowledged.

REFERENCES

1. Adamek, M., Roth, K., and Stepankova, M., *Oesterr. Z. Erforsch. Bekgemff. Krebskrankh.* **26**, 192–200 (1971).
2. Albert, A. S., Kobozeva, S. A., Maximov, I. A., and Trakhtenberg, A. K., *Riga, Govt. Ed.* pp. 535–536 (1968).
3. Alberto, P., *Cancer Chemother. Rep., Part 3* **4**, 199–206 (1973).
4. Alberto, P., Brunner, K., Martz, G. *et al., Proc. Cancer Congr., 10th, 1970* p. 469 (1971).
5. Band, P., Ross, C. A., and Holland, J. F., *Cancer Chemother. Rep.* **57**, 79–82 (1973).
6. Bates, M., Hurt, R., Levison, V. *et al., Lancet* **1**, 1134–1135 (1974).
7. Batinov, I. N., Thesis, University of Moscow (1970).
8. Ben-Asher, S., *Amer. J. Med. Sci.* **27**, 162–168 (1949).
9. Bergsagel, D. E., Jenkins, R. D. T., Pringle, J. F. *et al., Cancer* **30**, 621–627 (1972).
10. Bleehen, N. M., *Brit. Med. Bull.* **29**, 54–59 (1972).
11. Bleehen, N. M., *Postgrad. Med. J.* **49**, 723–728 (1973).
12. Blum, R. H., Carter, S. K., and Agre, K., *Cancer* **31**, 903–914 (1973).
13. Bodey, G. P., Gottlieb, J. A., Livingston, R. *et al., Cancer Chemother. Rep., Part 3* **4**, 227–230 (1973).
14. Bonadonna, G., *Cancer Chemother. Rep., Part 3* **4**, 231–238 (1973).
15. Bonadonna, G., Monfardini, S., Oldini, C. *et al., Tumori* **55**, 277 (1969).
16. Broder, L., and Hansen, H. H., *Eur. J. Cancer* **9**, 147–152 (1973).
17. Brouet, G., Flamant, R., and Hayat, M., *Eur. J. Cancer* **4**, 129–132 (1968).
18. Brouet, G., Flamant, R., and Hayat, M., *Eur. J. Cancer* **4**, 437–445 (1968).
19. Brunner, K. W., Marthaler, T. H., and Müller, W., *Eur. J. Cancer* **7**, 285–294 (1971).
20. Brunner, K. W., Marthaler, T. H., and Müller, W., *Cancer Chemother. Rep., Part 3* **4**, 125–132 (1973).
21. Bychkov, M. B., Thesis, University of Moscow (1966).
22. Carter, S. K., *Cancer* **30**, 1402–1409 (1972).
23. Carter, S. K., *Cancer* **30**, 1543 (1972).
24. Carter, S. K., *Cancer Chemother. Rep., Part 3* **4**, 109–118 (1973).
25. Chalmers, T. C., *Cancer Chemother. Rep.* **16**, 463–465 (1962).
26. Cliffton, E. E., *Cancer* **23**, 1151–1157 (1969).
27. Cooper, E. H., *Schweiz. Med. Wochenschr.* **104**, 275–276 (1974).

28. Cortes, E. P., Takita, H., and Holland, J. F., *Cancer* **34**, 518–525 (1974).
29. Coy, P., *Cancer* **26**, 803–807 (1970).
30. Creasey, W. A., Capizzi, R. L., and DeConti, R. C., *Cancer Chemother. Rep.* **54**, 191–194 (1970).
31. Crosbie, W. A., Kamdar, H. H., and Belcher, J. R., *Brit. J. Dis. Chest* **60**, 28–35 (1966).
32. Curreri, A., *Cancer Chemother. Rep.* **16**, 123–124 (1962).
33. Cutler, S. J., "End Results in Cancer," Rep. No. 3. U.S. Dept. of Health, Education and Welfare, Public Health Service, Washington, D.C., 1968.
34. Djerassi, I., Kim, J. S., and Suvansri, U., *Proc. Amer. Ass. Cancer Res.* **15**, 78 (1974).
35. Djerassi, I., Rominger, C. J., Kim, J. S. *et al., Cancer* **30**, 22–29 (1972).
36. Eagan, R. T., Carr, D. T., Coles, D. T. *et al., Cancer Chemother. Rep.* **58**, 913–918 (1974).
37. Edmonson, J. H., and Lagakos, S. W., *Proc. Amer. Ass. Cancer Res. and Amer. Soc. Clin. Oncol.* **15**, 180 (1974).
38. Elias, E. G., *Proc. Amer. Ass. Cancer Res.* **14**, Abstr. No. 26 (1973).
39. Falkson, G., van Dyk, J. J., van Eden, E. B. *et al., Cancer* **35**, 1141–1144 (1975).
40. Frikman, H. A., Mendez, F. L., Maurer, E. R. *et al., J. Amer. Med. Ass.* **196**, 5–10 (1966).
41. Gamsu, G., Weintraub, R. M., and Nadel, J. A., *Amer. Rev. Resp. Dis.* **107**, 214–224 (1973).
42. Garin, A. M., *Vop. Onkol.* **16**, 43–48 (1970).
43. Gehan, E. A., *J. Chronic Dis.* **13**, 346–354 (1961).
44. Godfrey, T. E., and Wilbur, D. W., (1972). *Cancer* **29**, 1647–1652 (1972).
45. Goffin, J. C., *J. Belge Radiol.* **55**, 415–423 (1972).
46. Goldin, A., *Cancer Chemother. Rep., Part 3* **4**, 189–198 (1973).
47. Goldin, A., Venditti, J. M., Kline, I. *et al., Nature (London)* **212**, 1548 (1966).
48. Gollin, F., Ansfield, F., Curreri, A. *et al., Cancer* **15**, 1209–1217 (1962).
49. Gollin, F., Ansfield, F., and Vermund, H., *Cancer Chemother. Rep.* **51**, 189–192 (1967).
50. Green, R. A., Humphrey, E., Close, H. *et al., Amer. J. Med.* **46**, 516–524 (1969).
51. Grinberg, R., and Abdelazim, M. I., *Proc. Amer. Ass. Cancer Res.* **14**, Abstr. No. 46 (1973).
52. Hansen, H. H., and Selawry, O. S., Carr, D. T., Sealy, R., and Simon R. *Proc. Int. Cancer Congr., 11th, 1974* **3**, 592.
53. Heyes, J., and Catherall, E. J., *Nature (London)* **247**, 485–487 (1974).
54. Higgins, G., *Cancer* **30**, 1383–1387 (1972).
55. Hoest, H., *Cancer Chemother. Rep., Part 3* **4**, 161–164 (1973).
56. Holland, J. F., Scharlau, C., Gailani, S. *et al., Cancer Res.* **33**, 1258–1264 (1973).
57. Holsti, L. R., *in* "Modern Radiotherapy in Carcinoma of the Bronchus" (T. J. Deeley, ed.), pp. 222–240. Butterworth, London, 1971.
58. Holsti, L. R., *Cancer Chemother. Rep., Part 3* **4**, 164–170. (1973).
59. Horowitz, H., Wright, T. L., and Perry, H., *Amer. J. Roentgenol. Radium Ther. Nucl. Med.* [N.S.] **93**, 615–637 (1965).
60. Israel, L., and Chahinian, P., *Eur. J. Cancer* **9**, 799–802 (1973).
61. Israel, L., Depierre, A., and Chahinian, P., *Proc. Amer. Ass. Cancer Res.* **15**, Abstr. No. 42 (1974).
62. Karnofsky, D. A., Abelmann, W. H., Craver, L. F. *et al., Cancer* **1**, 634–656 (1949).

63. Karrer, K., Pridun, N., and Zwintz, E., *Cancer Chemother. Rep., Part 3* **4,** 207–213 (1973).
64. Kaung, D. T., Wolf, J., Hyde, L., and Zelen, M., *Cancer Chemother. Rep.* **58,** 359–364 (1974).
65. Kenis, Y., *Eur. J. Clin. Biol. Res.* **16,** 103–107 (1971).
66. Kenis, Y., and Levy, P., (1971). *Eur. J. Cancer* **7,** 477–478 (1971).
67. Kenis, Y., and Stryckmans, P., *Cancer Chemother. Rep.* **56,** 151 (1972).
68. Khan, A., and Hill, J. M., *Transplantation* **13,** 55–57 (1972).
69. Kingra, G. S., Comis, R., Olsen, K. B. *et al., Cancer Chemother. Rep., Part 1* **55,** 281–283 (1971).
70. Korman, N. P. *et al., Vop. Onkol.* **11,** 35–40 (1971).
71. Košut, V., Hornova, J., and Smekal, M., *Neoplasma* **18,** 123–129 (1971).
72. Kurita, S., Nishimura, M., Ogawa, M. *et al., J. Jap. Soc. Cancer Ther.* **8,** 119–127 (1973).
73. Kurnick, N. B., Paley, K. R., Fieber, M. M. *et al., Ann. Intern. Med.* **30,** 974–1003 (1949).
74. Lahin, S. R., and Prasad, S. C., *Proc. Amer. Ass. Cancer Res.* **15,** 101 (1974).
75. Landgren, R. C., Hussey, O. H., Samuels, M. L. *et al., Ther. Radiol.* **108,** 403–406 (1973).
76. Lee, B. Y., Trainor, F. S., Schulz, R. Z. *et al., Surg., Gynecol. Obstet.* **132,** 3–6 (1971).
77. Matthews, M. J., *Semin. Oncol.* **1,** 175–182 (1974).
78. Maurer, L. H., Tulloh, M., Eagan, R. *et al., Cancer Chemother. Rep., Part 3* **4,** 171–176 (1973).
79. Mayo, J. G., Laster, W. R., Andrews, C. M. *et al., Cancer Chemother. Rep.* **56,** 183–195 (1972).
80. Miller, A. B., *Brit. Med. J.* **2,** 421 (1971).
81. Miller, A. B., Fox, W., and Tall, R., *Lancet* **2,** 501–502 (1969).
82. Mountain, C. F., *Cancer Chemother. Rep., Part 3* **4,** 307–310 (1973).
83. Neuman, S., and Hansen, H. H., *Cancer Chemother. Rep.* **57,** 101 (1973).
84. Neyazaki, T., Ikeda, M., Seki, Y. *et al., Cancer* **24,** 912–922 (1969).
85. Nissen, N. I., Larsen, V., Hansen, H. H. *et al., Proc. Int. Cancer Congr., 11th, 1974* **1,** 373.
86. Nyiredy, G., and Gevai, E., *Bronches* **21,** 202–206 (1971).
87. O'Bryan, R. M., Luce, J. K., Talley, R. W. *et al., Cancer* **32,** 1–8 (1973).
88. Oka, S., Sato, K., Nakai, Y. *et al., Sci. Rep. Res. Inst., Tohoku Univ.* **16,** 1–2 (1969).
89. Oka, S., Sato, K., Nakai, Y. *et al., Sci. Rep. Res. Inst., Tohoku Univ.* **17,** 3–4 (1970).
90. Oka, S., Sato, K., Nakai, Y. *et al, Sci. Rep. Res. Inst., Tohoku Univ.* **19,** 1–12 (1972).
91. Pereslegin, I. A., Sarkisian, R. S., and Savina, E. B., *Med. Radiol.* **15,** 3–7 (1970).
92. Perevodchikova, N. I., and Bychkov, M. B., *Cancer Chemother. Rep. Part 3* **4,** 251–255 (1973).
93. Perez, C. A., *Cancer Chemother. Rep., Part 3* **4,** 145–152 (1973).
94. Perloff, M., Muggia, F., and Ackerman, C., *Cancer Chemother. Rep.* **58,** 421–424 (1974).
95. Primack, A., (1974). *Semin. Oncol.* **1,** 235–244 (1974).
96. Ramirez, G., Wilson, W., Grage, T. *et al., Cancer Chemother. Rep.* **56,** 787–790 (1972).
97. Richards, F., Pajak, T. F., Cooper, M. R. *et al., Cancer Chemother. Rep.* **57,** 419–422 (1973).

98. Rossof, A. H., Slayton, R. E., and Perlia, C. P., *Cancer* **30,** 1451–1456 (1972).
99. Saccomano, G., *Cancer* **33,** 256–270 (1974).
100. Saito, T., Ohira, S. *et al., Jap. J. Cancer Clin.* **17,** 806–818 (1971).
101. Sandison, A. G., Falkson, G., Fichardt, T. *et al.,* (1967). *S. Afr. J. Radiol.* **5,** 21–27 (1967).
102. Sartorelli, A. C., and Creasey, W. A., *in* "Cancer Medicine" (J. F. Holland and E. T. Frei, eds.), pp. 707–717. Lea & Febiger, Philadelphia, Pennsylvania, 1973.
103. Scheef, W., *Pap., Int. Chemother. Congr. 7th* (1972).
104. Scheurlen, H., Drings, P., Vollhaber, M. M. *et al., Strahlentherapie* **143,** 154–158 (1972).
105. Selawry, O. S., *Cancer Chemother. Rep., Part 3* **4,** 177–188 (1973).
106. Selawry, O. S., *Cancer Chemother. Rep., Part 3* **4,** 215–225 (1973).
107. Selawry, O. S., *Semin. Oncol.* **1,** 259–272 (1974).
108. Selawry, O. S., and Hansen, H. H., *in* "Cancer Medicine" (J. F. Holland and E. T. Frei, eds.), pp. 1473–1518. Lea & Febiger, Philadelphia, Pennsylvania, 1973.
109. Selawry, O. S., Hansen, H. H., Carr, D. T. *et al., Proc. Amer. Ass. Cancer Res.* **15,** 118 (1974).
110. Shields, T. W., *Cancer Chemother. Rep., Part 3* **4,** 119–124 (1973).
111. Siering, H., and Reinhardt, M., *Arzneim.-Forsch.* **18,** 1182–1191 (1968).
112. Simecek, C., *Bronches* **21,** 181–185 (1971).
113. Skipper, H. E., Hutchinson, D. J., and Schabel, F. M., *Cancer Chemother. Rep.* **56,** 493–498 (1972).
114. Skipper, H. E., and Schabel, F. M., *in* "Cancer Medicine" (J. F. Holland and E. T. Frei, eds.), pp. 629–650. Lea & Febiger, Philadelphia, Pennsylvania, 1973.
115. Slack, N. H., *Cancer* **25,** 987–1002 (1970).
116. Smith, F. E., Lane, M., and Hudgins, P. T., *Cancer* **33,** 47–57 (1974).
117. Stähelin, H., *Eur. J. Cancer* **6,** 303–311 (1970).
118. Straus, M. J., *Semin. Oncol.* **1,** 167–174 (1974).
119. Svanberg, L., *Bleomycin Int. Symp.* pp. 115–126 (1973).
120. Takita, H., Brugarolas, A., Marabella, P. *et al., J. Thorac. Cardiov. Surg.* **66,** 427–477 (1973).
121. Takita, H., Brugarolas, A., Mittelman, A. and Vincent, R. *Cancer Chemother. Rep., Part 3* **4,** 257–260 (1973).
122. Takita, H., and Didolkar, M. S., *Cancer Chemother. Rep.* **58,** 371–374 (1974).
123. Tate, C. F., Viamonte, M., and Agnew, J. R., *Amer. Rev. Resp. Dis.* **97,** 685–693 (1968).
124. Tucker, R. D., Sealy, R., van Wyk, C., Soskolne, C. L., and Le Roux, P. L. M. *Cancer Chemother. Rep., Part 3* **4,** 157–158 (1973).
125. Tucker, R. D., Sealy, R., van Wyk, C. Le Roux, P. L. M., and Soskolne, C. L. *Cancer Chemother. Rep., Part 3* **4,** 159–160 (1973).
126. Vietti, T., Eggerding, F., and Valeriote, F., *J. Nat. Cancer Inst.* **47,** 865–870 (1971).
127. Wilson, K. S., Ricci, J. A., and Grobmeyer, A. J., *Cancer Chemother. Rep.* **54,** 243–244 (1970).
128. Wilson, W. L., Weiss, A. J., and Frelick, R. W., *Proc. Amer. Ass. Cancer Res.* **15,** 746 (1974).
129. Wolf, J., *Ann. Thorac. Surg.* **1,** 25–32 (1965).
130. Zelen, M., *Cancer Chemother. Rep., Part 3* **4,** 317–319 (1973).

Chapter 12

Palliative Surgery in Lung Cancer

Olivier Monod

A surgeon performs palliative surgery whenever he undertakes an operation fully conscious that there is no chance for long-term survival or when he performs a technically inadequate operation.

Palliative surgery may be undertaken for a number of reasons: to prolong life beyond the probable survival time, to pave the way for other therapeutic procedures, or to suppress pain or other subjective or objective disturbances. Excision may be incomplete (palliative) only from a surgical standpoint but may form part of a therapeutic strategy aimed at complete cure.

We shall begin by examining the reasons for undertaking surgery in certain assumably hopeless cases. We shall also discuss the objections to this type of surgery and we shall review the clinical situations in which this palliative surgery is indicated. In each case, the purely surgical tactics should be clearly differentiated from the therapeutic strategy. This means determining the role of surgery in the therapeutic program as a whole. We shall then briefly follow the evolution of ideas and of surgical attitudes that have undergone profound changes over the past 40 years. New ways of treating lung cancer are becoming necessary; we shall discuss them briefly.

I. JUSTIFICATION FOR PALLIATIVE OPERATIONS

A. Widening of Anatomical Indications

Surgery may already be considered palliative when circumstances require extensive pericardial resection that should be replaced by a prosthetic plate to prevent cardiac dislocation. The same is true when part of the left atrium together with the entrance to one or both pulmonary veins have to be removed or when part of the diaphragm is excised. The latter may be replaced by a prosthetic plate if required.

Also, the left pulmonary artery may have to be sutured at its very origin and both the section and the suture may encroach upon the trunk of the pulmonary artery itself. In a personal communication, Toty told me that he performed a pneumonectomy under extracorporeal circulation in order to resect the entrance to the left pulmonary veins safely.

The tumor may involve the esophagus. Not uncommonly, a few longitudinal esophageal muscle fibers have to be excised together with the cancer and in some cases even a small area of the muscle wall is removed. On only two occasions have I resected a noncircular part of the entire esophageal wall, including the mucosa.

Between 1966 and 1969 Naef and Kocher [1] operated on 85 cases of lung cancer which included 8 exploratory thoracotomies and 31 adequate resections using old procedures (lateral suture of the pulmonary artery, left atrium, etc.). Partisans of excision at any cost, their operative mortality rate attains 10%, while the percentage of long-term survivals is low. One factor in favor of this attitude is the good subjective quality of survival. In accordance with general opinion, these authors recognize that survival is less dependent on the surgical procedure than on prevailing biological conditions.

B. Tumor Volume Reduction

Certain oncologists have recommended extending the anatomic indications in lung cancer surgery. Very briefly, this attitude is based on the principle that it may be logical to excise the bulk of the tumor even if some tumor fragments cannot be removed, since this tumor volume reduction can help to increase the effectiveness of nonsurgical procedures. Thus, if complete cure cannot be hoped for, survival may at least be prolonged.

These extended operations do, however, have anatomical limitations that should be determined by the surgeon in the course of exploratory thoracotomy. The bulk of the tumor may be excised leaving extensions in the mediastinum, the intercostal spaces, the vertebrae, the esophagus, and contralateral lymph nodes. This implies great confidence in nonsurgical therapeutic procedures.

Smith [2] has reported several survivals after palliative resection. This possibility is well known to all thoracic surgeons as is the possibility of long-term survival after simple exploratory thoracotomy. I have personally observed two unquestionable cases. Similarly, Smith [2] observed a case of secondary regression of remaining cancer tissue in a patient who previously underwent palliative surgery and who died accidentally (autopsy control). Moreover, Everson [3] collected 176 cases of complete spontaneous regression of cancer in world medical literature. These included several cases of lung cancer.

C. Surgery for Pain

Operations designed to supress pain are the most common and the most justified form of palliative surgery. Intercostal neuralgia may result from involvement of an intercostal nerve at any point along its length.

Extension to the thoracic wall is a frequent occurrence in peripheral tumors. An upper lobe tumor, for example, may invade the third, fourth, and fifth intercostal spaces, destroying the ribs. The surgical procedure may consist of alcoholization of intercostal nerves under short-term general anesthesia. The needle is inserted posteriorly, 35 mm from the midline just lateral to the transverse process, thus making contact with the lower edge of the rib. The needle is then displaced downward slightly and inserted 2 mm beyond the rib edge after which 2 to 3 ml of isopropyl alcohol are injected. This procedure is performed in the neuralgic intercostal space or spaces and repeated in the overlying and underlying spaces.

Another possibility is severing the intercostal nerves at their origin after incision and resection of 2 cm of one or two ribs.

If pain due to chest wall involvement accompanies a resectable tumor, both the cancer (lung or lobe) and the involved chest wall (ribs and intercostal spaces) should be removed together. The ribs should preferably be dearticulated with their heads while the intercostal vessels and nerves should be severed at their spinal emergence. The lymph node often found in front of the rib's neck should be removed. I also prefer to remove mediastinal lymph nodes, even when only performing lobectomy.

Intercostal neuralgia occurring after excision may be due to either cicatricial sclerosis, in which case it can be easily managed by alcoholization or by severing the nerves, or to the cancer itself in which case the alternatives are palliative surgery or radiotherapy.

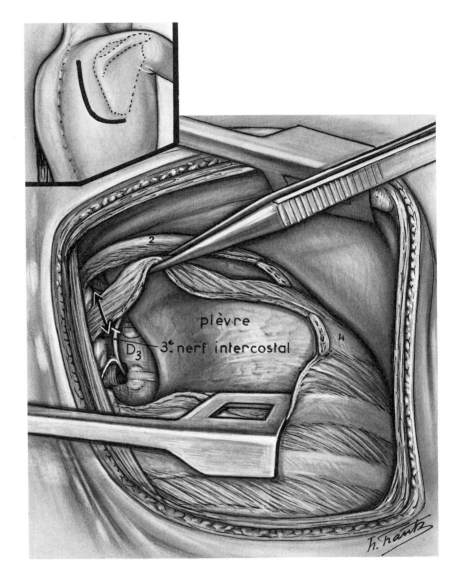

Fig. 1. Thoracotomy showing the operative field after dearticulation of the third and fourth ribs, including the head. The intercostal spaces have been incised and extrapleural cleavage performed prior to possible resection. Plèvre, pleura; nerf intercostal, intercostal nerve. D_3 equivalent to T.

Superior sulcus tumors give rise to the most intolerable and refractory pains. In some cases the radicular syndrome predominates with pain in the anterior chest wall and the upper extremity (medial aspect of the arm, forearm, and hand), often involving the regions supplied by the eighth cervical and first thoracic roots. It is in these cases that suppression of pain is most easily achieved through surgery.

The first step in the operation is upper lobectomy or pneumonectomy. Then, the first 4 (or 5) ribs are removed and the heads of the first, second (and third) ribs are dearticulated (Fig. 1). This provides good exposure of the supra- and retropleural fossae as well as of the supraclavicular fossa seen from below. The first three primary trunks and the secondary trunks of the brachial plexus may be dissected (Fig. 2). Tumor fragments often

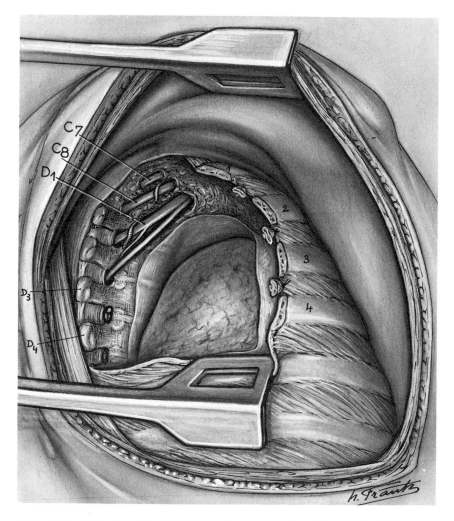

Fig. 2. The first four ribs (1–4) have been resected and dearticulated. The three last primary trunks of the brachial plexus have been dissected. The first intercostal nerve is visible at the lower part of the brachial plexus (pleura open). D_1, D_3, D_4 equivalent to T_1, T_3, T_4.

wind their way between nerve and vascular trunks but rarely penetrate them. All organs can be separated from the tumor by a somewhat long and careful, but not really difficult, dissection.

In some cases there is involvement of supraclavicular and/or cervical lymph nodes. In these cases surgical technique is the same as described above with dissection of the lower roots and the secondary trunks of the brachial plexus. The thoracotomy is closed, and classic neck dissection for removal of cervical lymph nodes is performed.

Sometimes a Claude–Bernard–Horner syndrome occurs early with involvement of rib necks and vertebrae. In these cases the operation is less often successful, and cobalt therapy and operations on the central nervous system are preferred. In any case, whether surgery is undertaken or not, radiotherapy and chemotherapy may be used to advantage.

These painful syndromes often persist or recur after cobalt therapy. In this case, operations on the central nervous system are the only way of relieving pain.

D. Mediastinal Compression

Although compression of the superior vena cava is more commonly related to malignant tumors of connective tissue than to bronchogenic squamous cell carcinoma, the latter is responsible in some cases. It has been possible to perform operations aimed at freeing a compressed superior vena cava when the venous wall was not invaded. I have used vertical sternotomy in five cases to excise malignant tumors (sarcomas) that compressed the superior vena cava without invading it.

If the vessel wall is involved, with intraluminal growths, the only surgical way of providing the patient with temporary relief is by a bypass to restore venous return. A synthetic tube is used to join the right heart chambers either to the left brachiocephalic vein or to the left subclavian vein. The tube should be solid enough not to collapse because of the low venous pressure. The lower junction is best achieved in the atrium, since the auricle bends or collapses easily. The patient feels considerably relieved after this bypass, and his outward appearance is radically transformed within a few short hours of the operation. I have performed this operation in 14 cases, but the results are marred by a high incidence of thrombosis. However, if the operation is performed under moderate heparinization and if calcium heparinate administration is continued immediately following the operation, the success rate improves appreciably. The chances of a successful bypass are much greater when stenosis of the vena cava results from constrictive fibrosis following cobalt therapy. I have witnessed two lasting successes in such cases.

I have also noticed that simple decompressive sternotomy considerably relieved impairment of venous return.

E. Respiratory Insufficiency

Respiratory insufficiency is one of the conditions least accessible to palliative surgery. Nevertheless, some benefit may be derived in certain cases of obstructive insufficiency and in some cases of poor general health: obesity and cardiovascular disturbances.

A typical example of such a case is described below:

A well-known actor was referred to me one day for cancer of the right lower lobe. He was in a state of serious respiratory distress, his chronic obstructive respiratory insufficiency having suddenly taken a turn for the worse. In this overweight patient, respiratory insufficiency was further aggravated by an enormous, long-standing xiphoumbilical eventration usually held in by a belt. Chest roentgenograms showed a shadow in the entire right lower lobe. Bronchoscopy revealed complete obstruction of the right lower lobe bronchus by a neoplastic growth (keratinizing cancer). Bilateral enlarged hilar lymph nodes were present.

To improve the patient's respiration, I removed the obstruction in the lower lobe bronchus by electrocoagulation of the tumor (1971). Bronchial permeability was completely restored, the roentgenogram became clear and the patient's relief was such that 3 weeks later he undertook a long tour of performances in the country. All respiratory function tests improved markedly as did oxygen saturation of hemoglobin.

A year later, the patient's respiratory state once again worsened suddenly. I repeated the same treatment, as I did for a third time in April 1973. Each time he felt great relief. However, contralateral extension and mediastinal compression led to death shortly thereafter. In short, the patient survived and, most important, continued acting and leading a normal life for $1\frac{1}{2}$ years thanks to this palliative operation.

I have performed this operation again on several occasions either to improve respiratory function or to evacuate secretions in preparation for radical resection. The surgeon should be careful to take accurate bearings in the bronchus and he should not overcoagulate in places where the pulmonary arteries are in contact with the bronchi or where they cross the latter. The operation is done under general anesthesia with oxygen administration. However, when coagulation is about to be effected, excess oxygen should be rapidly removed. We have had a special bronchoscope made which, in addition to its oxygen ventilation system, is fitted with an electrode adjustable for both length and direction.

Surgery of *involved lymph nodes* may also be considered palliative since it delays the final outcome. When performing right pneumonectomy the surgeon may be tempted to pursue removal of lymph nodes up to and including the nodes situated on the left side of the lower trachea and the left main bronchus.

On several occasions I have removed supraclavicular lymph nodes and sometimes even cervical nodes. The operations on lymph nodes may be performed at the same time as pneumonectomy or a long time afterward, when lymph node involvement appears as a local, clinically isolated metastasis. In such cases I feel that these operations are fully justified.

Metastases from primary lung cancer may be treated surgically when they are isolated and accessible. Tumors growing on the operative cicatrix (3 personal cases) or in the area draining this cicatrix can be removed without difficulty. Removal of single brain tumors sometimes results in remarkably long survival.

In many cases a lung tumor is thought to be secondary to a cancer situated elsewhere: out of a total of 3452 cases, I encountered 242 cases of secondary, or presumably secondary, cancer. The initial tumor was situated in the colon in 7 cases, pancreas 6, kidney 13, prostate 6, uterus 6, ovary 4, thyroid gland 9, breast 2, maxillary sinus and pharynx 3, larynx 4. In 43 cases the initial site was assumed to be the gastrointestinal tract and in 10 cases the genitourinary tract, but the primary tumor was not actually demonstrated. In 129 cases cancer was assumed to be secondary and was of undetermined origin.

In 1927 and 1930, Divis [4] and Thorek [5] reported several cases of resection of a single pulmonary metastasis. Choksi *et al.* [6] operated on 75 patients with a single metastasis in the lung. Six of these patients underwent surgery twice, thus bringing the total number of operations to 81. Out of a total of 229 pulmonary metastases from various primary sites, Fallon and Roper [7] reported that resection of a single lesion was possible in 12% of cases.

In principle, surgery is indicated for pulmonary metastases if only one lesion is present or if only one lobe is involved. Non-surgical therapeutic procedures should, however, always be associated.

Crile [8] remarked that thyroid carcinoma most commonly metastasized to the lung, and he achieved good results with thyroid extract (2.5 mg daily) in 12 cases out of 19. Mean survival was 11 years. Total thyroidectomy is an essential prerequisite. In pulmonary metastases from breast cancer, surgery should be complemented by castration, androgen therapy, chemotherapy, and even hypophysectomy in women of child-bearing age, and estrogens or progesterone-like drugs after menopause [9].

Pulmonary metastases from hypernephromas should be treated primarily with progesterone (6 gm monthly), surgery being an accessory. In pulmonary metastases from ovarian [10] or endometrial cancer [11] progesterone-like drugs should be added. Surgery is rarely indicated in metastatic prostate cancer [12]. The efficacy of radiotherapy in pulmonary metastases from bone tumors, seminomas, and nephroblastomas is a well established fact [13]. The lung is the most common origin of cerebromeningeal metastases (25 to 30%). Approximately one-third are single, surgically accessible lesions [14].

On several occasions I have performed lobectomy or limited resection of a lung nodule combined with removal of another organ, often in the course of the same operation: uterus, kidney, thyroid gland, and especially the colon. In a few cases, the patients survived several years.

F. Rapidly Growing Tumors

With rapidly growing tumors, which include cancer in young patients and anaplastic or oat cell carcinomas, the surgeon is faced with the same dilemma. He cannot reasonably hope for prolonged survival, and if he undertakes surgery he knows that he is merely performing a palliative operation. Thus, in my opinion, surgery is not indicated initially. I tend to proceed in the following manner: cobalt therapy on the lung lesion and systematic simultaneous irradiation of the liver and brain combined with chemotherapy and immunotherapy. Only if the lung tumor regresses should surgical removal be attempted while continuing chemotherapy and immunotherapy. In many cases, the course of these rapidly growing tumors is slowed down by the simultaneous use of these different procedures. I have observed survivals of several years in cases of oat cell carcinoma treated in this fashion (including one of 8 years).

I have operated on 1592 patients with cancer over a 10-year period, from 1964 to 1974. These included 37 cases of oat cell carcinoma (2.2%) 17 of which were diagnosed before operation. The percentage of oat cell carcinomas varied from one year to the next (0.8% in 1968, just over 4% every year since 1969). I have been less reluctant to accept these cases over the past few years. One such patient has survived for 8 years (histologic diagnosis confirmed). Out of the 161 cases of oat cell carcinoma reported by Takita [15], 35 underwent surgery, but in only two cases was resection adequate or "curative." One of these patients died after 47 months with no signs of recurrence, and the other died after 77 months because of recurrence following chemotherapy and radiotherapy [8].

Kato et al. [16] observed 138 cases of oat cell carcinoma out of 1386 surgical cancer patients. Of these 138 cases, 27% were surgically resectable. In two cases survival reached 7 years (5.4% of surgically resectable cases, 1.4% of the total number of cases).

Lennox *et al.* [17] performed 1773 thoracotomies for lung cancer in 15 years. These included 275 oat cell carcinomas (several different pathologists examined the specimens). Out of these 275 thoractomies, the tumor was resected in 58% of cases. The mean 2-year survival rate was 10.6%. The mean 2-year survival rate in patients who underwent lobectomy was 32%; the mean 5-year survival rate was 18%. However, these investigators concluded that "surgery cannot be said to influence survival."

Miller *et al.* [18] treated 144 patients with oat cell carcinoma. These patients were randomized between surgery and radiotherapy. Of the 71 patients randomized to the former group, 4% survived for 2 years and 3% survived for 4 years. Resection was performed in 48% of cases, 34% underwent exploratory thoracotomy, and the remaining 18% received no treatment. Of the 73 patients randomized to the radiotherapy group, 10% survived for 2 years, 7% for 4 years, and 4% for 5 years. The 5-year survivors all belonged to the radiotherapy group.

As a rule, recurrence in the remaining lobe should be treated surgically. Recurrence in the other lung may be treated surgically, especially if the initial operation was a lobectomy. Jensik [19] operated on 14 patients who had already had a tumor removed from the other lung. He reported 4 survivals exceeding 2 years and one of 7 years. These cases of recurrence may also be treated by radiotherapy, but the doses required for curative radiotherapy are the equivalent of physiologic lobectomy.

Furthermore, these cases may be likened to cases in which a *new primary cancer* of another organ is observed after resection for lung cancer [1]. Shields [20] reported 35 such primary malignant tumors in 535 5-year survivors out of 2371 surgical patients.

Intraarterial chemotherapy has been attempted either by injection into the bronchial arteries during the operation or by intraaortic injections. Using the latter route, Freckmann [21] reported two regressions of pulmonary metastases from hypernephromas with survivals of 28 and 42 months. However, the course of hypernephromas is even more erratic than that of other cancers [3].

Cryotherapy has been used in a few trials. Cooper [22] used liquid nitrogen ($-196°C$) injected through a cannula as the source of cooling. A thermoelectric couple was used for monitoring. He treated 500 cases of various disorders including cancer in this manner, without specifying the organs affected.

Performing palliative surgery means hoping to slow down the course of the disease, to make other therapeutic procedures more effective, and often to enable death to result from cerebral metastases, which is less trying than gradual suffocation or the agonizing pain associated with a superior sulcus tumor.

II. OBJECTIONS TO PALLIATIVE SURGERY

Long survival is observed in less than 40% of cases even when the indications for surgery are carefully selected (T1 or T2 and N0 M0). This percentage becomes derisive when the indications are extended (T3 or N2 or M1).

The number of operative deaths is very small in good risk cases (2.5% in T1 or T2, N0 cases) but rises in palliative operations (18% being the overall figure in my series).

Uncertainty always exists as to the duration of the course of the disease and the development of metastases. Thus, one can never be sure that palliative surgery, aided by other therapeutic procedures, does in fact slow down the course of the disease.

Finally, *the difficulties in applying* nonsurgical therapeutic procedures (without which palliative surgery cannot be conceived), the side effects of these procedures, their constraints, and various other disadvantages constitute serious drawbacks that limit the possibilities of palliative surgery.

III. THE LIMITS OF INDICATIONS FOR SURGERY

From what has been said it is apparent that schematically speaking two equally justified and equally respectable surgical attitudes are possible in the face of lung cancer. Both of these attitudes are based on philosophical and ethical criteria, since there is no strictly scientific guideline for the management of these patients.

Some surgeons are of the opinion that an operation should be attempted only if there is a good chance of long-term survival, i.e., localized tumor, no involvement of contralateral lymph nodes confirmed by mediastinoscopy, no liver metastases confirmed by laparotomy, and satisfactory cardiovascular function. The desire not to inflict an operation that may only prolong life by a few short months, the concern for avoiding a vital risk in a patient who may have several years to live, and the uncertain duration of the spontaneous course justify this attitude, which may be summed up in one phrase—respect for human life.

In contrast, some surgeons are of the opinion that in view of the other complementary therapeutic procedures available surgery may be justified even in cases where a radical "curative" operation is impossible. The decision to operate depends largely on personal factors involving the surgeon, the patient, and his family. Randomized trials and advances in therapeutic procedures may eventually reduce the influence of the surgeon's personal tendancy in the indication for surgery.

The very title of this chapter is a clear indication that I have no hesitation in performing this palliative surgery, which is not spectacular and hardly glorious but which is often appreciated by the patients themselves. I have been operating on patients with lung cancer since 1938, and have performed almost 4000 operations in all. Over the years I have repeatedly revised not only the indications for surgery, but its very significance as well.

In this chapter I have put forth my own ideas. I have done so without reserve or reticence, and I have done so without the support of detailed statistics. Indeed, even if I were to confine my figures to the period 1960–1970 they would have little significance in view of the fact that the cases and the circumstances varied widely, not to mention the interference of adjuvant therapies.

Furthermore, our decisions are invariably influenced by day to day experience. While a run of successful operations or a long follow-up period after excision of a metastasis may encourage greater audacity, a few unsuccessful cases invariably lead to greater conservatism.

To quote an example, here are a few figures reflecting the variations in surgical indications. From 1963 to 1972 (10 years) I performed 1592 operations, 25% of these being exploratory thoracotomies. This is the overall percentage and the annual percentages varied considerably: 39% in 1963, 9.8% in 1970, 21% in 1973. The percentage of lobectomies or segmental resections as compared to pneumonectomies was 45% in 1960, 51% in 1963 and 60% in 1968 (but these partial resections usually included removal of mediastinal lymph nodes).

These hesitations on the part of the surgeon with regard to the operative decision call for an explanation. *The reasonable limits* of resection must be well defined (involvement of the trachea, the superior vena cava, the esophagus, supraclavicular lymph nodes, the phrenic nerve, the atrial wall, and in most cases the left recurrent laryngeal nerve); other contraindications were anaplastic or oat cell carcinoma, multiple metastases, bilateral involvement, and contraindications stemming from poor general health or inadequate respiratory function. Young patients or rapidly progressive tumors were borderline cases.

On the other hand, the notion that surgery alone could enable long-term cure was a firmly established one, hence the temptation to perform as extensive a resection as possible. This led to a high percentage of exploratory thoracotomies and a poor reflection in our statistics. Another consequence was the high percentage of pneumonectomies as compared to limited resections and a high percentage of mediastinal lymph node excisions, even in lobectomies.

Many of these notions have since been questioned in view of the possibilities of cobalt therapy and high frequency irradiation, and of the hopes raised by chemotherapy and immunotherapy.

Surgical indications have been extended with the advent of other therapeutic methods that have encouraged greater audacity in widespread cancer, in secondary cancer, in single metastases or metastases confined to one organ, in cases with supraclavicular lymph nodes, in young patients, and in bronchogenic carcinoma of the oat-cell variety. Surgical and nonsurgical methods may be used successively or concomitantly.

Physicians are often more pessimistic than surgeons are about nonsurgical methods of treatment. Perhaps this is because they see a large number of advanced cases that are not even referred to the surgeon and in which death ensues despite radiotherapy and chemotherapy.

When cobalt therapy is suggested, it is often accepted half-heartedly and without optimism. Moreover, irradiation is usually confined to the thorax and is rarely directed against the liver or brain. Chemotherapy and immunotherapy are rarely prescribed, and when they are, the dosage, schedule and duration are not always adequate.

The family physician, the family, and the patient are often apprehensive about the adverse effects of these therapeutic methods (various side effects of chemotherapy, multiple abscesses resulting from immunotherapy) or the constraints imposed by the supervision and regular pursuit of such a program. However, treatment can after all be initiated and later modifications made if tolerance proves to be poor. As for the regularity, perseverance, and constraints necessary, their acceptance is not difficult to obtain if the patient and his family are informed of the diagnosis.

An opposite stand may be taken, however, and one may be tempted to limit the indications of surgery as the initial procedure even in clearly operable cases. If one goes by the indications advocated by the supporters of the TNM classication, cobalt therapy should be the first step in squamous cell carcinomas exceeding 3 cm in diameter when growth involves the main bronchus less than 2 cm from the tracheal bifurcation (T3) without involvement of mediastinal lymph nodes (N0–M0). Similarly, anaplastic and oat cell carcinomas should be initially treated with cobalt and possibly simultaneous chemotherapy. If volume reduction is achieved, the surgeon may then intervene.

It is my opinion that in 1974, and until present notions are revised through advances in immunotherapy, virology and other branches, we should use all the available therapeutic procedures of proved or putative efficacy. These procedures should be individually adapted and modulated according to the patient's reactions.

However, it is no mean task to make a patient accept radiotherapy, antimitotic agents, and repeated immunotherapy with all the constraints and adverse effects that this program entails. When a patient is aware of the diagnosis, treatment is usually better understood and accepted. Of course a patient should not be informed lightly, and this should only be done with the consent of the family and the family physician. Many patients are aware of their diagnosis without having to be told, while others do not discuss the diagnosis but negligently ask whether chemotherapy is effective against metastases. There is increasing awareness among the general public, and I feel that stubborn refusal to confirm what the patient already suspects is pointless, backward, and an impediment to treatment.

IV. GENERAL STRATEGY

When considering general therapeutic strategy we should use clear language and accurate definitions, acquired through personal discipline, in order to compel ourselves to analyze all the factors in any given case. This would result in more reliable statistics and more fruitful international exchange of experience.

We are fully aware of the fact that 85 to 90% of all cases detected are beyond hope of surgical cure. A review of international statistics shows the following overall results: at the most, 50% of patients undergo thoracotomy—15% without resection, 5% with palliative tumor resection, and 30% with surgically adequate resection. The operative mortality rate is 4 to 9%, and long-term survival is around 7 to 8%. Later postoperative deaths are due to cerebral metastases in 50% of cases and to liver metastases in 25% of cases.

Nonsurgical therapeutic procedures have done little to improve long-term survival but have given us a better understanding of the theoretical problems involved. Chemotherapy and immunotherapy have encouraged further research in this direction [23].

Thus, to speak a common language concerning the anatomical extension of a cancer, we should adopt the international TNM classification (tumor–nodes–metastases) discussed at length by Mountain in Chapter 6. Indeed, accurate assessment of anatomical extension may have as much bearing on the management of a patient as the tumor's histologic type [24].

In this regard, we would like to appeal to pathologists to adopt the World Health Organization's classification. Even though this classification is sometimes criticized by our colleagues, it does have the advantage of existing and making unequivocal agreement possible in the vast majority of cases. Together with anatomic extension and histologic type, the third essential factor to be taken into account when weighing the decision to operate is the tumor's growth rate. If one accepts the implications of doubling time, the influence of palliative surgery on survival is quite evident.

To go a little beyond the scope of our subject, we shall just mention that our therapeutic strategy [18] is that recommended by Clifton Mountain [25] with a few minor modifications resulting from the palliative reasoning that I have discussed above.

There is no doubt that more extensive use of cytology as an early diagnostic tool may increase the number of long-term survivals considerably [26–28], but this is only related to palliative surgery from a prophylactic standpoint.

There is no longer any justification for treating patients in a haphazard and dispersed fashion—the surgeon deciding whether or not to operate, patients refused by the surgeon being referred to the radiotherapist who decides whether or not to undertake radiotherapy, chemotherapy being administered according to the poorly informed physician's personal views and in an irrational manner.

Therapeutic strategy should be established jointly by the physician, the surgeon, and the radiotherapist who should determine the various procedures to be undertaken, their timing, and the necessary changes. A well-organized secretarial staff will enable regular supervision of patients, a small point perhaps but an important one nevertheless.

The need for profound changes in our reasoning habits has become imperative. Too many physicians hesitate to make the inevitable diagnosis and delay initiation of effective therapy by irrationally pursuing test treatment or by adopting a "wait and see" policy. If we work toward this goal, accumulating scientifically significant data, we shall add another few percent to long-term survival figures while waiting for chemistry, virology, genetics, and immunology to clear the road leading to effective treatment of lung cancer. The poor results achieved up to now are hardly surprising, since we have approached the problem at a stage when disease was so advanced that permanent cure could not reasonably be expected. The true answer undoubtedly lies at the root of the problem, that is in the molecular biology of the cancer cell [29].

REFERENCES

1. Naef, A. P., and Kocher, A., La chirurgie radicale du cancer bronchique avancé. *Schweiz. Med.* **43,** 1848 (1970).
2. Smith, R. A., Long term clinical follow-up after operation for lung carcinoma. *Thorax* **25,** 62 (1970).
3. Everson, T. C., and Cloe, W. H., "Spontaneous Regression of Cancer," Vol. 1, pp. 11–27. Saunders, Philadelphia, Pennsylvania, 1966.

4. Divis, G., Ein Beitrag zur operativen Behandlung der Lungenschwultse. *Acta Chir. Scand.* **62,** 329 (1927).
5. Thorek, F., The surgical management of solitary pulmonary metastasis. *Arch. Surg., (Chicago)* **21,** 1416 (1930).
6. Choksi, M. B., Takita, M. D., and Vincent, M. D., The surgical management of solitary pulmonary metastasis. *Surg., Gynecol. Obstet.* **134,** 479–482 (1972).
7. Fallon, R. H., and Roper C. L., Operative treatment of metastatic pulmonary cancer. *Ann. Surg.* **166,** 263–265 (1967).
8. Crile, G., "The Endocrine Dependency of Papillary Carcinomas of the Thyroid," p. 269. Livingstone, Edinburgh, 1970.
9. Juret, P., L'hormonothérapie des métastases cancéreuses. *Gaz. Med.* **80,** 1285–1292 (1973).
10. Ward, H. W. G., Progestogen therapy for ovarian carcinoma. *J. Obstet. Gynecol. Brit. Common.* **79,** 555 (1972).
11. Muller, P., and Levy, G., "Hormones et cancers génitaux de la femme, in problems actuels d'endocrinologie et de nutrition," p. 269. L'Expansion, 1969.
12. Couvelaire, R., Les indications respectives de la chirurgie et de l'hormonothérapie dans le traitement du cancer de la prostate. *Presse Med.* **67,** 217 (1961).
13. Eschwege, F. *et al.,* Radiothérapie des métastases cancéreuses. *Gaz. Med. Fr.* **80,** 1305–1307 (1973).
14. Constans, J. P., Tumeurs métastatiques et Neurochirurgie. *Gaz. Med. Fr.* **80,** 1309–1316 (1973).
15. Takita, H., Brugarolas, A., Marabella, P., and Vincent, R. G., Small cell carcinoma of the lung. Clinicopathological studies. *J. Thorac. Cardiov. Surg.* **66,** 472–477 (1973).
16. Kato, Y., Ferguson, T. L., Bennett, D., and Burford, T. H., Oat cell carcinoma of the lung. *Cancer* **23,** 517 (1969).
17. Lennox, S., Flavell, G., Pollok, D., Thompson, D., and Wilkins, J., Results of resection post oat cell carcinoma of the lung. *Lancet* **2,** 925 (1968).
18. Miller, A. B., Fox, W., and Tall, R., Five year follow-up of the comparative trial of surgery and radiotherapy for the primary treatment of small-cell carcinoma of the bronchus. *Lancet* **2,** 501 (1969).
19. Jensik, R. J., Faber, L. P., Milloy, F. J., and Monson, D. O., Segmental resection for lung cancer. A fifteen year experience. *J. Thorac. Cardiov. Surg.* **66** (4), 563–572 (1973).
20. Shields, T. W., Long term survivors after resection of bronchial carcinoma. *Surg. Gynecol. Obstet.* **136,** 759–762 (1973).
21. Freckmann, H. A. *et al.,* Chemotherapy for lung cancer by intra aortic infusion. *J. Amer. Med. Ass.* **196,** 5–10 (1966).
22. Cooper, I. S., Cryogenic surgery. *N. Engl. J. Med.* **268,** 743–749 (1963).
23. Mountain, C. F., Carr, D. T., Selawry, O. S., Israel, L., Shields, T., Mathews, M., Tucker, R. D., Bonadonna, G., and Takita, H., *Cancer Chemother. Rep.* **4,** No. 2 (1973).
24. Carr, D., Keynote address on diagnosis, staging, and criteria of response to therapy for lung cancer. *Cancer Chemother. Rep.* **4,** No 2, p. 17 (1973).
25. Mountain, C. F., The surgeon's viewpoint on collaborative research on lung cancer. *Cancer Chemother. Rep.* **4,** No. 2, 307–309 (1973).
26. Lukeman, M., Reliability of cytologic diagnosis in cancer of the lung. *Cancer Chemother. Rep.* **4,** No. 2, 79 (1973).

27. Kreis, B., Le dépistage cytologique systématique du cancer du poumon. *Rev. Tuberc. Pneumol.* **35,** No. 5 (1971).

28. Gallouedec, C., La précession cytologique dans le diagnostic des cancers des voies aériennes. *Rev. Tuberc. Pneumol.* **36,** No. 1 (1972).

29. Higgins, G. A., Chemotherapy and lung cancer. *Ann. Thorac. Surg.* 809–811 (1965).

Chapter 13

The Role of Anticoagulation Chemotherapy in Lung Carcinoma

Elias G. Elias

I. INTRODUCTION

Chemotherapy is directed toward the cell kill. This has been successful in inducing remission in leukemia, but is very seldom successful in solid tumors. The difference lies in the fact that solid tumors form lumps that consist of cells in a matrix. It seems then that the lumps of solid tumors defeat the action of chemotherapy and immunosurveillance more so than the microcolonies.

A. The Tumor Matrix

O'Meare [22] reported on tumor growth and showed that fibrin had to grow or precipitate around the tumor mass to provide a new matrix for the dividing tumor cells. Wood, in the same year, reported on the mechanism of development of metastases and found that the tumor microcolonies had to stick to the wall of the blood vessel and form a clot before division can take place [27]. Day *et al.* [8] and Hiramoto *et al.* [13] using the radioimmune assays and fluorescein label techniques, proved the presence of fibrin

259

and fibrinogen in a variety of human and animal tumors. However, electron microscopic studies by Jones et al. [14] and others suggested that a loose reversible platelet–protein aggregate, rather than fibrin, forms rapidly around the tumor cells in experimental metastases. Laki and Yancy [17] reported on the possible presence of thrombin and factor XIII (fibrinase) in some animal tumors. In addition, the work of Folkman [11] indicated the importance of the capillary formation in the tumor matrix. Therefore, it seems that the final stages of the clotting mechanism can be carried out at the tumor site. This process may reflect itself on the peripheral blood in the form of a hypercoagulable state. Miller et al. [19] and Davis et al. [7] reported on the hypercoagulability in cancer patients and showed: short bleeding time; decreased silicone coagulation time and partial thromboplastin time; increased tolerance to heparin; marked elevation of plasma factor I, II, V, VIII, IX and XI; acceleration of thromboplastin generation; and elevation of platelet count in the untreated cancer patients with metastases.

Since coagulation seemed to have such a vital role for the tumor growth and metastases, it should be possible to interfere with such growth or metastases by affecting the clot formation. Therefore, to prevent capillary formation, we have to prevent fibroblast proliferation by preventing clot formation at the tumor site. Also, if ongoing coagulation at the tumor site could be halted, the fibrinolytic mechanism—whether the physiological or the tumorous (as suggested by Unkeless et al. [26])—will hopefully be adequate to remove the recently deposited fibrin and thereby deny the tumor cells their matrix. This may also reduce the incidence of hypercoagulability in cancer state and its complications.

B. The Effects of Chemotherapy on Hemostasis

Chemotherapy has a nonspecific cytotoxic action, i.e., it destroys all types of cells and creates tissue damage. Hidalgo et al. [12] showed that tissue damage can increase plasma fibrinogen, possibly due to thromboplastin release from the damaged tissue. Davis et al. observed the presence of disseminated intravascular coagulopathy (DIC) in the subclinical level after chemotherapy and related that to the release of thromboplastic material from tumor destruction. Leavy et al. [18] and Brodsky and Conroy [5] reported on DIC due to chemotherapy in leukemia that was treated successfully with heparin.

It appears then that chemotherapy can cause elevation in plasma fibrinogen, thromboplastins, or thromboplastin-like material that all lead to hypercoagulable states and may result in more fibrin clot, fibrinogen–fibrin coagulum, or a protein aggregate of some sort for the tumor mass. This clot, coagulum, or aggregate may play two roles: (1) It may coat the viable tumor cells and increase their stickiness and make them hibernate under possibly anoxic conditions. On one hand, the increase of stickiness can lead to an increase in the metastases and/or the survival of these cells at the site of the original tumor lump or matrix. On the other hand, the anoxic condition could make these cells more resistant to the chemotherapeutic effect, a condition that is similar to that described with irradiation. (2) That created clot, coagulum, or aggregate may also help in the formation of the new tumor matrix for the dividing tumor cells that survived the chemotherapeutic effect, which lasts from minutes to a few hours.

Hypercoagulability can also lead to other complications, namely, thromboembolism and DIC. Therefore, it seems that further investigation of the role of anticoagulation in the control of cancer is in order.

C. Anticoagulation

1. ANIMAL EXPERIMENTATION

The extensive work of Agostino and Cliffton [1–4, 6], Ryan *et al.* [24, 25], and Kudrjashov *et al.* [16] showed definite effect of anticoagulation on animal tumors. This could be summarized in that different anticoagulants and fibrinolytic agents prevented, reduced, or retarded tumors. It should be pointed out that in these experiments, the anticoagulants and fibrinolytic agents were utilized alone and not in combination with irradiation or chemotherapy, yet these were significantly effective.

2. HUMAN EXPERIMENTATION

The first approach was to utilize anticoagulation as adjunct to chemotherapy to induce remission in metastatic cancer. The purpose of using anticoagulation in this approach was not to anticoagulate peripherally the patient, but to halt the coagulation mechanism at the tumor site to a minimum, and allow the fibrinolytic mechanism to go on and affect or hopefully to lyse the tumor matrix. Of course, to attempt to block the coagulation at the tumor site, in most instances, the patient had to be systematically anticoagulated. Anticoagulation had to be established and maintained, then followed by the chemotherapy that would be directed toward the cell kill.

Anticoagulation of the cancer patients should not be too worrisome, as most of these patients were presumably hypercoagulable and liable to develop thrombi and emboli, and this might even prove to be beneficial to them in preventing such complications.

The possibility of increasing metastases was thought of, but because anticoagulants were administered in combination with chemotherapy, it seemed it would be safe but should be watched for. Another important point was that tumor cells need to stick to the blood vessel wall to develop into metastases. This stickiness was to be prevented by anticoagulation, and if the microcolonies did not lodge and develop into metastases, these would die mechanically, immunologically, and by the chemotherapeutic agents.

Hypercoagulability, whether secondary to the tumor or to the chemotherapy, might protect the viable tumor cells and anticoagulation might enhance the effect of chemotherapy by maintaining this process to a minimum.

In a pilot study, heparin was chosen for the following reasons: (1) Heparin is an anticoagulant that is relatively safe, since its effect can be reversed immediately if so desired. It also blocks thrombin, i.e., it interferes with the final stages of the clotting mechanism. (2) It has been shown that heparin has some inhibitory effects on the growth of some experimental tumors [23] and it may prolong the mitotic (M) phase in cell kinetics [21] and therefore, may make the cells more amenable to chemotherapy. (3) Heparin as a polyanion may change the cell surface, or make the cells metabolically active, and, in either case, they become an easy target to chemotherapy. (4) Heparin, a lipoprotein labelizer, may affect the lipoprotein in the cell membrane or exhibit a lysosomal labelizing effect [20], causing partial or complete cell damage. Based on the above, the following pilot study was carried out.

II. HEPARIN AS ADJUVANT TO CHEMOTHERAPY—PILOT STUDY

A. Patients and Methods

Twenty-eight patients with metastatic carcinoma of the lung—that had no evidence of brain metastases, history of bleeding, or peptic ulcers— were treated by a multiple chemotherapeutic program, outlined below. Most of these patients had comparable extent of disease and all had previously failed to respond to conventional chemotherapy or radiotherapy. The first 14 patients received the multiple chemotherapy only, while the rest of the patients received aqueous heparin intravenously (i.v.) until they became adequately anticoagulated (see below) and then were treated with the same chemotherapeutics.

The multiple chemotherapy program (chemotherapy) in this study consisted of cyclophosphamide 700 mg i.v. on day one; 5-fluorouracil 500 mg orally (p.o.)/day on days 2, 3, and 4; 6-thioguanine 1 mg/kg/day p.o. on days 2 through 8; methotrexate 5 mg p.o./day on days 2 through 8; and vincristine 50 μg/kg i.v. (not to exceed 3 mg) on day 9. This course of chemotherapy was repeated every 2 weeks.

Aqueous heparin was administered as 150 IU/kg i.v. bolus followed by 600 IU/kg per 24 hours as continuous i.v. infusion (using a battery operated pump) to obtain a one tube 37°C whole blood clotting time to 3 times the baseline and to maintain it for at least 48 hours. Heparin was then continued while the multiple chemotherapeutics were administered over the next 9 days. Daily whole blood clotting time, plasma fibrinogen levels, and complete blood counts were carried out. Twice weekly, blood chemistries (12 profiles) were obtained. Coumadin therapy was initiated 2 days before the end of each course of heparin and chemotherapy and maintained and adjusted to keep the patients' prothrombin time in the therapeutic range of 20% ($\pm$5%) during the following 2 weeks of rest, i.e., no chemotherapy.

B. Results

For the purpose of this presentation, the results will be limited to the tumor response. The chemotherapeutic toxicity has been reported by Elias et al. [10]. No tumor regression was noted in any of the first groups of patients who received 2–5 courses of chemotherapy alone. On the contrary, all of them showed tumor progression and subsequently 12 succumbed to their disease in less than 6 months. The other 2 patients were shifted to the heparin–chemotherapy program (after they had failed the same chemotherapy program alone) and subsequently both patients did respond with a significant tumor regression.

In the second group, 14 patients received heparin and the same chemotherapeutics. Of these, 7 patients had over 50% tumor regression. The initial response was noted after 1 to 3 courses of heparin and chemotherapy. In this group, the duration of response varied between 4 months to over 1 year. Two patients who received heparin–chemotherapy are living and well for over 19 and 16 months, respectively, since the initiation of this therapy. The first one belongs to the over 50% tumor regression group (patient 17), while the second one has less than 20% tumor regression and was considered no change (patient 16) (Table I). Of the other 6 patients who were considered failures on the heparin–chemotherapy program, one died of heart attack after 2 courses, while the rest of the patients showed slow progression of the disease 3–4 months since the initiation of this therapy. Table I summarizes these results.

During the period of heparinization (with or without chemotherapy)

TABLE I
Tumor Response[a]

Patients treated with chemotherapy only		Patients treated with heparin–chemotherapy	
Patient number	Tumor response	Patient number	Tumor response
1	Progression noted after 2 courses	15	Regression after 1 course and maintained it for 4 months
2	Progression noted after 2 courses	16	No change for 16 months, living with no change
3	Progression noted after one course		
4	Progression, after 3 courses	17	Regression after 2 courses, maintained it for 19 months, no progression, alive
5	Progression, after 5 courses		
6	Progression, after 5 courses	18	Regression after 2 courses, maintained it for 4 months, no progression, alive
7	Progression, after 5 courses		
8	Progression, after 1 course		
9	Progression after 1 course	19	Regression after 3 courses, maintained it for 4 months
10	Progression, after 2 courses		
11	Progression, after 4 courses	20	Regression after 1 course, maintained it for 6 months
12	Progression, after 2 courses		
13	Progression, after one course	21	Regression after 1 course, maintained it for 4 months
14	Progression after 2 courses		
		22	Regression after 3 courses, maintained it for 4 months
		23	Progression after 4 courses
		24	Progression after 6 courses
		25	Progression after 6 courses
		26	No change after 2 courses, died of heart attack
		27	Progression after 2 courses
		28	Progression after 4 courses

[a] From Elias et al. [10].

there was no evidence of hemorrhage or bleeding in any of the patients, except occasional hemoptesis that stopped spontaneously when the cough crisis ceased. At no time did heparinization have to be reversed. All the patients showed resistance to heparin anticoagulation, i.e., they did not show adequate anticoagulation for 4–14 days with the continuous heparin infusion alone. In two patients, the amount of heparin had to be increased over a period of 2 weeks to $1\frac{1}{2}$ times the recommended dose, before adequate anticoagulation could be obtained (Figs. 1 and 2).

After adequate anticoagulation was established, the administration of

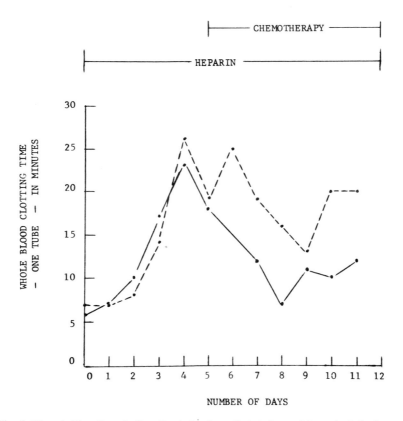

Fig. 1. The clotting time in 2 patients to show that 4 days of heparin infusion were needed to obtain anticoagulation. Then, notice the effect of chemotherapy in shortening the clotting time in spite of continuing heparin infusion. From Elias *et al.* [10].

the chemotherapeutics with the heparin did not result in any untoward effects. There were no evidences of bleeding or increased toxicity from the drugs. On the contrary, most of the patients showed a decline in the whole blood clotting time 24 hours after the initiation of chemotherapy, with a slow return to their previously established anticoagulation levels, over the next few days while still on heparin (Fig. 1).

Another interesting phenomenon noted in two of our patients, was that during their first period of heparin and chemotherapy, some lesions enlarged in size, but then regressed during the following weeks (Fig. 3), i.e., after the first course of heparin–chemotherapy. One of these patients had skin metastases that were amenable to clinical evaluation and biopsy. These lesions enlarged and became erythematous (not hemorrhagic) but subsided shortly after the first course. Biopsies obtained before and 2

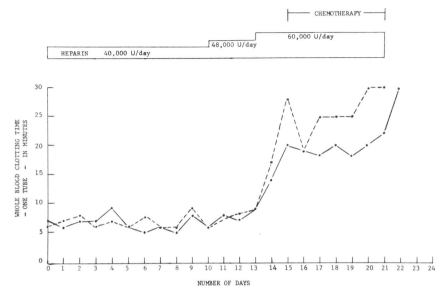

Fig. 2. Two patients that showed resistance to heparin anticoagulation in the form of longer periods of heparin infusion (14 days) and larger doses of heparin to bring on anticoagulation. Again, notice the effect of chemotherapy. From Elias *et al.* [10].

weeks after a single course of heparin–chemotherapy showed massive tumor necrosis and a large number of lymphocytes and plasma cells infiltrating the tumor (Fig. 4).

During heparin anticoagulation, there was no clinical or biochemical evidence of increased incidence of metastases. This was evident in the two long survivals and in those patients who failed to respond to this regimen; the disease progressed slowly, and at autopsy no new metastases were noted.

III. DISCUSSION

In a previous study (E. Elias, unpublished), the multiple chemotherapeutic regimen was administered simultaneously with heparin, and no tumor regression was noted. When the above study was started, utilizing heparin alone initially increased resistance to heparin anticoagulation which was clearly demonstrated in Figs. 1 and 2. Four to 14 days of continuous heparin infusion and occasionally large doses of heparin were required to obtain adequate anticoagulation. This could be part of the hypercoagulable state that had been reported to accompany malignant diseases in man.

The administration of chemotherapy after establishing adequate anti-

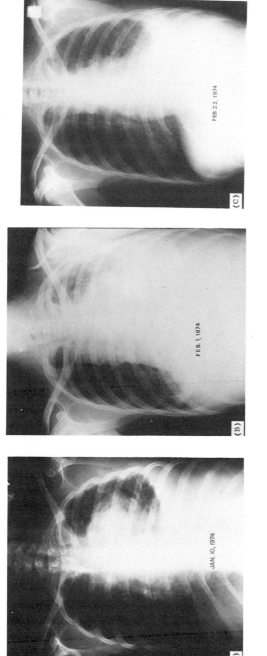

Fig. 3. Chest X-ray of patient 18. (A) Before initiating heparin–chemotherapy, showing adenocarcinoma of left lung with mediastinal metastases. (B) At the end of the first course of heparin–chemotherapy. Note the enlargement in tumor size and development of pleural effusion. (C) Few days later. Note the significant tumor regression following one course of therapy.

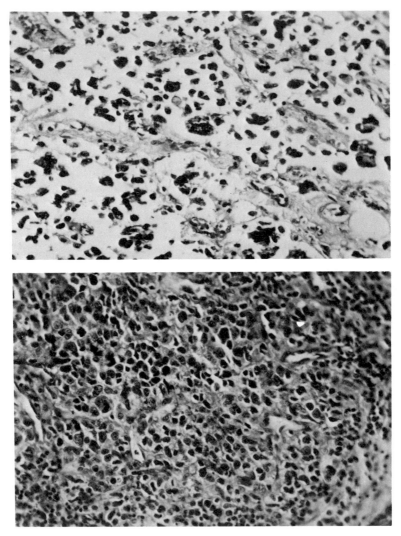

Fig. 4. Histological sections of lymph node obtained from patient 15. Bottom, before heparin–chemotherapy. Top, after one course of heparin–chemotherapy, to show the massive tumor necrosis and the lymphocyte and plasma cells infiltrating the lesion; ×400; hematoxylin and eosin stain.

coagulation again resulted in a shorter clotting time. This could suggest that a secondary hypercoagulable state was created by the chemotherapy as hypothesized earlier. Also, this might indicate that the combination of anticoagulants and chemotherapy was a safe clinical approach.

The group of patients that were treated with heparin–chemotherapy program showed better response, in the form of tumor regression and longer survivors (2 patients over 1 year), than the group that received the same chemotherapy alone. This was further demonstrated in the two patients that showed tumor progression while receiving chemotherapy only, yet their tumors regressed when they received the same chemotherapy after heparinization. During an earlier study, Coumadin was not used between courses of heparin–chemotherapy. However, two patients (in another study) died with massive pulmonary emboli 10 and 14 days, respectively, after discontinuation of heparin at the end of a chemotherapeutic course. Coumadin maintenance was then initiated to prevent this probable "rebound" or "tertiary" hypercoagulable phenomenon, and no further overt thrombotic episodes was seen in any of the patients.

The enlargement in the size of some lesions during the first course of heparin and chemotherapy could be explained on the basis of edema rather than progression of the disease. This is because these lesions regress so fast, i.e., in a matter of days, to a much smaller size than the original mass (Fig. 3).

The few histological sections that were studied revealed that not only massive tumor necrosis but also lymphocyte and plasma cell infiltrating these tumor sites (Fig. 4). This might indicate that heparin anticoagulation enabled the immune survey to penetrate the tumor lump [9]. This was further supported by the report of Kiricuta et al. [15] that heparin anticoagulation and immunostimulation had significantly reduced (not only delayed) tumors in an animal model.

Some of the patients that were treated with heparin–chemotherapy regimen had repeated plasma fibrinogen determinations, and it was interesting to find that all of them were hyperfibrinogenemic prior to therapy. After therapy, all responders, i.e., showing tumor regression, also showed a significant fall in plasma fibrinogen levels, most to the normal range as seen in Table II. It was of utmost importance also to note that there was no clinical, radiological, or laboratory evidence that anticoagulants increased the incidence of metastases in this group of patients. This was further confirmed pathologically, since almost all the patients were followed until death, and the autopsies did not reveal miliary or new metastases.

Finally, on two occasions, attempts were made to maintain partial tumor regression by anticoagulants alone (namely, Coumadin) but failed and chemotherapy had to be resumed.

Therefore, it seems that anticoagulants and/or disruption of tumor matrix may play an important role in cancer control. The future plans should include randomized studies on the clinical and experimental levels to study

TABLE II

The Correlation of Plasma Fibrinogen with Tumor Growth and Regression

Patient No.	Plasma fibrinogen[a] (mg%) Before therapy	During response	Extent of tumor regression	Plasma fibrinogen[a] (mg%) at time of tumor progression
1	687	337	> 50%	Died of pneumonia 11 days later
2	522	412	> 50%	589
3	918	342	> 50%	Maintained same
4	607	313	> 50%	Refused further therapy
5	742	387	> 50%	665
6	748	201	25%	Died of emphysema
7	455	333	25%	637
8	468	337	Complete regression of cervical lymph nodes, but minimal regression in lung lesion	633
9	592	652	< 20%	Maintained same
10	909		Tumor progression	1166
11	586		No change, progression	768
12	565		No change	585

[a] Plasma fibrinogen, normal range 200–400 mg%.

1. Anticoagulants such as heparin and Coumadin
2. Defibrinating agents such as Arvin
3. Fibrinolytic agents
4. Anti-factor XIII (when available)
5. Anti-platelet aggregation
6. Combinations of the above

in conjunction with all modalities of cancer therapy, namely, (a) surgery, (b) immunotherapy, (c) chemotherapy, and (d) radiotherapy.

These approaches would enable us to utilize all available means of cancer therapy to its utmost.

REFERENCES

1. Agostino, D., and Cliffton, E. E., Anticoagulants and the development of pulmonary metastases. *Arch. Surg.* (*Chicago*) **84**, 87–91 (1962).
2. Agostino, D., and Cliffton, E. E., Trauma as a cause of localization of blood

born metastases. Preventive effect of heparin and fibrinolysin. *Ann. Surg.* **161,** 97–102 (1965).

3. Agostino, D., and Cliffton, E. E., Fibrinogen levels and pulmonary metastases in rats. *Arch. Pathol.* **87,** 141–145 (1969).
4. Agostino, D., Grossi, C. E., and Cliffton, E. E., Effect of heparin on circulating Walker 256 carcinosarcoma cells. *J. Nat. Cancer Inst.* **27,** 17–24 (1961).
5. Brodsky, I., and Conroy, J. F., The effects of chemotherapy on hemostasis. *In* "Cancer Chemotherapy II. The 22nd Hahnemann Symposium" (I. Brodsky, S. B. Kahn, and J. H. Moyer, eds.), pp. 85–92. Williams & Wilkins, Baltimore, 1972.
6. Cliffton, E. E., and Agostino, D., The effects of fibrin formation and alterations in the clotting mechanism on the development of metastases. *J. Vasc. Dis.* **2,** 43–52 (1965).
7. Davis, R. B., Theologides, A., and Kennedy, B. J., Comparative studies of blood coagulation and platelet aggregation in patients with cancer and non-malignant diseases. *Ann. Intern. Med.* **71,** 67–80 (1969).
8. Day, E. D., Planinsek, J. A., and Pressman, D., Localization in vivo of radio-iodinated anti-rat fibrin antibodies and radioiodinated rat fibrinogen in Murphy rat lymphosarcoma and in other transplantable rat tumors. *J. Nat. Cancer Inst.* **22,** 413–431 (1959).
9. Elias, E. G., and Brugarolas, A., The role of heparin in the chemotherapy of solid tumors. Preliminary clinical trial in carcinoma of the lung. *Cancer Chemother. Rep.* **56,** 783–785 (1972).
10. Elias, E. G., Shukla, S. K., and Mink, I. B., Heparin-chemotherapy in the management of inoperable lung carcinoma. *Cancer* **36,** 129–136 (1975).
11. Folkman, J., Tumor angiogenesis: Therapeutic implications. *N. Engl. J. Med.* **258,** 1182–1186 (1971).
12. Hidalgo, J., Fowell, A. H., and Ralls, R. J., The effect of tissue damage on the plasma fibrinogen level. *Surg., Gynecol. Obstet.* **95,** 661–664 (1952).
13. Hiramoto, R., Bernecky, J., Jurandowski, J., and Pressman, D., Fibrin in human tumors. *Cancer Res.* **20,** 592–593 (1960).
14. Jones, D. S., Wallace, A. C., and Fraser, E. E., Sequence of events in experimental metastases of Walker 256 tumor: Light, immunofluorescent and electron microscopic observations. *J. Nat. Cancer Inst.* **46,** 493–504 (1971).
15. Kiricuta, I., Todorutiu, C., Muresian, T., and Risca, R., Prophylaxis of metastases formation by unspecific immunologic stimulation associated with heparin therapy. *Cancer* **31,** 1392–1396 (1973).
16. Kudrjashov, B. A., Kalishevskaya, T. M., and Kolomina, S. M., Blood anticoagulating system and malignant tumors. *Nature (London)* **222,** 548–550 (1969).
17. Laki, K., and Yancy, S. T., Fibrinogen and the tumor problem. *In* "Fibrinogen" (K. Laki, ed.), Chapter 16, pp. 359–367. Dekker, New York, 1968.
18. Leavy, R. A., Kahn, S. B., and Brodsky, I., Disseminated intravascular coagulation—a complication of chemotherapy in acute myelomonocytic leukemia. *Cancer* **26,** 142–145 (1970).
19. Miller, S. P., Sanchez-Avalos, J., Stefanski, T., and Zuckerman, L., Coagulation disorders in cancer. *Cancer* **20,** 1452–1465 (1967).
20. Nitani, H., Taniguchi, T., Inagaki, J., and Kimura, K., Labelizing effect of lipoprotein lipase on lysosomes of tumor cells. *Gann* **62,** 61–63 (1971).
21. Norrby, K., Effect of heparin on cell population kinetics, mitosis and topoinhibition. *Virchows Arch., B* **9,** 292–310 (1971).

22. O'Meara, R. A. Q., Coagulative properties of cancers. *Ir. J. Med. Sci.* [6] pp. 474–479 (1958).
23. Regelson, W., (1968). The antimitotic activity of polyanions. *Advan. Chemother.* **3**, 303–315.
24. Ryan, J. J., Ketcham, A. S., and Wexler, H., Reduced incidence of spontaneous metastases with long-term coumadin therapy. *Ann. Surg.* **168**, 163–168 (1968).
25. Ryan, J. J., Ketcham, A. S., and Wexler, H., Warfarin treatment of mice bearing autochthonous tumors: Effect on spontaneous metastases. *Science* **162**, 1493–1494 (1968).
26. Unkeless, J. C., Tobia, A., Ossowski, L., Quigley, J. P., Rifkin, D. B., and Reich, E., An enzymatic function associated with transformation of fibroblasts by oncogenic viruses. *J. Exp. Med.* **137**, 85–126 (1973).
27. Wood, S., Jr., Pathogenesis of metastasis formation observed in vivo in the rabbit ear chamber. *AMA Arch. Pathol.* **66**, 550–568 (1958).

Chapter 14

Nonspecific Immune Stimulation with Corynebacteria in Lung Cancer

Lucien Israel

Very few studies have been devoted to nonspecific immunostimulation in lung cancer. Existing studies have been recently reviewed by Hersch *et al.* [7]. As for the current investigations of the EORTC* lung group, they have been dealt with in a separate chapter of this book. This chapter is devoted to the investigations conducted by us since 1967 with *Coryne-bacterium parvum* in advanced cases of cancer and to the facts that may be deduced from our results.

* EORTC, European Organization for Research and Treatment of Cancer; Lucien Israel, Chairman of EORTC Lung Group.

I. A BRIEF SUMMARY OF THE EXPERIMENTAL
PROPERTIES OF *Corynebacterium parvum*

Killed bacterial material of various strains of corynebacteria (*C. parvum, C. granulosum, C. anaerobium*) behaves as a nonspecific immune adjuvant. It is capable of activating macrophages, stimulating the reticuloendothelial system, and enhancing the secondary antibody response to antigenic challenge [1, 7, 13, 14]. In terms of antitumor effect, these properties are reflected in preventing certain tumor grafts from taking, as well as possibly causing rejection of established tumors [4, 5, 11, 17]. Moreover, corynebacteria work synergistically with cytotoxic agents [2, 12]. They are also capable of increasing the level of colony-stimulating factor, thus countering bone marrow depression induced by chemotherapy or radiotherapy [3, 6, 17]. Finally, recent investigations have shown that these properties may be related to stimulation of macrophages and B lymphocytes, since the antitumor effect was maintained in animals after thymectomy or administration of anti-lymphocyte serum [18].

II. STUDY PROTOCOL

This study involved patients with either squamous cell or oat cell bronchogenic carcinoma, all of whom had distant metastases from the outset or recurrences after initial surgery or radiotherapy. Each cell type was separately randomized into two subgroups, one receiving chemotherapy alone, the other receiving the same chemotherapy plus *Corynebacterium parvum*.

A. Patient Population

Seventy-five patients with bronchogenic squamous cell carcinoma were treated with only chemotherapy, while 68 patients were treated with a combination of chemotherapy and *C. parvum*. In the oat cell carcinoma group there were 30 patients in each subgroup. No patient was excluded from the study on the grounds of too extensive lesions, and even patients with cerebral metastases were included on the condition that their life expectancy was assessed to exceed 1 month. None of the patients were given cortisone or other antiinflammatory agents. Only patients with evaluable or measurable tumors were included in the study.

B. Administration of *Corynebacterium parvum*

Corynebacterium parvum (Merieux strain) is supplied in ampules containing 4 mg of heat-killed material suspended in 2 ml of saline and 2% formaldehyde. Patients were given regular weekly injections of 1 ampule administered subcutaneously in the deltoid region. In some cases the contents of the ampule were mixed with 1 ml of Xylocaine. The onset of fever in the hours following the injection is a common occurrence and is the only significant side effect we have observed in our 7-year experience. Patients are advised not to take aspirin.

C. Chemotherapy

Patients in the squamous cell group and those in the oat cell group were given the same chemotherapy. This chemotherapy, administered by intravenous infusion every 2 weeks, included cyclophosphamide, 15 mg/kg; methotrexate, 0.7 to 1 mg/kg; flourouracil, 15 mg/kg; vinblastine, 0.1 mg/kg, and streptonigrin, 0.003 mg/kg. If the white cell count dropped below $4000/mm^3$ or if the platelet count dropped below $100,000/mm^3$ chemotherapy was postponed until return to these levels while *C. parvum* was continued. Treatment was pursued indefinitely.

D. Study Parameters

A blood count, chest X-ray, and clinical examination were performed each week. Levels of blood urea nitrogen, blood sugar, transaminases, and serum creatinine were determined twice monthly. Skin responsiveness to purified protein derivative of tuberculin (PPD) was tested in all patients before initiation of therapy and every 2 months thereafter. Only a small group of patients underwent more thorough skin testing (candidin, streptokinase, sensitization to dinitrochlorobenzene).

III. RESULTS IN SQUAMOUS CELL CARCINOMA

Results are shown in Table I. The difference in mean survival between the group receiving *C. parvum* plus chemotherapy and the group receiving only chemotherapy is significant $(p < 0.001)$. This difference is also re-

TABLE I
Comparison of Survival in Two Randomized Groups of Patients with Bronchogenic Squamous Cell Carcinoma

Group[a]	Median survival (months)	Range (months)	Mean survival (months)	Difference
Chemotherapy only (75)	4	1–28	5.6	$p < 0.001$
Chemotherapy + *C. parvum* (68)	9	2–38	9.8	

[a] Number of patients in parentheses.

TABLE II

Comparison of Survival in Two Randomized Groups of Patients with Bronchogenic Oat Cell Carcinoma

Time from onset of therapy (months)	% survivors (30 patients on chemotherapy only)	% survivors (30 patients on chemotherapy + C. parvum)	Significance
3	70	100	
6	26	73	
9	13	40	$p < 0.05$
12	3	30	
15	3	24	
18	0	24	

flected in median survival and the distribution of survival values. Survival from the time of initiation of therapy was almost twice as long when *C. parvum* was added to chemotherapy. This result was due chiefly to an increase in the duration of response, since the response rate was similar in both groups, around 50%.

IV. RESULTS IN OAT CELL CARCINOMA

Table II shows that the results are very similar to those obtained in squamous cell carcinoma, and the results are statistically significant despite the small number of patients. In short, the addition of *C. parvum* doubles survival, mainly by prolonging the response in patients who responded.

V. RESULTS ACCORDING TO PRETHERAPEUTIC IMMUNE STATUS

In this study we confirmed our earlier findings [9–11]. In the chemotherapy group, patients with positive delayed hypersensitivity reactions, as reflected in skin tests, did better than those with a negative response. The same was true in the chemotherapy plus *C. parvum* group. The best overall results were obtained in patients with positive pretherapeutic skin tests who were on chemotherapy plus *C. parvum*.

VI. CHANGES IN SKIN TESTS
DURING TREATMENT

Considerable care should be taken in analyzing these changes, since conversion to negative may be due to both cytotoxic chemotherapy and to progression of the tumor itself, although different mechanisms are involved. Moreover, as mentioned earlier, *C. parvum* is chiefly a B cell stimulant and therefore cannot be expected to directly convert negative delayed hypersensitivity reactions to positive. The findings in these two studies, which have been substantiated by simultaneous investigations in other types of cancer may be briefly summarized as follows: In nonresponders, and even more so in cases of progression, *C. parvum* appears incapable of converting initially negative tests to positive. It does, however, appear to delay conversion of initially positive tests to negative. In responders, *C. parvum* maintains positive skin tests that have a tendency to become negative in patients on chemotherapy alone. Furthermore, more patients in the *C. parvum* group converted negative tests to positive than in the chemotherapy group.

VII. LEUKOPENIA AND INFECTION

A remarkable finding in this study was the protection conferred by *C. parvum* against both microbial and viral infections (viral hepatitis, herpes zoster) which were relatively common in the group on chemotherapy alone. We were not able to obtain data concerning opportunistic lung infections, but we have reason to believe that they followed the same tendency.

With regard to leukopenia, leading to discontinuation of therapy, patients on chemotherapy alone had twice as many such episodes and these lasted twice as long as in patients on both chemotherapy and *C. parvum*. Consequently, patients on *C. parvum* received a higher dose of cytotoxic drugs per unit time than patients in the control group.

VIII. TOXICITY

Subcutaneous *C. parvum* Merieux strain, given weekly as we have just described, is not a toxic agent. No fatalities have been seen, neither have anaphylactic reactions nor liver, kidney, or bone marrow damage—even after years of administration. Local morbidity may be seen, manifesting as pain and swelling for a few hours and very rarely as more long lasting inflammation or suppuration.

General morbidity consists of fever, rarely up to 40°C, usually about 38.5C°, lasting for a few hours and spontaneously receding. It has been noted by several investigators that it usually tends to decrease with time.

IX. DISCUSSION AND INTERPRETATION
OF RESULTS

Apart from the unquestionably beneficial effect of nonspecific immunostimulation with *C. parvum* on survival, we feel that the analysis of our results leads to the following deductions.

Nonspecific tumor-induced immunodepression and drug-induced immunodepression are related to different underlying mechanisms. Only the latter appears to be countered by *C. parvum*.

Corynebacterium parvum has proved to be effective in reducing the leukopenic effect of cytotoxic drugs and in controlling consequent infections. This finding is consistent with experimental data on the colony-stimulating factor. This property of *C. parvum* means that it works synergistically with cytotoxic drugs and may be used with the latter. This is contrary to the dogma that immunotherapy should be administered after chemotherapy and not simultaneously. Another consequence of the stimulation of bone marrow stem cells is an increased production of immunocytes (lymphocytes, macrophages), which may play a decisive role when considered from the all important, but often underestimated, quantitative angle: immunocytes/target cell ratio.

In view of the two points discussed above, it is not really surprising that *C. parvum* has been able to exert a detectable effect on disseminated tumors. This phenomenon is contrary to the dogma that immunotherapy can only be of use in cases of minimal residual disease. It is encouraging to find that immunotherapy is useful in all clinical situations, including the most unfavorable.

In addition, taking into account the special frequency of opportunistic infections of various origins in lung cancer patients, the use of a nonspecific immune stimulant able to prevent or reduce these infections is of special interest. Attempts at stimulating alveolar macrophages by means of aerosol treatment with *C. parvum* are being made in our unit.

Having found that *C. parvum* is effective both in disseminated tumors and in association with chemotherapy is one thing; learning to apply this knowledge in the most effective manner possible is another. Trials to determine the best dose, the most appropriate timing in relation to chemotherapy, and the most effective route of administration are now under way. It is quite obvious that only acquisition of this knowledge will make it possible to achieve real progress in the efficacy of our therapeutic efforts. Moreover, reliable immunological monitoring methods must be developed and applied in order to establish accurate assay of the biological effects of *C. parvum.*

In conclusion, we would simply like to mention that our latest investigations, as yet uncompleted, indicate that the intravenous route is clearly more effective than the subcutaneous route, although tolerance is more of a problem because of the high fever induced by the former. With intravenous *C. parvum,* we have witnessed several partial regressions without chemotherapy, and we have observed that an increase in immunoglobulin levels and a decrease in the C3 fraction of complement attended these regressions (N. Dimitrov, unpublished data).

We may conclude at the present time that nonspecific immunostimulation is of definite use in the field of lung cancer, as has been proved by the studies reported here. We feel that the time has come to include immunotherapy with *C. parvum* in all lung cancer protocols and in all combined modality procedures.

REFERENCES

1. Castro, J. E., The effect of *Corynebacterium parvum* on the structure and function of the lymphoid system in mice. *Eur. J. Cancer* **2**, 115 (1974).
2. Currie, G. A., and Bagshawe, K. D., Active immunotherapy with *Corynebacterium parvum* and chemotherapy in murine fibrosarcomas. *Brit. Med. J.* **1**, 541 (1970).
3. Dimitrov, N., in "International Symposium on Experimental and Clinical Effects of *Corynebacterium parvum,*" p. 173. Springer-Verlag, Berlin and New York, 1974.
4. Fisher, J. C., Grace, W. R., and Mannick, J. A., The effect of non-specific immunostimulation with *Corynebacterium parvum* on patterns of tumor growth. *Cancer* **26**, 1379 (1970).
5. Halpern, B. N., Biozzi, G., Stiffel, C., and Mouton, D., Inhibition of tumor by administration of killed *Corynebacterium parvum*. *Nature* (*London*) **212**, 853 (1966).
6. Halpern, B. N., Prévot, A. R., Biozzi, G., Stiffel, C., Mouton, D., Morard, J. C., Bouthillier, Y., and Deucresefond, C., Stimulation de l'activité phagocytaire du système réticuloendothélial provoquée par *Corynebacterium parvum*. *J. Reticuloendothel. Soc.* **1**, 77 (1964).
7. Hersch, E. M., Gutterman, J. V., and Mavligit, G. M., Perspectives in immunotherapy of lung cancer. *Cancer Treat. Rev.* **1**, 65 (1974).
8. Israel, L., Preliminary results of non specific immunotherapy for lung cancer. *Cancer Chemother. Rep., Part 3* **4**, 283 (1973).
9. Israel, L., La stimulation immunitaire des cancéreux par les corynébactéries. *Entretiens Bichat-Ther.* p. 23 (1973).

10. Israel, L., and Halpern, B., Le *Corynebacterium parvum* dans les cancers avancés. *Nouv. Presse Med.* **1,** 19 (1972).
11. Milas, L., and Mujavic, H., Protection by *Corynebacterium parvum* against tumour cells injected intravenously. *Eur. J. Clin. Biol. Res.* **17,** 498 (1972).
12. Pearson, J. W., Pearson, G. R., Gibson, W. T., Cherman, J. C., and Chirigos, M. A., Combined chemo-immunostimulation therapy against murine leukemia. *Cancer Res.* **32,** 904 (1972).
13. Raynaud, M., Konznetzova, B., Bizzini, B., and Cherman, C., Etude de l'effet immunostimulant de diverses espèces de corynébactéries anaérobies et de leurs fractions. *Ann. Inst. Pasteur, Paris* **122,** 695 (1972).
14. Scott, M. T., Biological effects of the adjuvant *Corynebacterium parvum.* Evidence for macrophage–T-cell interaction. *Cell. Immunol.* **5,** 459 (1972).
15. Toujas, L., Dazord, L., Le Garrec, Y., and Sabolovic, D., Modification du nombre d'unités formatrices de colonies spléniques par des bactéries induisant l'immunostimulation non spécifique. *Experientia* **28,** 1223 (1972).
16. Wolmark, N. and Fisher, B. The effect of a single and repeated administration of *Corynebacterium parvum* on bone marrow macrophage colony production in syngeneic tumor-bearing mice. *Cancer Res.* **34,** 2869–2872 (1974).
17. Woodruff, M. F. A., and Boak J. L., Inhibitory effects of injection of *Corynebacterium parvum* on the growth of tumour transplants in Isogenic hosts. *Brit. J. Cancer* **20,** 345 (1966).
18. Woodruff, M. F. A., Dunbar, N., and Ghaffar, A., The growth of tumours in T-cell deprived mice and their response to treatment with *Corynebacterium parvum. Proc. Roy. Soc., Ser B* **184,** 97 (1973).

Chapter 15

Presentation of the Current EORTC Lung Group Protocols for Immunostimulation with BCG in Lung Cancer

Lucien Israel

In view of the possible benefit to be derived from immunostimulation in cases of lung cancer after surgical or radiotherapeutic tumor reduction, the EORTC lung group activated two protocols in 1973 which made provision for immunostimulation in these clinical situations. The immunostimulant chosen was BCG, owing to the fact that distribution of homogenous batches of *Corynebacterium parvum* to all participating European institutions was impossible at the time. We felt it would be useful to briefly describe these protocols and to discuss the questions that they will ultimately answer.

I. ADJUVANT POSTSURGICAL PROTOCOL

This protocol (see Fig. 1) was designed for cases of squamous cell carcinoma having undergone adequate resection of the tumor and dependent lymph nodes, irrespective of the surgical procedure used. Patients are then stratified according to whether pathologic examination shows lymph node involvement or not. Initial randomization allocates patients either to a postoperative radiotherapy group (4500 to 5500 rads to the mediastinum and tumor bed) or to a control group. Further randomization allocates

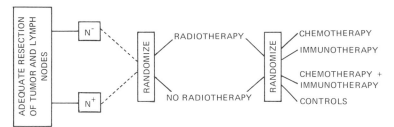

Fig. 1. Mechanics of study in the adjuvant postsurgical protocol.

all patients to one of four groups, namely, (a) a control group; (b) a group receiving monthly chemotherapy consisting of methotrexate 40 mg/m^2, cyclophosphamide 1 gm/m^2, CCNU 70 mg/m^2; (c) a group receiving monthly BCG, 0.2 ml (2 × 10^6 bacilli) of rehydrated freeze-dried BCG Pasteur injected intradermally at the upper part of each extremity; (d) a group receiving both chemotherapy and immunotherapy as described above. All patients are skin tested with recall antigens and with DNCB before treatment and every 2 months.

This protocol thus includes 8 subgroups, and even 16 subgroups if stratification is taken into account, a number that may appear somewhat ambitious. However, the questions that this protocol hopes to answer are numerous. Not only does it compare chemotherapy and immunotherapy with a control group, but it also seeks to determine the effects of combining the two and to establish whether the efficacy of this combination is influenced by prior radiotherapy. Is there any advantage to be gained by adding immunotherapy to radiotherapy or chemotherapy in order to prevent the possible detrimental effects of the latter on immune status? Does postoperative radiotherapy exert a beneficial influence? Is radiotherapy combined with chemotherapy more effective than chemotherapy alone?

These are just some of the questions that will be answered by investigating survival, disease-free interval, local recurrence, and distant metastases in each group.

II. PROTOCOL FOR LOCAL UNRESECTABLE CARCINOMA

This protocol (Fig. 2) is also designed exclusively for cases of squamous cell carcinoma, and it includes cases that are deemed unresectable, prior to surgery, for oncological reasons. Cases with distant metastases are excluded.

The protocol provides for radical cobalt irradiation of the tumor and mediastinum in all patients, who are then randomized to the same four groups as in the previous protocol.

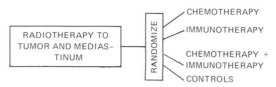

Fig. 2. Mechanics of study in the protocol for local unresectable lung cancer.

Patients who show progression or no response after radiotherapy are not included in the randomization, the aim being to determine which of the four arms is most apt to prolong the local beneficial effect achieved by radiotherapy and to prevent the development of detectable distant metastases. The questions that this protocol will ultimately answer, the study parameters, and the end points are exactly the same as in the adjuvant postsurgical protocol.

III. DISCUSSION

In this brief discussion we shall not include criteria for dosage modifications, exclusion criteria, etc. The aim of this chapter is simply to inform specialists of the goals and essential modalities of trials now in progress. For practical purposes, BCG is administered on the same day as chemotherapy in patients that are randomized to the immunotherapy group. In my opinion there should be no theoretical objections to such a procedure, since BCG-induced suppuration usually lasts several weeks and hence so does the immune stimulation produced by the latter. Cicatrization takes place without any remarkable events, leaving a round scar of 1 cm in diameter that becomes less and less pronounced with time.

The chemotherapeutic regimen chosen was in fact a compromise. It is probably not the most effective combination possible, but we took into account the fact that patients should lead as normal a family and social life as possible. Methotrexate and cyclophosphamide were chosen because of their recognized relative efficacy as single agents in bronchogenic squamous cell carcinoma, while CCNU was chosen chiefly because of its ability to cross the blood–brain barrier and hence possibly to prevent the development of cerebral metastases.

In both protocols discussed above an underlying hypothesis submitted to trial is that immunotherapy and chemotherapy work synergistically. This problem has been discussed in Chapter 14 analyzing the results of immunochemotherapy in disseminated disease. Other relevant problems will be discussed in Chapter 16.

Problems in Designing Postoperative Strategies with Respect to Immune Status, Kinetics, and Resistance

Lucien Israel

There is conflicting data about the results of adjuvant chemotherapy in lung cancer [1, 2, 4, 15]. As always, medical opinion has been more impressed by the negative results of the Swiss group that reported a detrimental effect of long-term Cytoxan versus no therapy. Unfortunately no data are given about the specific characteristics of the patients in these trials, and, furthermore, only partial actuarial results have been published.

Data derived from our earlier studies and from the analysis of other relevant publications lead us to discuss how trials for adjuvant postsurgical therapy of lung cancer are designed at present and to suggest different methods both for stratification and for therapeutic programs.

I. ADJUVANT THERAPY AND IMMUNE STATUS

From the data included in Chapter 7, it is quite clear that immune status must be taken into account in the design of an adjuvant study. If it is assumed, as our data show, that "positive" patients live longer than "negative" patients, and that patients who convert to positive after surgery live longer than those who remain negative, it follows that prior to randomization patients should be stratified into three groups, namely, positive, negative, and spontaneous conversion from negative to positive after resection. It is possible that only one of these groups will show a detrimental or a beneficial effect with adjuvant therapy, and if this is true the fact has not emerged in studies published so far.

Immune status prior to therapy is not the only important parameter, and patients should be monitored throughout the entire study. It is not known from available data whether therapeutic schedules now used depress immune responsiveness in previously positive patients, whether a detrimental effect is observed only in patients whose immune status is already poor (iatrogenic or tumor-induced), whether recurrence and metastases appear after conversion to negative of previously positive patients, etc. It would be of considerable interest to determine the relationships between pretherapeutic immune status, therapy, posttherapeutic changes in immunity and disease-free interval. Until these relationships have been determined, interpretation of presently available data will be problematical.

If such relationships are ultimately proved, and our studies suggest they will be, it is evident that an attempt to protect or restore immune competence should be included in adjuvant trials, not only as an isolated procedure but also in combination with chemotherapy. Indeed, our studies with *Corynebacterium parvum* in advanced cases have revealed that this type of nonspecific immunotherapy affords more effective protection against drug-induced immune depression than against tumor-induced depression.

The EORTC protocol for postoperative adjuvant situations, referred to in Chapter 15, is designed in this way, i.e., it randomizes patients to four groups, namely, immunotherapy, chemotherapy, and immunochemotherapy.

For the time being, and until such data becomes available, we are somewhat sceptical about prolonged, unchanged adjuvant chemotherapy. We shall develop this idea later; suffice it to say that such treatment probably loses its effectiveness after a few months because of resistance, while it retains its ability to destroy immunocytes for as long as it is administered.

It can be said then that:

1. Any adjuvant postoperative treatment should be evaluated according to the immune status, by means of stratification of subgroups before randomization.

2. Cooperative trials should be designed in order to answer questions as to whether immune stimulation induces any benefit in "negative" patients, or in "positive" ones, whether it should be started prior to immune-sup-

pressive chemotherapy in same categories of patients, whether it should be prolonged after discontinuation of immune suppressive drugs according to the immune status of the host.

3. Calculations should be made, from available experimental and clinical data, in an attempt to estimate at what time the sensitive tumor cell part of the residual disease have been killed by the adjuvant chemotherapy. As I have said, after that time, therapy is just exerting an immunosuppressive and detrimental effect without tumor cell killing as a counterpart. It is obvious that duration should be shorter when single drugs are being used than when combinations of non-cross-resistant drugs are employed.

II. ADJUVANT THERAPY AND KINETICS

In a previous study [11], we showed that growth fraction, cell losses, resistance, and optimal schedule are linked by mathematical relationships. Consideration of these relationships has shown that better results could be obtained by simultaneous rather than sequential administration of drugs without cross-resistance and by shortening the interval between courses. The need for shorter therapeutic intervals was deduced from a model in which it was assumed that after a course of chemotherapy, the growth fraction returned to preadministration levels by the next course, or could even exceed this level if the recruitment phenomenon was taken into account. A second course of chemotherapy administered during the phase when the growth fraction is temporarily elevated would be particularly effective.

It was then shown in another study, on the mathematical conditions of eradication [12], that the above parameters are also linked to the total number of tumor cells, but in a nonlinear fashion. This means that when the initial number of tumor cells is small, eradication may be achieved with a far less effective combination in terms of resistance. This same study showed that given the optimal relationship between growth fraction, resistance, and number of residual cells, the ideal interval between therapeutic courses varied considerably from one tumor to another according to the spontaneous doubling time, whereas the total number of courses needed to achieve eradication was mathematically linked to the growth fraction. Without going into mathematical details, it is obvious that the optimal schedule of any given treatment is definitely related to the growth rate of the tumor to be treated, and that a schedule capable of achieving eradication in tumors of a defined growth rate will be totally ineffective in other cases.

As already mentioned, it is not always possible to determine the doubling time of a tumor prior to resection. However, it should at least be possible, by using Feinstein's classification [3] to divide patients into two categories, namely, fast and slow growth rates, the border between the two being 55 days, which is the median value [7].

Rather than stratifying patients according to spontaneous growth rate, this classification would lead to different schedules for each group: fewer courses with shorter intervals between courses for fast-growing tumors and more courses but longer intervals between courses for slow-growing tumors.

This may appear overly sophisticated but the only way of improving adjuvant therapy is to take advantage of all the differences in cell kinetics between different patients. From a clinical standpoint the least we can do is to take into account the growth rate. We have shown that this parameter, however approximate it may be, is critical.

The above holds true, obviously, for the treatment of advanced disease. However, as the strategies designed for adjuvant situations are likely to be more successful, one should not overlook the kinetic factor in such studies. It is, again, not acceptable, on theoretical grounds, to treat in the same way tumors with a doubling time of 20 days and tumors with a doubling time of 200 days. Whether such a statement would hold true on clinical grounds remains to be shown. The only way to find out would be to randomize patients with fast-growing tumors (before resection) to two different schedules—the conventional one and an experimental one with shorter intervals between courses—the doses of cytostatic drug being given at the maximum tolerated dose within the frame of the new schedule. It should not be necessary to wait 10 years to activate such studies. It is hoped that, in 10 years, more active drugs will erase the difference. It is now that we have to take advantage of such differences, if possible.

III. ADJUVANT THERAPY, RESISTANCE AND SPREAD OF DISEASE

The importance of resistance in eradication strategies has been thoroughly investigated in the study described above (12). However, several facts of strategic importance have also been learned from clinical studies involving measurable tumors of known doubling time and their response to chemotherapy [5, 8, 13]. The knowledge relevant to eradication thus acquired over many years may be summarized as follows.

The lower the growth fraction, the lower the resistance against the total drug combination to be used must be. As an example, we have been able to show that for a growth fraction of 25% and a total cell number of 10^7 cells for each residual metastasis (i.e., a tumor of roughly 2 mm in diameter), the total resistance encountered should not exceed 10^{-9}, whereas for the same growth fraction and residual metastases of 10^9 cells (1 cm in diameter), the drug combination should not encounter a resistance risk exceeding 10^{-14}. If residual metastases contain only 10^3 cells, the drug combination may encounter a resistance of 10^{-4} and still terminate in eradication. In our experience, this is feasible with two drugs. From the above data it can be deduced that combinations are always needed in adjuvant therapy and that they should include more drugs in stage II than in stage I patients. Furthermore, a greater number of drugs should be administered to eradicate slow-growing tumors than to eradicate fast-growing ones.

Maximum regression and total resistance occur in very close succession. When optimal schedules are being used in terms of cell killing, susceptible tumor cells are being destroyed while resistant cells keep growing at the same undisturbed rate. As soon as all susceptible cells have been killed, the tumor resumes its previous growth rate [4].

Maximum response in clinically detectable tumors is observed in a matter of weeks with single agents. If 3 to 5 effective agents are used in combination, maximum regression is achieved in 4 to 6 months and is invariably closely followed by resistance [4].

At this point we may make some assumptions, keeping in mind that every assumption must be tested by means of controlled trials. The first assumption is that residual undetectable metastases contain no more than 10^8 cells (10^9 being the size of the smallest detectable visceral tumor). In an adjuvant situation such a tumor should be managed by a three-drug combination given at the optimal not at the maximum schedule with regard to toxicity. If we extrapolate the data acquired by us through detectable lung tumors, we can then assume that after 3 months there would be 10^4 resistant cells left. If the first three-drug combination is then replaced by another three-drug combination without cross-resistance, eradication could be achieved in another 3 months. However, if the initial growth fraction was low, there would be 10^6 cells left after 3 months and 10^3 after 6 months. In this situation, it would be wiser to administer a two-drug combination for another 2 months. We have deliberately omitted discussing problems related to recruitment, synchronization, etc., since our purpose is simply to consider drugs in terms of their spectrum of resistance. Using three drugs without cross-resistance which show effectiveness against bronchogenic carcinoma, we would advocate the following schedule: three drugs for the first 3 months, three other drugs for the next 3 months, and two other drugs for the last 2 months. As we mentioned earlier, when a given drug or combination of drugs has eliminated all susceptible cells and only resistant cells are left, not only is there no benefit to be derived from continuing treatment, but only a detrimental effect can be expected, namely, immunodepression. Therefore, in view of the kinetics of resistance it is clear that adjuvant therapy should be of relatively short duration, but should include more drugs, when lung cancer is the tumor under consideration.

Evaluating resistance in individual clinical cases is another matter that still remains highly speculative. However, there appears to be a probable relationship between resistance and spread of disease. Statistically speaking, the probability of encountering large numbers of resistant clones is higher for stage II tumors with lymph node involvement than for T1 N0 cases, which is due of course to the fact that the percentage of resistant cells being the same their absolute numbers are greater in large tumors, and also to the fact that the greater the number of tumor cells, the greater the chances are that mutations leading to resistance will appear. This probability remains of the same order for undetectable tumor cells after resection of all detectable disease. It would, therefore, appear logical to employ more drugs, administered for a longer period of time in postoperative strategies for stage II tumors than for stage I tumors, a hypothesis that must, of course, be tested by means of controlled trials.

IV. HYPOTHESES ON DIFFERENT THERAPEUTIC SUBGROUPS

Contrary to what might have been expected, we did not observe any correlation between immune status, spread of disease, and growth rate [9, 14], particularly in lung cancer. In view of this finding, when differentiating prognostic subgroups and designing clinical trials, one must formulate the hypothesis that these three factors are at least partly independent of one another. If this is indeed true, and if the prognostic incidence of each of these factors is defined as either poor or good, there are eight different situations to be considered. These are listed in the tabulation below.

Good immune status	Slow growth	Stage I
Good immune status	Slow growth	Stage II
Good immune status	Fast growth	Stage I
Good immune status	Fast growth	Stage II
Poor immune status	Slow growth	Stage I
Poor immune status	Slow growth	Stage II
Poor immune status	Fast growth	Stage I
Poor immune status	Fast growth	Stage II

From the above discussion, it is evident that optimal adjuvant strategies would differ in each of these groups. In patients with poor immune status, no effort should be spared to restore immune competence; slow-growing tumors should be treated by prolonged chemotherapy with longer intervals between courses, and stage II disease would require more drugs than stage 1 disease. These considerations lead to discussing the design of current clinical trials.

V. HOW SHOULD POSTSURGICAL
TRIALS BE DESIGNED?

Considering the eight categories described above and the theoretical reasons why they should behave differently both spontaneously and on any given therapy, one may make at least two proposals.

a. The less ambitious and more conservative of these proposals concerns stratification. If it is recognized that immune status, growth rate, and anatomical spread do indeed bear prognostic significance, then patients should at least be stratified into eight different subgroups. If a cooperative group agrees on a given therapy, for example, a chemotherapeutic agent, patients would be stratified into the eight subgroups previously mentioned prior to randomization between a treated group and a control group. This would amount to 16 subgroups submitted for final analysis. Such a program may appear ambitious but it is the only way by which something might be learned about why any given individual does better than another. The author feels that the time has come to go one step further than merely accepting the fact that four patients have to undergo surgery in order to register one 5-year survival without being able to predetermine which of the four will survive these 5 years [6, 10]. In this respect, cooperative groups that are not willing to accept the approach described below should at least stratify their patients in order to analyze all available prognostic factors and their interactions. At the present time this means dividing patients into at least eight subgroups.

b. There is of course another way to achieve progress which might be proposed to more aggressive cooperative groups. This would consist of adapting different therapeutic programs to meet expected differences between different prognostic subgroups, the ultimate goal being not to determine why some cases are failures but to avoid these failures. This could be done in keeping with "scientific" principles, simply by considering each subgroup as a separate entity to be submitted to different randomized trials. To be more specific each of these subgroups will now be discussed separately.

1. Patients with a good immune status, slow growth rate, and very limited disease are the most likely candidates for 5-year survival and hence potentially dangerous procedures should not be used in this situation. One possibility would be to compare nonspecific immune stimulation and follow-up without treatment. An alternative would be to compare three groups, namely, controls, a group on immunotherapy, and a group on both immunotherapy and chemotherapy with one or two agents administered for a short period of time.

2. For good immune status, slow growth but stage II a 3-arm study could be envisaged, comparing controls to immunochemotherapy, using two different schedules of chemotherapy, for example, three drugs for 8 months versus three drugs for 4 months, and another 3 drugs for 4 additional months.

3. Good immune status, stage I, rapid growth calls for more aggressive chemotherapy and shorter intervals between courses. Here again immunotherapy alone would not be included and we could suggest immunochemotherapy as in situation (1) compared to controls and to immunochemotherapy using the same cytostatic drugs but administered in doses closer to the maximum tolerated dose and with shorter intervals between courses.

4. Good immune status, rapid growth, stage II should be treated with aggressive chemotherapy both in terms of regimen and schedule. This chemotherapy could be compared to immunochemotherapy using a nonspecific immune stimulant.

5. The group with poor immune status, slow growth rate, and stage I disease is very similar to group 1 and could be submitted to the same protocol or to a protocol comparing "light" and "heavy" immunotherapeutic procedures.

6. For poor immune status, slow growth, stage II, both immunostimulation and "heavier" chemotherapy are theoretically required. A regimen including nonspecific immune stimulation and two consecutive combinations of two or three drugs administered at long intervals could be compared to the same immunotherapy plus a single three-drug combination administered according to the same schedule.

7. Poor immune status, stage I, rapid growth could be submitted to trials along the same lines, namely, comparison of immunotherapy plus a two-drug combination administered at short intervals and immunotherapy plus the same chemotherapy with longer intervals between courses.

8. Finally, the poorest prognostic group, namely, poor immune status, fast growth rate, stage II would call for immune stimulation and aggressive chemotherapy using consecutive combinations of more drugs with shorter intervals between courses. We would suggest that in this group the only variable be different chemotherapeutic agents.

It is evident that the above proposals can be easily criticized. It might well be that a control group, receiving no therapy, would be necessary in each of the situations described. Furthermore, different priorities could lead to different designs and different therapies in any of these situations, and we are the first to recognize that the views expressed in this chapter are purely speculative. However, speculation must be considered as a pressing necessity in a field in which no successful therapeutic program has been developed during the past 20 years. One of the most promising attitudes in lung cancer at present is the attempt to define prognostic subgroups along the lines discussed above. It should also be kept in mind that stratification according to prognostic differences is not the best way to investigate differences in survival simply because these prognostic differences should entail different therapeutic approaches. General agreement should be reached all the more so on this principle for lung cancer, a disease for which current therapeutic procedures are not very effective and consequently for which any slight differences between patients or particular characteristics of the disease should be fully exploited. As for the contents of any given protocol, they should of course remain open to discussion and should probably include as many approaches as can be reasonably undertaken.

REFERENCES

1. Brunner, K. W., Marthaler, T., and Muller, W., Unfavorable effects of long-term adjuvant chemotherapy with Endoxan in radically operated bronchogenic carcinoma. *Eur. J. Cancer* **7**, 285 (1971).
2. Curreri, A. R., Nitrogen mustard as an adjuvant to pulmonary resection in the treatment of carcinoma of the lung. *Cancer Chemother. Rep.* **16**, 123 (1962).
3. Feinstein, A. R., Symptoms as an index of biologic behavior and prognosis in human cancer. *Nature (London)* **209**, 241 (1966).
4. Higgins, G. A., Humphrey, E. W., Hugues, F. A., and Keehn, R. J., Cytoxan as an adjuvant to surgery for lung cancer. *J. Surg. Oncol.* **1**, 221 (1969).
5. Israel, L., L'évaluation des traitements anticancéreux dans les tumeurs mesurables. *In* "The Design of Clinical Trials in Cancer Therapy." Editions Scientifiques Européennes, Bruxelles, 1972.
6. Israel, L., and Chahinian, P., De l'impossibilité de guérir les cancers bronchiques par la chirurgie seule. Données statistiques. Raisons théoriques. Déductions thérapeutiques. *Presse Med.* **77**, No. 11, 389 (1969).
7. Israel, L., and Chahinian P., Absence de corrélation entre la vitesse de croissance et le degré de différenciation des cancers bronchiques. *Presse Med.* **79**, No. 35, 1567 (1971).
8. Israel, L., Chahinian, P., Accard, J. L., Choffe, C., Combes, P. F., Danrigal, A., Guermouty, J., Migueres, J., Schaerer, R., and Sotto, J. J., Growth curve modification of measurable tumors by 75 mg/m^2 of CCNU every 3 weeks. *Eur. J. Cancer* **9**, 789 (1973).

9. Israel, L., Chahinian, P., and Depierre, A., Response of 65 measurable epidermoid bronchogenic tumors of known spontaneous doubling-time to four different chemotherapeutic regimens—strategic deductions. *Med. Pediat. Oncol.* **1,** No. 2, 83–93 (1975).

10. Israel, L., and Depierre, A., La problématique du pronostic dans les cancers bronchiques opérés. *Rev. Tuber. Pneum.* **35,** 291 (1971).

11. Israel, L., and Duchatellier, M., Growth fraction, resistance, schedule-doubling time relationship sequential versus simultaneous combinations, as evaluated by a mathematical model of response to chemotherapy. *Eur. J. Cancer* **7,** 545 (1971).

12. Israel, L., and Duchatellier, M., A strategy of chemotherapeutic eradication based upon correlative variations in total cell population, growth fraction and resistance. *Eur. J. Cancer* **8,** 263 (1972).

13. Israel, L., Duchatellier, M., and Chahinian, P., Predictability models for drug resistance. *Advan. Antimicrob. Antineoplast. Chemother. Proc. Int. Congr. Chemother., 7th, 1971* Vol. 2, p. 775 (1972).

14. Israel, L., Mugica, J., and Chahinian, P., Prognosis of early bronchogenic carcinoma survival curves of 451 patients after resection of lung cancer in relation to the results of the preoperative tuberculin skin test. *Biomedicine* **19,** No. 2, 68 (1973).

15. Karrer, K., Kombinierte chirurgishe und cytostatische therapie des bronchialcarcinoms. *Muenchen. Med. Wochenschr.* **109,** 24 (1967).

Chapter 17

A Discussion of Current Strategies for Limited Unresectable Squamous Cell Carcinoma and Adenocarcinoma of the Lung

Lucien Israel

The generally accepted method for treating limited unresectable lung cancer is radiotherapy to the tumor, mediastinum, and possibly, supraclavicular areas. The purpose of this chapter is to present possible alternatives for consideration by cooperative groups.

I. IS RADIOTHERAPY A SAFE AND USEFUL PROCEDURE?

To the best of my knowledge, there is no available data comparing radiotherapy and abstention in limited unresectable disease. This is hardly surprising, since radiotherapy may induce impressive tumor regression as well as subjective improvement, and it is legitimately felt that patients should be given the benefit of any effective procedures medicine has to offer.

However, there are several theoretical objections to radiotherapy, and these will be listed below if only to illustrate that nothing in this field is simple.

Radiotherapy has been shown to induce a state of immune depression, especially when directed against the thymus area [1–3, 7]. Furthermore, radiotherapy for breast cancer has been reported to increase the incidence of distant metastases [4]. In view of these findings it is not unreasonable to ask whether radiotherapy for lung cancer might induce a state of immune depression leading to an increased incidence of distant metastases and shorter survival. In any case, this aspect of the problem certainly warrants investigation. This could be approached by the following:

1. Monitoring immune changes in patients submitted to radiotherapy and attempting to demonstrate a possible correlation between such changes and survival
2. Evaluating the survival and determining the cause of death in patients who could not be irradiated for any reason
3. Comparing radiotherapy alone and radiotherapy plus immune protection by nonspecific immune stimulation. This might be the most significant investigation, since if immune stimulation was shown to improve survival in patients having undergone radiotherapy, this would tend to prove that the latter may be detrimental to the host's immune defense mechanisms

Radiotherapy may also exert a detrimental effect on blood vessels and myocardium. It may facilitate pulmonary embolism, which is not an infrequent cause of death in lung cancer patients. A clinical trial of interest would be radiotherapy alone versus radiotherapy plus anticoagulation. Interpreting the results of such a trial would not be simple, since anticoagulants have been shown to decrease the incidence of distant metastases [8]. From an empirical viewpoint, however, such a trial would be very informative.

Finally, it has not yet been convincingly demonstrated that radiotherapy in limited disease induces higher response rates and longer responses than adequate chemotherapy. For obvious reasons, cytostatic agents without radiotherapy are used only in disseminated cases. As discussed in Chapter 11 of this book, these agents can induce impressive regressions, including regression of the primary tumor, and there is no reason to think that they could not achieve a similar result in limited disease. If it were shown that irradiation is in any way detrimental, then it would be necessary to compare the following strategies: "conventional" radiotherapy alone, "conventional" radiotherapy plus immune stimulation, "conventional" radiotherapy followed by chemotherapy with immune stimulation, radiotherapy in decreased doses followed by chemotherapy with or without immune stimulation, chemotherapy without radiotherapy with or without immune stimulation. Such a program may appear ambitious, but so many patients are irradiated and not included in any clinical trials that it would probably not take very long to obtain answers if only a small percentage were assigned to randomly chosen therapeutic procedures.

At this point I would like to make it clear that the purpose of this discussion is not to discredit radiotherapy, which is obviously beneficial. It is simply my aim to draw attention to the fact that, at the present time, radiotherapy is probably not being used in the safest and most effective way. It may well be that some simple procedures, such as prophylactic anticoagulation and/or immune stimulation, could considerably improve end results of radiotherapy without adding any toxic effect. It may also ultimately be shown that lower doses of radiotherapy plus chemotherapy are more effective and safer than "conventional" radiotherapy alone or followed by "conventional" chemotherapy.

II. CONCOMITANT NONMYELOTOXIC CHEMOTHERAPY AND RADIOTHERAPY

Simultaneous administration of cytostatic agents and radiotherapy is a dangerous undertaking, and at least 2 weeks should be allowed to elapse after completion of radiotherapy before initiating a chemotherapeutic program. This means that for a period of 8 weeks the patient will be receiving treatment for regional disease while he is known to have systemic disease. If the tumor is fast growing, this loss of time may have detrimental consequences. This is why we undertook pilot studies with nonmyelotoxic chemotherapy administered from the beginning of radiotherapy. The chemotherapeutic regimen was the same for all cell types and included dehydroemetine [5, 6] 3 mg/kg, vincristine 0.8 mg/m², and bleomycin 10 mg/m². These three drugs were administered at weekly intervals throughout the entire duration of radiotherapy and were followed by cytostatic agents according to various protocols. In the 68 patients thus treated so far no myelotoxic effect or respiratory insufficiency have been encountered, and in every case it was possible to put the patient on a "conventional" chemotherapeutic program without major hematological problems. No attempt was made to compare this procedure with radiotherapy alone after randomization. Such a procedure would call for a very careful work-up of patients prior to treatment in order to ensure that there were no clinically undetectable metastases that could be demonstrated by more refined procedures.

However, this pilot study being terminated, a cooperation randomized trial may now be undertaken. The purpose of this trial would be to compare the degree and rate of local response and the rate of appearance of distant metastases in the two groups. Our preliminary results show that

no distant metastases have been documented within 3 months of completion of radiotherapy in the 68 consecutive cases mentioned above.

III. SURGERY IN "UNRESECTABLE" DISEASE

It may appear paradoxical to discuss surgery in the context of what is
commonly referred to as unresectable disease. However, this paradox
serves to emphasize that unresectable is certainly not an adequate term to
use in many circumstances and that it has unconsciously become synonymous of "disease that should not be resected in view of the poor results to
be expected."

However, not only is the prognostic value of preoperative classification
subject to error, but, furthermore, this prognostic value was deduced from
patients who were not given any other form of therapy or, in any event,
not the best available form of therapy. It might ultimately be shown that
patients with supraclavicular lymph nodes, classified as M1, do better with
surgery, radiotherapy, and chemotherapy (or chemotherapy, surgery, and
radiotherapy) than with only radiotherapy and chemotherapy. The time has
come to recognize that the prognostic groups established by surgeons at a
time when no effective medical therapy was available should be reevaluated. The concept of adjuvant surgery is gaining popularity in other fields
of oncology, and it is my opinion that this approach should be given
serious consideration in lung cancer.

IV. CONCLUSION

Cases of so-called limited unresectable disease are more common than
resectable cases and therefore warrant more imaginative attitudes and
closer attention that they usually receive. These cases constitute an ideal
situation for considering combined modality approaches, since they call for
aggressive therapeutic procedures and since every available procedure is
probably more advantageous than detrimental in this situation, which is not
necessarily the case for resectable lung cancer. This situation has made it
necessary to review current methods of employing radiotherapy and chemotherapy, to discuss ways of attenuating undesirable side effects of radiotherapy and of controlling systemic disease while regional disease is being
irradiated. Finally, surgery in cases that are not truly unresectable should
be given careful reconsideration.

From our various personal attempts at improving the results in this situation, the best sequence seems to be (a) immunotherapy plus conven-

tional combination chemotherapy, (b) radiotherapy plus nonmyelotoxic chemotherapy, and (c) resumption of immunotherapy plus conventional chemotherapy. In addition surgery can be done in some cases, usually between (a) and (b). Again a conflict arises between the rigidity of fixed protocols and the necessity in order to achieve the best results in any individual patient, to combine modalities in a flexible way, according to the individual characteristics of the case, and to the results of every previous therapeutic step.

REFERENCES

1. Braeman, J., and Deeley, T. J., Radiotherapy and the immune response in cancer of the lung. *Brit. J. Radiol.* **46,** 446 (1973).
2. Check, J. H., Damsker, J. I., Brady, L. W., and O'Neill, E. A., Effect of radiation therapy on mumps-delayed type hypersensitivity reaction in lymphoma and carcinoma patients. *Cancer* **32,** 580 (1973).
3. Cosimi, A. B., Brunstetter, F. H., Kemmerer, W. T., and Miller, B. N., Cellular immune competence of breast cancer patients receiving radiotherapy. *Arch. Surg.* (*Chicago*) **107,** 531 (1973).
4. Getzen, L. C., and Riffenburgh, R. H., A statistical analysis of radical mastectomy with adjuvant therapy in the initial treatment of carcinoma of the breast. *Amer. J. Surg.* **123,** 278 (1972).
5. Israel, L., and Depierre, A., Boutiller, J., and Chahinian, P., Activité anticancéreuse de l'Emétine. *Nouv. Presse Med.* **2,** No. 13, 1147 (1973).
6. Israel, L., Depierre, A., and Chahinian, P., Dehydroemetin in 50 disseminated carcinomas unresponsive to other drugs. *Proc. 10th Annu. Meet. Amer. Soc. Clin. Oncol., 1974* (1974).
7. Jenkins, V. K., Olson, M. H., and Ellis, H. N., In vitro methods of assessing lymphocyte transformation in patients undergoing radiotherapy for bronchogenic cancer. *Tex. Rep. Biol. Med.* **31,** No. 1, 19 (1973).
8. Ketcham, A. S., Sugarbaker, E. V., Ryan, J. J., and Orme, S. K., Clotting factors and metastasis formation. *Amer. J. Roentgenol., Radium Ther. Nucl. Med.* [N.S.] **3,** No. 1, 42 (1971).

Chapter 18

A Discussion of Current Strategies for Disseminated Lung Cancer

Lucien Israel

This chapter is written in the hope that patients with disseminated disease will no longer be used as clinical material for evaluating only chemotherapeutic agents in cooperative trials. The present situation is understandably different from that which prevailed 20 years ago when nothing more than a minor palliative effect was expected from chemotherapy, and in any case nothing else could be done. Today more effective chemotherapeutic agents are available, at least in terms of response rates if not yet in terms of duration of response. In view of this prevailing situation, it is conceivable that greater efforts should be made from the onset in an attempt to control disease. Some investigators may feel that the difficulty in evaluating response rates to a given therapy because of "interference" by another therapeutic procedure is frustrating or even "anti-scientific." However, it is equally frustrating, if not more so, to think that patients may be deprived of the possible benefit of such a "nonscientific" approach. A few examples of what could be done will help clarify the concepts underlying this attitude.

I. DISSEMINATED DISEASE, IMMUNITY AND NONSPECIFIC IMMUNE STIMULATION

In Chapter 14, devoted to immune stimulation with *Corynebacterium parvum,* we showed that when added to chemotherapy this agent is definitely able to prolong survival of patients with lung cancer. This finding is consistent with current knowledge on the prognostic significance of immune depression in these patients. Furthermore, it is well known that after a given chemotherapeutic regimen has failed, a second regimen produces a lower response rate than when administered before any other chemotherapy. Our data (unpublished) indicate that this phenomenon may be accounted for by the immunodepression induced both by the initial treatment and by progression of the disease.

These findings lead us to a first conclusion, namely, that disseminated disease should no longer be treated by chemotherapy alone but by a combination of chemotherapy and immunotherapy (provided our results are confirmed by other studies).

II. DISSEMINATED DISEASE AND RADIOTHERAPY

Cooperative protocols usually call for dropping of patients on chemotherapy if radiotherapy is also applied, since the interpretation of results becomes difficult, if not impossible. However, is it unreasonable to refuse a patient the benefit of an effective procedure on these grounds?

Patients with disseminated disease have numerous tumor masses that could be effectively and safely irradiated using narrow beams, thus probably producing less undesirable systemic effects than chemotherapy while achieving a beneficial reduction in the tumor cell burden. According to the number, location, and radiosensitivity of the various tumors, programs could be designed using different combinations of nonmyelotoxic agents, reduced doses of standard agents, and/or "palliative" rather than maximum regimens of radiotherapy. In all cases, immunostimulation should be added as a means of protecting host defenses. Such a program should be tested first in oat cell carcinomas, because of their well-known radiosensitivity.

III. DISSEMINATED DISEASE AND SURGERY

It has been shown that resection of isolated metastases with long doubling times is of unequivocal benefit in terms of survival [3]. However, this attitude is not popular in patients with disseminated lung cancer except for resection of a single cerebral metastasis following irradiation of an unresectable primary tumor. It has been our constant policy to consider that metastases arrested in their growth by chemotherapy should be managed in the same way as spontaneously slow-growing tumors and removed, provided that the chemotherapy was well tolerated and could be continued. Metastases in the brain, lung, and liver have been thus removed whenever possible, namely, when they were resectable and controlled by treatment. In many cases radiotherapy was performed postoperatively using submaximal doses, and chemotherapy was resumed as soon as possible. However, these are isolated cases that cannot be presented in terms of response rates and duration of response to a single procedure, but this situation will arise more and more often if cancer patients are to be treated by what is called a combined modalities approach. It will become the task of biostatisticians to learn how to evaluate these procedures. It is unreasonable to expect therapists to conform to what biostatisticians are presently able to evaluate.

IV. DISSEMINATED DISEASE AND SEQUENTIAL CHEMOTHERAPEUTIC COMBINATIONS

As we have shown previously [1, 2], clinical resistance is encountered very early in disseminated lung cancer even when combinations are used. In the time that elapses between maximal regression and assessment of progression (progression being defined as an increase of 25% of the product of 2 diameters over the lowest value of this product), the drugs kill more immunocytes than tumor cells and are therefore detrimental. This is why waiting to assess the duration of response, as is currently done in all cooperative groups, is probably the worst procedure in disseminated cases. Our studies show that the best results are achieved by changing the combination as soon as there is no further improvement. This approach also gives the best results with regard to anticancer effects versus undesirable effects. Such data should at least lead to protocols designed to test the underlying idea. One way of doing this might be to assign patients with disseminated lung cancer randomly to one group in which combination B would follow combination A after documented progression and to another group in which B would follow A as soon as maximum regression had been documented.

As for nonresponders, it has been our constant experience that they can be identified at most after the second course of chemotherapy. When a response is to occur, it generally occurs after the first course. It is not necessary then to waste time by waiting for a progression to at least 50% before changing the chemotherapeutic regime.

V. CONCLUSION

We have discussed several ways in which current therapeutic approaches for disseminated lung cancer could be improved. This could be achieved with relative ease if it is accepted that combined modalities approaches are no longer reserved only for resected cases and that the current habits of biostatisticians should not dictate the design of clinical trials. As a matter of fact, the association of immunotherapy, palliative radiotherapy of a maximum of identifiable deposits, and sequential combinations of chemotherapy administered as soon as there is no more regression obtained from the previous one, should be the standard treatment of disseminated lung cancer.

REFERENCES

1. Israel, L., Chahinian, P., and Le Bourgeois, J. P., Evaluation du délai d'apparition de la résistance aux chimiothérapies anticancéreuses. Comparison des courbes de croissance tumorale en fonction de trois schémas thérapeutiques différents. *Ann. Med. Interne* **121,** No. 4, 415 (1970).
2. Israel, L., Duchatellier, M., and Chahinian, P., Les tumeurs mesurables bronchopulmonaires comme moyen d'évaluation de la chimiorésistance et du coefficient de prolifération cellulaire. Conséquences thérapeutiques. *Presse Med.* **78,** No. 25, 1137 (1970).
3. Joseph, W. L., Morton, D. L., and Adkins, P. C., Prognostic significance of tumor doubling time in evaluating operability in pulmonary metastatic disease. *J. Thorac. Cardiovasc. Surg.* **61,** 23 (1971).
4. Israel, L., Chahinian, P., and Depierre, A., Response of 65 measurable bronchogenic tumors of known spontaneous doubling time to four different chemotherapeutic regimens. Strategic deductions. *Med. Pediat. Oncol.* **1,** No. 2, 83–93 (1975).

Subject Index

A 6
B 7
C 8
D 9
E 0
F 1
G 2
H 3
I 4
J 5